The CRA's Guide to Monitoring Clinical Research

Elizabeth Weeks-Rowe

SIXTH EDITION

CenterWatch
A WCG Company

The CRA's Guide to Monitoring Clinical Research, Sixth Edition
Elizabeth Weeks-Rowe

300 N. Washington St., Ste. 200
Falls Church, VA 22046
www.centerwatch.com

Printed in the United States.

ISBN: 978-1-60430-217-2

TABLE OF CONTENTS

	Introduction	**ix**
1	**What Is a CRA?**	**1**
	GCP Role and Responsibilities	1
	Changes to Clinical Research and the CRA Role	7
	The COVID Impact	10
	Current CRA Roles and Collaborative Positions	18
	The CRA Personality	20
	Career Preparation	24
	In the Future	29
	Your Value	31
	Key Takeaways	31
2	**The History Behind the Regulations**	**33**
	Regulation and Human Subject Protection Milestones	34
	Summary	42
	Key Takeaways	43
3	**Regulations and GCPs**	**45**
	FDA Regulations for Clinical Trials	45
	ICH Guidelines for Good Clinical Practice	46
	FDA Guidances and Information Sheets	47
	FDA Compliance Program Guidance Manuals	48
	NIH-Regulated Research	49
	FDA Bioresearch Monitoring Program	49
	Good Clinical Practice	50
	Contacting the FDA	51
	Key Takeaways	52

4 Roles and Responsibilities in Clinical Trials **53**
Sponsors 53
Institutional Review Boards (IRBs) 56
Clinical Investigator 57
Other Research Partners 59
Managing Relationships 60
Key Takeaways 61

5 The Research Process **63**
Preclinical Research 64
The IND Application 68
Clinical Trials 70
Key Takeaways 76

6 Devices and Biologics **79**
Biologics and Vaccines 82
COVID Vaccine Development 85
Key Takeaways 86

7 Globalization of Clinical Trials **87**
Managing Multinational Trials 88
Key Takeaways 91

8 Institutional Review Boards and Data Safety Monitoring Boards **93**
Types of IRBs 94
IRB Responsibilities 96
IRB Review of Proposed Research 100
IRB Membership 105
IRB Operations 106
Conflict of Interest 106
IRB Registration 106
FDA Guidance Documents for IRBs 107
Scientific Review Committee 107
Additional Review Committees 108
Data Safety Monitoring Boards 108
Key Takeaways 110

9 **Informed Consent** **113**
Monitoring Informed Consent 114
Obtaining Informed Consent 121
The Consent Process 123
Exceptions to Consent 126
Electronic Informed Consent 129
Conclusion 134
Key Takeaways 135

10 **Preparing for a Study** **137**
Study Design 137
Statistical Significance 140
Control Groups Used in Clinical Trials 140
Common Study Designs 145
Other Statistical Issues 149
Summary 150
Key Takeaways 151

11 **Preparing for a Study** **153**
Developing a Protocol 153
Case Report Forms 168
Electronic Data Capture 173
Summary 177
Key Takeaways 178

12 **Clinical Investigators** **181**
Investigators and Their Responsibilities 181
Types of Investigative Sites 189
Locating Potential Investigators 193
Key Takeaways 207

13 **Study Initiation** **209**
Study Initiation Documents 209
Financial Disclosure 210
The Investigator Meeting 212
Study Initiation Meetings 223
Grants and Contracts 232
Key Takeaways 236

14 Study Monitoring **239**
The Monitoring Plan 239
Preparing for a Monitoring Visit 253
Site Monitoring Visits 256
Electronic Source 272
Risk-Based Monitoring: Remote and Central Monitoring Practices 275
Errors, Queries and Corrections 286
Good, High-Quality Data 288
Investigational Product (Drug, Biologic, Device) 289
Confidentiality 297
Follow-up Letter to the Investigator 301
Conclusion 304
Key Takeaways 306

15 Adverse Events and Safety Monitoring **309**
Regulations and Definitions 309
Adverse Events in Clinical Trials 314
Key Takeaways 323

16 Recruitment, Retention and Compliance **325**
Recruitment of Study Subjects 325
Established, Successful Recruitment Strategies 334
Retention of Study Subjects 342
Subject Compliance 347
Key Takeaways 354

17 Study Closeout **357**
Reasons for Study Closeout 357
Closeout Procedures 359
Key Takeaways 363

18 Quality Management **365**
Site Metrics 368
Key Takeaways 373

19 Audits **375**
Sponsor Audits of Investigative Sites 375
IRB Audits of Investigative Sites 378
FDA Inspections 378
Site Preparation 381
The Audit Process 383
After the Audit 386
Consequences 388
Key Takeaways 394

20 Errors, Misconduct and Fraud **397**
Definitions 397
Errors 397
Misconduct 401
Fraud 402
Suspicion of Misconduct or Fraud 408
Consequences of Fraud 409
Key Takeaways 410

21 The Future for CRAs **411**
Impact of Technology 411
Increased Responsibility 413
Impact of Diversity on the Clinical Trial Landscape 414
Regional Monitoring 415
Conclusion 416
Key Takeaways 416

Appendices **419**
A Resources 419
B Hints and Tips 423
C Sample Forms, Checklists and Logs 427
D Job Descriptions and Academic Programs 463

Index **469**

INTRODUCTION

The most important goal I had for the 2023 release of *The CRA's Guide to Monitoring Clinical Research* was to effectively document the changes to the clinical research industry we have experienced over the past five years, including the impact of COVID on the clinical trials infrastructure, the working paradigm and the role of the CRA, the technological advancements that are integral to data reporting and analysis, the importance of diversity in clinical trial populations, and integrating clinical trials into patient care.

This guide continues to evolve and stay relevant with industry advancements/innovations but the core content is timeless and consistent with the CRA's responsibilities. Each update brings a fresh perspective while staying true to the fundamentals of patient safety, study ethics and the guidelines that govern trial conduct. *The CRA's Guide* still serves as the industry reference for experienced and new clinical researchers, whether endeavoring to confirm established knowledge or enhance their learning with new information.

I have been involved in the updates to the CRA's Guide since 2016 and am so grateful to be able to contribute to the very guidebook that helped me learn the CRA role and obtain CRA certification at the start of my career. I am especially grateful to the original authors, Karen Woodin and John Schneider, for providing the original framework and timeless content for this important work.

–Elizabeth Weeks-Rowe

Elizabeth Weeks-Rowe

Elizabeth Weeks-Rowe, LVN, CCRA, has 23 years of diverse clinical research experience, as a study coordinator, CRA, CRA trainer and CRA manager. A frequent speaker at clinical research industry conferences, she has developed CRA training content and delivered classroom and field training to new and experienced CRAs for several CROs. She has written numerous articles for clinical research publications and authored a monthly clinical research column for *CenterWatch Weekly* from 2011-2018 about life as a traveling CRA. She authored the 2016 and 2019 updates to *The CRAs Guide to Monitoring Clinical Research* and the 2019 update to *The PI's Guide to Conducting Clinical Research.* Inspired by the study coordinators with whom she has worked over the years, she also self-published a clinical research novella, entitled *Clinical Research Trials and Triumphs*, about a nurse entering the field of clinical research. She is a staff trainer for a prominent clinical research training company and works as an independent clinical research consultant, providing training, content creation and clinical operations support services. She has been an Association of Clinical Research Professionals (ACRP) Certified Clinical Research Associate (CCRA) since 2004.

CHAPTER 1

What Is a CRA?

There is surprising diversity in what Clinical Research Associates (CRA) say their jobs and duties are. This is due to the great variation in their experience and in the organizations for which they work. There are also many people who are not CRAs who want to get a better feel for the clinical research process by understanding what CRAs do and how they do it.

The purpose of this chapter is threefold: to give the reader who is already a CRA a portrait of what a typical CRA "looks like," to highlight the changes to the CRA role (and the clinical research landscape) over the past 25 years to illustrate the impact of the COVID pandemic on the CRA role and the overall clinical research industry, and to provide non-CRA readers with a concise description of CRAs and an overview of what they do.

GCP Role and Responsibilities

The acronym CRA has evolved into a catchall title in the pharmaceutical industry and has become the universal term for anyone involved in monitoring clinical trials. According to section 5.18 of the International Council for Harmonization (ICH) guideline E6(R2) Good Clinical Practice (GCP):

> The purposes of trial monitoring are to verify that:
>
> (a) The rights and well-being of human subjects are protected.
>
> (b) The reported trial data are accurate, complete and verifiable from source documents.
>
> (c) The conduct of the trial is in compliance with the currently approved protocol/amendment(s), with GCP and with applicable regulatory requirement(s).

It continues in section 5.18.2 Selection and Qualifications of Monitors:

(a) Monitors should be appointed by the sponsor.

(b) Monitors should be appropriately trained and should have the scientific and/or clinical knowledge needed to monitor the trial adequately. A monitor's qualifications should be documented.

(c) Monitors should be thoroughly familiar with the investigational product(s), the protocol, written informed consent form and any other written information to be provided to subjects, the sponsor's SOPs, GCP and the applicable regulatory requirement(s).

Section 5.18 also delineates a monitor's primary responsibilities:

The monitor(s), in accordance with the sponsor's requirements, should ensure that the trial is conducted and documented properly by carrying out the following activities when relevant and necessary to the trial and the trial site:

(a) Acting as the main line of communication between the sponsor and the investigator.

(b) Verifying that the investigator has adequate qualifications and resources and these remain adequate throughout the trial period; that facilities, including laboratories and equipment, and staff are adequate to safely and properly conduct the trial and remain adequate throughout the trial period.

(c) Verifying, for the investigational product(s):

(i) That storage times and conditions are acceptable, and that supplies are sufficient throughout the trial.

(ii) That the investigational product(s) are supplied only to subjects who are eligible to receive it and at the protocol specified dose(s).

(iii) That subjects are provided with necessary instruction on properly using, handling, storing and returning the investigational product(s).

(iv) That the receipt, use and return of the investigational product(s) at the trial sites are controlled and documented adequately.

- (v) That the disposition of unused investigational product(s) at the trial sites complies with applicable regulatory requirement(s) and is in accordance with the sponsor.

(d) Verifying that the investigator follows the approved protocol and all approved amendment(s), if any.

(e) Verifying that written informed consent was obtained before each subject's participation in the trial.

(f) Ensuring that the investigator receives the current Investigator's Brochure, all documents, and all trial supplies needed to conduct the trial properly and to comply with the applicable regulatory requirement(s).

(g) Ensuring that the investigator and the investigator's trial staff are adequately informed about the trial.

(h) Verifying that the investigator and the investigator's trial staff are performing the specified trial functions in accordance with the protocol and any other written agreement between the sponsor and the investigator/institution and have not delegated these functions to unauthorized individuals.

(i) Verifying that the investigator is enrolling only eligible subjects.

(j) Reporting the subject recruitment rate.

(k) Verifying that source documents and other trial records are accurate, complete, kept up-to-date and maintained.

(l) Verifying that the investigator provides all the required reports, notifications, applications and submissions, and that these documents are accurate, complete, timely, legible, dated and identify the trial.

(m) Checking the accuracy and completeness of the [case report form (CRF)] entries, source documents and other trial-related records against each other. The monitor specifically should verify that:

- (i) The data required by the protocol are reported accurately on the CRFs and are consistent with the source documents.
- (ii) Any dose and/or therapy modifications are well documented for each of the trial subjects.
- (iii) Adverse events, concomitant medications and intercurrent illnesses are reported in accordance with the protocol on the CRFs.

(iv) Visits that the subjects fail to make, tests that are not conducted and examinations that are not performed are clearly reported as such on the CRFs.

(v) All withdrawals and dropouts of enrolled subjects from the trial are reported and explained on the CRFs.

(n) Informing the investigator of any CRF entry error, omission or illegibility. The monitor should ensure that appropriate corrections, additions or deletions are made, dated, explained (if necessary) and initialed by the investigator or by a member of the investigator's trial staff who is authorized to initial CRF changes for the investigator. This authorization should be documented.

(o) Determining whether all adverse events (AEs) are appropriately reported within the time periods required by GCP, the protocol, the IRB/IEC, the sponsor and the applicable regulatory requirement(s).

(p) Determining whether the investigator is maintaining the essential documents.

(q) Communicating deviations from the protocol, SOPs, GCP and the applicable regulatory requirements to the investigator and taking appropriate action designed to prevent recurrence of the detected deviations.

Section 5.18.5 Monitoring Procedures is also clear that the "monitor(s) should follow the sponsor's established written SOPs, as well as those procedures that are specified by the sponsor for monitoring a specific trial."

Most CRAs have a bachelor's or master's degree in one of the health, natural or medical sciences; many of them are nurses. There are also some CRAs with a bachelor's or master's degree in areas other than the medical or health sciences, such as business, sociology or liberal arts. They have had to take adjuvant medical terminology or health courses to supplement the missing medical/health education from their nontraditional college degree. In rare circumstances, there are CRAs who do not have a bachelor's or master's degree. These CRAs have specific medical training or certification (medical assistants, licensed vocational or practical nurses, respiratory therapists, pharmacy technicians, etc.), have worked as study coordinators, data managers or research pharmacy staff at an investigational site/institution and were able to advance to the CRA role due to their cumulative clinical research work experience and medical training being considered a sufficient equivalent in lieu of a degree.

Independent vs. In-House CRAs

CRAs can be field monitors working regionally, or they can be based in-house at a sponsor or other organization. Some CRAs are employees of pharmaceutical companies developing a new drug or of contract research organizations (CRO) hired by pharmaceutical companies to help with drug development projects. Other CRAs work as independent contractors (1099 or W-2 contractor). W-2 contractors typically work for a staffing company that provides health benefits/401k options. The staffing company withholds social security tax, income tax, Medicare tax and any state income taxes for the benefit of the employee. Pharmaceutical companies/CROs work with these staffing companies to fill resourcing gaps/CRA needs. W-2 contract CRAs still have the advantage of higher pay and independence that comes with being a contractor, though not to the degree of a 1099 contractor as they are employees of the staffing company. 1099 contractors are truly independent in that they form their own corporation/business entity to support the 1099 status. They are responsible for paying for federal and state taxes themselves. They need to enlist the help of an accountant to structure their business and understand the tax burden, obtain health and employee insurance, learn to invoice and complete all tasks that are normally taken care of for full-time employees. However, 1099 contract CRAs traditionally charge a high enough hourly rate to offset these additional expenses.

When contractors work for pharmaceutical companies/CROs, they are assigned to a project just as an organizational CRA is and even report to a CRA line manager. However, the similarities traditionally stop there. There is an expectation that contract CRAs are very experienced and therefore should assimilate at a faster pace than a "regular" CRA. They are required to complete organizational standard operating procedure (SOP) and systems training and start project work at an accelerated pace, which is why most contract CRAs have worked as traditional CRAs for a number of years before transitioning to a contractor role. Contract CRAs typically juggle several projects at a time; they may work on projects for one or more pharmaceutical companies and/or CROs concurrently.

Most contract CRAs once worked as CRAs for large medical or pharmaceutical organizations before making the transition to a contract CRA role. Some CRAs prefer the independence of contract CRA work. They relish the autonomy of picking their own projects and of essentially being their own boss. They

Potential CRA activities

Study planning

- Write and edit protocols for clinical studies.
- Assist/coordinate protocol review.
- Write and review patient informed consent.
- Identify and evaluate CROs that may assist in a development program.
- Identify and evaluate central labs for a study.
- Identify and evaluate vendors for a study, (e.g., central lab vendor, recruitment vendor, interactive web response/voice response systems (IVRS and IWRS) vendor, patient-reported outcomes (PRO) vendor, central imaging vendor, electronic trial master file (TMF) vendor).
- Assist in overall drug development planning.

Development

- Write or review sections of the trial design and contribute to content development of case report forms (CRF) and electronic case report forms (eCRF).
- Help design and contribute to content development of patient reported outcomes (PRO)—paper or electronic—such as patient diaries, quality-of-life surveys and questionnaires.
- Help write, assemble and distribute investigator brochures.
- Write and assemble study/eCRF/CRF instruction manuals.
- Prepare and submit documents required to meet regulatory, GCP and SOP requirements.
- Determine, order, ship and track investigational drug supplies.
- Create feasibility questionnaires for site completion based on critical protocol elements.
- Contact sites for feasibility purposes, provide feasibility questionnaires and follow up with interested sites to obtain completed questionnaires.
- Evaluate and select investigators (sites).
- Conduct pre-study visits at investigative sites.
- Help plan investigator meetings and/or present sessions.
- Review investigator contracts.
- Develop study budgets and grant payment schedules.

Study conduct

- Write and review annual investigational new drug (IND) reports.
- Update investigator brochures.
- Conduct study initiation visits.
- Conduct routine monitoring visits.
- Maintain oversight of CRO activities.
- Maintain and track study data (enrollment, eCRF/CRF collection).
- Assist in data review and correction (eCRF/CRF entries/queries, diary entries/queries, lab entries/queries, etc.).
- Review, assess and interpret study data.

- Review regulatory documents.
- Review and help manage site enrollment.
- Assist in resolving site training and communication issues.
- Monitor and report protocol deviations.
- Monitor and report serious adverse events (SAE)/adverse events (AE) and ensure timeliness and accuracy of documentation, data and reporting.

Closeout

- Conduct study closeout visits.
- Perform post-study follow-ups.

Post-study

- Write and review final study reports.
- Archive study files.
- Assist with writing and reviewing sections of the new drug application (NDA).
- Assist in response to any FDA site inspections.

Miscellaneous

- Train and mentor new people.
- Act as a project manager (PM) or clinical trials manager (CTM).

would never return to being an organizational employee unless they had to. Other CRAs become contractors but ultimately return to the organizational "fold" as they are uncomfortable with the sometimes inconsistent project and financial parameters of contract work (dictated by outside factors, such as economic or organizational climate) and prefer a consistent paycheck/work environment.

Although CRAs perform a variety of clinical operations and monitoring activities, they traditionally are the people who meet with/visit, work and communicate with study sites on behalf of a company sponsoring the research. The CRA's main role is to help ensure proper study conduct, patient safety and the timely generation, review and retrieval of quality data.

Changes to Clinical Research and the CRA Role

Over the past 25 years, the field of clinical research has changed dramatically due to innovation in technology, fluctuations in the economy and therapeutic need/advancements. The clinical research industry must continually innovate to stay relevant, and that includes the evolution of the CRA role to support these changes.

The early CRAs were true road warriors, traveling across the country to conduct monitoring visits at investigational sites as pharma/CRO companies had yet to formally adopt a regional model and assign CRAs sites in the region where they lived. These CRAs carried the earlier model laptops that were heavy and cumbersome to their monitoring visits to document activities and complete monitoring visit reports. They may also have had to bring a second laptop if the study was using an electronic data capture (EDC) system or eCRF system. The early EDC/eCRF systems required a separate laptop to utilize. Other common tools in the early CRA's arsenal for monitoring visits included a bevy of books in the days before electronic resources: books of common drugs and uses, ICH guidelines and FDA regulations, Title 21 of the Code of Federal Regulations (CFR). CRAs had to carry packing/shipping materials for retrieving and sending in paper CRFs to the data management department. They also had to bring paper copies of site folders for each investigational site they were assigned. These folders were thick and included monitoring worksheets, a listing of site essential documents and IRB approvals, printed site directions and demographic information that the CRA needed to have on hand. CRAs also had to bring study documents on monitoring visits, such as the printed protocol, CRF completion guidelines and monitoring plans. CRAs were also responsible for collecting and sending regulatory documents from the site.

CRAs would sometimes spend all week onsite, as virtually all monitoring activities had to be done at the site level and the paper CRFs retrieved manually. CRAs also had to dedicate more time onsite due to the traditional review model of 100 percent source data verification (SDV). CRAs also had to visit investigational sites at specific intervals according to the monitoring plan (usually every four to six weeks) to meet data review requirements. A high enrolling investigational site would require additional visits. Before the remote CRA role emerged, CRAs were responsible for all aspects of site monitoring and management in addition to their on-site responsibilities, including informed consent and regulatory document content review, queries, supplies inventory, and serving as the first contact to their investigational sites.

As technology developed and more studies transitioned to EDC/eCRF systems for data collection and reporting and to electronic PROs for study questionnaires and diaries and electronic regulatory systems, the CRA role expanded to include additional proficiency with computers, databases and Microsoft office programs. CRAs that refused to develop computer skills/expertise were left in the proverbial dust of the modern age as the days of fax machines and paper-based tools waned.

Monitoring practices were changing, to the discomfort of CRAs and sites accustomed to collecting, documenting and reviewing everything; if on-site monitoring had a motto back then, it would have been "100 percent data review, 100 percent of the time." That was the standard for monitoring practice and had been since the beginning of time. The concept of risk-based monitoring first made an appearance more than 11 years ago and was as questioned and doubted as much as the early EDC systems and ePROs were. Risk-based monitoring of clinical research studies was more targeted/focused on those trial processes that had the most effect on data credibility and patient safety. Study protocols had a risk analysis; and targeted endpoints/data points were the focus of review, accompanied by centralized monitoring and data analytics as an adjuvant form of data review to supplement traditional data review practices. This was a more holistic approach to monitoring that encompassed risk analysis and proactivity to address process failures and areas of concern that compromised patient safety and credible data. This approach would identify and address trends before negatively impacting study outcomes. Risk-based monitoring has become the accepted norm.

Technology is interwoven into the fabric of drug development; there are numerous technology platforms used to facilitate/complete study activities: IVRS/IWRS systems for patient randomization, study drug assignments, and tracking shipments and receipt; regulatory portals for investigational site staff to upload essential documents and for sponsor/CRO regulatory staff to make and communicate document changes and provide updated essential documents; central lab databases to log specimen receipt and for investigative sites to receive and review lab results; electronic source systems and video conferencing platforms to facilitate remote monitoring and remote SDV/review; and central IRB portals for sites to log in and see updated versions of approvals and documents. The role of the CRA has adapted as technology has firmly implanted itself in nearly every element of study conduct. The below list reflects additional CRA responsibilities that have evolved as a result of technology in clinical research.

- Review of IVRS/IWRS systems in between monitoring visits to track patient enrollment and randomization.

- Review of central lab portals to ensure patient screening activities/labs are completed correctly, biological specimens are shipped to the central lab and investigators are addressing lab results in a timely manner.
- Review of EDC systems and diary portals between monitoring visits to monitor site EDC and diary entry, queries and AE oversight.
- Review of regulatory portals/electronic TMF to monitor site startup activities/IRB approvals.
- Review of study portals and trackers to monitor site receipt of supplies, investigational product (IP) and systems access to facilitate scheduling of site initiation visits and start-up activities.
- Review of central IRB portals to track site essential documents.

The COVID Impact

The COVID pandemic changed the conduct and trajectory of the clinical research industry more than any event in recent history. It forced the adaptation of the CRA role to virtual monitoring activities/responsibilities that were necessary due to pandemic restrictions. Beyond our individual home and office lives, COVID-19 impacted the core infrastructure of the entire clinical trials community with operational pauses at both industry and institutional levels. Stay-at-home orders resulted in studies halting, institutions furloughing and brick-and-mortar offices uneasily transitioning to virtual workplaces to preserve safety. Everything and everyone were affected while ever-changing regulatory guidances complicated early efforts to rebound. There were radical alterations in traditional site management and monitoring practices. For example, video conferencing platforms replaced in-person meetings and facilitated critical industry conferences. Further, remote monitoring/data review became the new normal, with institutions providing remote electronic medical record access to CRAs and sites using portals and/or electronic source systems to create/upload source documents for remote review.

Investigational sites and institutions closed their doors to outside visitors due to pandemic restrictions and to protect their patients. As a result, traveling CRAs were forced off the road and back to their home offices for fully remote work. The good news with such a dramatic change was that most CRAs had been home-based for years and were already set up to work remotely; they would work at their home office on the days they were not traveling. The bad news, traveling CRAs who loved the nomadic lifestyle the monitoring role afforded, who thrived on the diversity and excitement of life on the road and were more productive in that environment, now had to dramatically change their work paradigm and learn how to do all on-site monitoring activities remotely. They had to learn new medical record/electronic source systems to review data remotely. They had to learn new video conferencing applications to perform monitoring visits and sometimes data review if a site did not have electronic records or the ability to upload source documents. CRAs would spend hours on a call with a site reviewing source documents with the "share screen" option of video conferencing platforms as part of remote monitoring during the pandemic. Both CRAs and site staff had to learn a "new trade" and exhibit extreme patience and understanding with the more challenging communication and execution of fully remote monitoring activities. Meanwhile, the lack of control and uncertainty with all of the role changes, furloughs, layoffs, studies stopping and starting, and the overall long-term impact the pandemic would have on the clinical research industry lurked in the background, resulting in anxiety/mental health issues for clinical researchers. However, a positive change was the realization of the importance of addressing mental health issues in the workplace and providing employees tools and therapy to cope. Many large organizations implemented change and introduced additional resources to support their employees in crisis.

In March 2020, the FDA issued the first version of a final guidance it would revise and update several times during the pandemic: Conduct of Clinical Trials of Medical Products During the COVID-19 Public Health Emergency. In section 3, the guidance discusses considerations for ongoing trials:

> Ensuring the safety of trial participants is paramount. Sponsors should consider each circumstance, focusing on the potential impact on the safety of trial participants, and modify study conduct accordingly. Study decisions may include those regarding continuing trial recruitment, continuing use of the investigational product for patients already participating in the trial, and the need to change patient monitoring during the trial. In all cases, it is critical that trial participants are kept informed of changes to the study and monitoring plans that could impact them.

Sponsors, in consultation with clinical investigators and Institutional Review Boards (IRBs)/Independent Ethics Committees (IECs), may determine that the protection of a participant's safety, welfare, and rights is best served by continuing a study participant in the trial as per the protocol or by discontinuing the administration or use of the investigational product or even participation in the trial. Such decisions will depend on specific circumstances, including the nature of the investigational product, the ability to conduct appropriate safety monitoring, the potential impact on the investigational product supply chain, and the nature of the disease under study in the trial.

Since trial participants may not be able to come to the investigational site for protocol-specified visits, sponsors should evaluate whether alternative methods for safety assessments (e.g., phone contact, virtual visit, alternative location for assessment, including local labs or imaging centers) could be implemented when necessary and feasible, and would be sufficient to assure the safety of trial participants. Sponsors should determine if in-person visits are necessary to fully assure the safety of trial participants (for example, to carry out procedures necessary to assess safety or the safe use of the investigational product appropriately); in making the decision to continue use or administration of the investigational product, the sponsor should consider whether the safety of trial participants can be assured with the implementation of the altered monitoring approach.

In some cases, trial participants who no longer have access to investigational product or the investigational site may need additional safety monitoring (e.g., on withdrawal of an active investigational treatment).

The need to put new processes in place or to modify existing processes will vary by the protocol and local situation. For example, this assessment could include consideration of whether it is appropriate to delay some assessments for ongoing trials, or, if the study cannot be properly conducted under the existing protocol, whether to stop ongoing recruitment, or even withdraw trial participants.

COVID-19 screening procedures that may be mandated by the health care system in which a clinical trial is being conducted do not need to be reported as an amendment to the protocol, even if done during clinical study visits, unless the sponsor is incorporating the data collected as part of a new research objective.

Changes in a protocol are typically not implemented before review and approval by the IRB/IEC, and in some cases, by FDA. Sponsors and clinical investigators are encouraged to engage with IRBs/IEC as early as possible when urgent or emergent changes to the protocol or informed consent are anticipated as a result of COVID-19. Such changes to the protocol or investigational plan to minimize or eliminate immediate hazards or to protect the life and well-being of research participants (e.g., to limit exposure to COVID-19) may be implemented without IRB approval or before filing an amendment to the investigational new drug (IND) or investigational device exemption (IDE), but are required to be reported afterwards. FDA encourages sponsors and investigators to work with their IRBs to prospectively define procedures to prioritize reporting of deviations that may impact the safety of trial participants.

The implementation of alternative processes should be consistent with the protocol to the extent possible, and sponsors and clinical investigators should document the reason for any contingency measures implemented. Sponsors and clinical investigators should document how restrictions related to COVID-19 led to the changes in study conduct and duration of those changes, indicate which trial participants were impacted, and how those trial participants were impacted.

Changes in study visit schedules, missed visits, or patient discontinuations may lead to missing information (e.g., for protocol-specified procedures). It will be important to capture specific information in the case report form that explains the basis of the missing data, including the relationship to COVID-19, for missing protocol-specified information (e.g., from missed study visits or study discontinuations due to COVID-19). This information, summarized in the clinical study report, will be helpful to the sponsor and FDA.

If scheduled visits at clinical sites will be significantly impacted, certain investigational products, such as those that are typically distributed for self-administration, may be amenable to alternative secure delivery methods. For other investigational products that are normally administered in a health care setting, consulting FDA review divisions on plans for alternative administration (e.g., home nursing or alternative sites by trained but non-study personnel) is recommended. In all cases, existing regulatory requirements for maintaining investigational product accountability remain and should be addressed and documented.

With respect to efficacy assessments, FDA recommends consultation with the appropriate review division regarding protocol modifications for the collection of efficacy endpoints, such as use of virtual assessments, delays in assessments, and alternative collection of research-specific specimens, if feasible. For individual instances where efficacy endpoints are not collected, the reasons for failing to obtain the efficacy assessment should be documented (e.g., identifying the specific limitation imposed by COVID-19 leading to the inability to perform the protocol-specified assessment).

If changes in the protocol will lead to amending data management and/or statistical analysis plans, the sponsor should consider doing so in consultation with the applicable FDA review division. Prior to locking the database, sponsors should address in the statistical analysis plan how protocol deviations related to COVID-19 will be handled for the prespecified analyses.

If planned on-site monitoring visits are no longer possible, sponsors should consider optimizing use of central and remote monitoring programs to maintain oversight of clinical sites.

In general, and if policies and procedures are not already in place for applicable trials:

Sponsors, clinical investigators, and IRBs should consider establishing and implementing policy and procedures, or revise existing policy and procedures, to describe approaches to be used to protect trial participants and manage study conduct during possible disruption of the study as a result of COVID-19 control measures at study sites. Changes to policy and procedures could address, but not be limited to, impact on the informed consent process, study visits and procedures, data collection, study monitoring, adverse event reporting, and changes in investigator(s), site staff, and/or monitor(s) secondary to travel restrictions, quarantine measures, or COVID-19 illness itself. Policy and procedures should be compliant with applicable (regional or national) policy for the management and control of COVID-19. Depending upon the nature of the changes described above, a protocol amendment may be required under the applicable regulations.

In the discussion of trials that were impacted by the COVID-19 public health emergency, the guidance says:

> Sponsors should describe in appropriate sections of the clinical study report (or in a separate study-specific document):
>
> 1. Contingency measures implemented to manage study conduct during disruption of the study as a result of COVID-19 control measures.
> 2. A listing of all participants affected by the COVID-19 related study disruption by unique trial participant number identifier and by investigational site, and a description of how the individual's participation was altered.
> 3. Analyses and corresponding discussions that address the impact of implemented contingency measures (e.g., trial participant discontinuation from investigational product and/or study, alternative procedures used to collect critical safety and/or efficacy data) on the safety and efficacy results reported for the study.
>
> Robust efforts by sponsors, investigators, and IRBs/IECs to maintain the safety of trial participants and study data integrity are expected, and such efforts should be documented. As stated above, FDA recognizes that protocol modifications may be required, including unavoidable protocol deviations due to COVID-19 illness and/or COVID-19 control measures. Efforts to minimize impacts on trial integrity, and to document the reasons for protocol deviations, will be important.

After nearly 14 months, pandemic restrictions eased and investigational sites began to welcome CRAs back for on-site monitoring visits, with additional rules to ensure safety. Masks were almost always required to be worn and some institutions required CRAs to show proof of vaccination or a negative COVID test ahead of monitoring visits. Additional permission was required to bring a second CRA for a co-monitoring visit. Monitoring visits were limited to one or two days, and some institutions would only allow on-site monitoring visits for data review purposes; at these institutions, clinic locations, lab and pharmacy did not open for on-site monitoring tours/confirmation until nearly two years after the pandemic first struck. Three years later, some institutions were still not allowing on-site monitoring activities of any kind. This creates a challenge when studies require on-site confirmation of facilities, equipment and in-person monitoring of source documents/medical records at investigational sites considered high risk due to multiple deviations or questionable data.

Several Microsoft Office programs emerged as integral to the CRA role in the remote/virtual monitoring paradigm.

Information storage: OneNote for continuous, historical documentation and tracking data; a singular, cohesive storage location if you will. OneNote enables the user to send emails, information and updates to the OneNote folder; imbed analytics and data; and insert tables, spreadsheets, data listings and links to websites. Study teams use OneNote for robust training requirements, multiple links and videos. CRAs use OneNote for study and investigational site folders for a more cohesive, singular location for information storage relative to site status and monitoring visits.

Data management: Excel spreadsheets, with their ability to import select study data from websites/portals, became critical for CRAs conducting remote data review or tracking. Such platforms as EDC, IVRS/IXRS and central lab portals allow for data exports to Excel spreadsheets and can make or break productivity in the event of system outages or internet connectivity issues.

Videoconferencing: Microsoft Teams and Zoom platforms were vital to conducting remote site evaluation, initiation, monitoring and closeout visits. The screen share function in both programs allows CRAs to review source documents/regulatory documents at the site remotely, collaborate with study team members and sites with document share and screen share slide presentations used in site evaluation and initiation visits.

Presentation: Almost all site evaluation and site initiation visits involve PowerPoint slide presentations, and CRAs must be familiar with PowerPoint requirements to facilitate remote study visit presentations/conduct.

Accelerated site activation and regulatory submission/approval timelines resulted in several vaccines created and distributed within a year of the virus's first occurrence. Pharmaceutical companies continue to develop treatments to prevent or treat the virus and emerging variants of concern; trial conduct continues to rise and there is a burgeoning resourcing problem as a result of the influx of COVID studies into the already-busy clinical trials landscape. There are literally more studies than CRAs to monitor them, and this gap spurred creative solutions to staffing problems. Most importantly, the collective industry realized it had to lessen the once-rigorous requirement for clinical research staff to have two years of research experience to be hired as a CRA. CRA training programs emerged at nearly every major CRO to answer the need for CRAs and the multitude of study nurses, coordinators and data managers applying for CRA jobs. Another positive result of the pandemic was the acceptance of diverse and alternative clinical research experience and the ability for site personnel to finally fulfil their career dreams of becoming a CRA.

Author's Story

Before the pandemic, I worked as a CRA conducting pre-study evaluation visits, traveling three to four days a week visiting sites across the country. I will never forget my last day on the road before a forced 14-month "grounding." I had conducted a pre-study evaluation visit at a site in Michigan on Tuesday and then travelled to Milwaukee, Wisc., for a pre-study evaluation visit scheduled for Thursday. I arrived at the hotel in Milwaukee late Tuesday evening and planned to work in the hotel on Wednesday and then conduct the pre-study evaluation visit at the site the next day. It saved time and considerable cost when visiting multiple cities in one week to work in the hotel in between site visits instead of flying home and then out again the next day.

Then, everything changed. On Wednesday, the study manager from the Milwaukee site contacted me and informed me that the university was on lock down and asked if we could conduct the pre-study evaluation visit remotely. I received approval from the study CTM for remote conduct and the evaluation occurred as planned, but via telephone instead of in person. I had done numerous telephone pre-study evaluation visits, so this change to visit conduct was not a big deal, except for the reason for the change. I don't know how I got through that telephone call, but the pre-study evaluation visit call was conducted successfully despite my anxiety level at 100 percent.

I went to the airport after the call and flew home without incident. The atmosphere on the airplane was surreal. People were quiet and nervous, with the rumblings of forced lockdowns and unknowns of the COVID-19 virus. Only a few passengers wore masks, but there were plenty of glares when someone coughed. I will never forget my last day of travel during the pandemic, March 13, 2020. I did not get on a plane again to conduct a site visit until May 2021.

–Elizabeth

Current CRA Roles and Collaborative Positions

In more recent years, the CRA's responsibilities—and in some cases title—have expanded to that of site manager, a fully dimensional role that encompasses the traditional monitoring activities of SDV/CRF review, regulatory binder review and drug accountability, as well as expanded duties of handling investigational site relations, developing and assisting with patient recruitment plans, site blinding plans, corrective and preventive actions (CAPA), protocol deviation reporting oversight and data management. With more emphasis placed on the CRA-site relationship as a partnership, as opposed to the previous CRA oversight dynamic, the trend of collaborative communication and problem-solving between CRAs and investigational site staff will help promote data credibility, study transparency and patient safety.

Technology is interwoven into clinical trials conduct as many platforms are used for study management and monitoring activities. This has resulted in additional monitoring responsibilities and burden upon the already heavy CRA workload. To supplement the trend of the CRA as the site manager and provide additional CRA-site support, the remote monitoring role emerged and continues to grow in importance. The remote monitor has added an additional layer of preparation and quality to the previously singular role of the CRA and monitoring visit conduct. Remote monitoring is a component of risk-based monitoring, as well as a stand-alone adjunct to traditional monitoring. It is a separate, specific role but can also be performed by a regional CRA.

The responsibilities of the remote monitor are very similar to the responsibilities of the CRA but are performed remotely. The remote monitor is the primary site contact, however, the CRA remains the overall site manager. No longer is SDV or CRF review limited to onsite monitoring visits. The prevalence of electronic CRF systems used in clinical trials, the opportunity for CRAs to review patient data almost immediately after entry via an EDC web portal or internet database (as opposed to onsite), the means for site staff to upload source documents and even paper CRFs to a cloud-based shared drive, enable faster and more efficient (remote) data review to prepare for onsite monitoring visits and to expedite data analysis between monitoring visits. This has streamlined study conduct and added this critical dynamic to assist the CRA role. The activities of the home- or office-based remote monitor include:

- Review of eCRF data entered by investigational sites to ensure data integrity and accuracy.
- Querying sites (via email and eCRF system tools) regarding data entry to question or confirm data completion.
- Conducting remote review of source documents/regulatory documents transmitted by sites (e.g., concomitant medication logs, adverse event logs, protocol deviation logs, enrollment logs, drug accountability logs, informed consent forms and various regulatory documents).
- Generating site payments for study patient visits and eCRF completion.
- Tracking and resolving data entry/queries during data analysis and as needed in between monitoring visits.
- Sending periodic study correspondence to sites with important study information/reminders/protocol amendments.
- Collaborating with sites on regulatory documents/activities for site activation prior to and during study conduct.
- Conducting weekly, biweekly or monthly site monitoring calls with investigational sites to discuss a variety of items, including regulatory activities, data entry, protocol deviations, SAEs, enrollment and any outstanding items from previous monitoring visits.
- Serving as the first line of contact for investigational site questions or issues.

The remote monitor and CRA work collaboratively in a site management model; the remote monitor supplements/supports the CRA with various site management activities between and during monitoring visits. He or she also helps the CRA prepare for site initiation/monitoring/closeout visits by retrieving outstanding data, regulatory documents and SAE line listings for CRAs to utilize during monitoring visits. In some models, the remote monitor is solely responsible for regulatory activities, allowing the CRA to concentrate on drug accountability, SDV/CRF review, site management and training and patient safety during monitoring visits. In other models, the role of the remote monitor and regional CRA overlap and they assist each other with completion of the above-referenced site monitoring and management tasks.

Another role to support site management activities and the traveling CRA is the clinical trials assistant or project assistant role. This role has been around for a while but has been revamped and redeveloped to be of more importance. Like the remote monitoring role, the clinical trials assistant/project assistant role is a bridge role to the remote or traveling CRA position and is much sought after.

Responsibilities of the clinical trial assistant/project assistant include:

- Mass study communications and updates to investigational sites.
- Protocol amendment communications/updates and document provision to sites.
- Collection of screening and enrollment logs from sites.
- Administrative support for the study team.
- Updating the clinical trials management system with site and staffing changes and contact information, enrollment updates, etc.
- Updating study trackers, training trackers.
- Miscellaneous administrative support tasks for the project team.

The remote monitor and clinical trials assistant roles are good starting points for clinical research professionals who want to move into the CRA role. Many pharmaceutical companies or CROs promote from within and have CRA bridge programs in which individuals hired into one role are promoted and internally trained as a CRA.

The CRA Personality

What type of person makes a good CRA? What skills are required to be successful?

A CRA should be someone who is detail-oriented, a self-starter with good interpersonal relationship skills and a good writer and speaker. A CRA must be self-confident, flexible and adaptable to a changing environment. He or she must also be focused, manage time well and follow through on problems and commitments.

As innovations in technology continue to influence and change the clinical trials landscape, CRAs must be adept with the various computer/technology platforms used to manage clinical trials. In the wake of the pandemic, CRAs must be able to adapt to working a hybrid of remote and onsite trials, to review data and conduct monitoring activities.

Above all else, a CRA must be professional. Respect is the cornerstone of the CRA-site relationship. The CRA must maintain a professional demeanor with site personnel despite the potential for chaos or crisis onsite. A positive CRA-site dynamic is the primary driver of study success at the site level. Most CRAs spend a significant amount of time working away from the office without close supervision. It can be very easy to involve yourself in any number of diversions when your supervisor isn't around. Good CRAs maintain the same discipline and work habits on the road as they do in the office.

Years ago, almost all CRAs were former regional sales managers. People in these positions were recruited and hired as CRAs because field experience and interpersonal relationship skills were considered of paramount importance. The assumption was that it would be much easier to teach the skills necessary to monitor clinical trials than to teach the personal skills necessary to work and interact successfully with the variety of situations and personalities that a CRA encounters when monitoring clinical trials. These former sales folks were some of the best CRAs in the industry. That same rationale applies to the current dynamic of medical professionals (physicians, nurses, health educators) being sought for entry-level CRA positions. Not only do these individuals have the medical terminology and clinical training critical to this role, they are skilled in the most fundamental elements of human interaction and can relate to investigational site staff on a variety of levels due to similar backgrounds.

Some people are simply never able to develop excellent people skills. You can have all the training and knowledge in the world regarding the conduct and monitoring of clinical trials, but if you cannot work or communicate with the people involved, you won't be a successful CRA.

If you're considering this profession, or if you are already a CRA and hope to improve your performance, you must ask yourself:

- Am I a team player?
- Do I interact positively and successfully with individuals from different cultures and all walks of life?
- Am I able to maintain poise and professional behavior even with difficult or challenging situations/personalities or when having a bad day?
- Do speaking and writing come easily to me?

- Do I have strong documentation and retention skills?
- Am I comfortable working remotely?
- Am I comfortable with various operating systems and computer platforms?
- Do I conduct an honest day's work, in or out of the office?
- Do I meet deadlines?
- Do I pay attention to details?
- Do I listen?
- Do I like to travel?
- Am I able to work in different environments (e.g., airport, exam room, hospital basement)?
- Do my personal commitments allow me to travel with a clear conscience?

Be honest with yourself. If you answer "no" to any of these questions, take action to improve.

The dynamics of the working relationships between the CRA, the sponsor/CRO and the investigative sites are complex. A CRA must maintain current information on each site that he or she is monitoring, including data on site performance, current enrollment status, problem resolution and corrections that must be made during the next visit. To maintain this information, the CRA must depend on other sponsor personnel—people who may be stressed, busy and working to meet deadlines.

At an investigative site there are similar problems, including the fact that your study may not enjoy the same priority at the site that it does at your company. Consequently, the CRA must be able to act as a cheerleader and coach as well as an enforcer. These are difficult roles to perform at the same time. Whether working with colleagues at the home office or site personnel, the CRA needs to employ all the skills mentioned above to avoid problems and get the job done.

A CRA must be a "Jack or Jill of all trades" if they plan to be involved in this line of work for any length of time because there are so many activities and tasks to be a part of.CRAs must also be able to work under adverse conditions, think on their feet and be away from home for days at a time. Travel today is strenuous, time-consuming, frustrating and stressful. Being alone under these conditions and in places unfamiliar to you may be unsettling.

In addition to the stress of travel and working conditions at sites that are often less than ideal, medical institutions and private-practice facilities rarely have enough room because clinical studies usually don't enjoy a very high priority with regard to space. Consequently, you might be doing various monitoring tasks in some pretty uncomfortable places. It's hard to work when you're balancing everything on your knees or leaning over an exam table between patient visits. However, as detailed in the travel scenarios noted in this chapter, the positives far outweigh the negatives for the brave individual who wants to tread the exciting and demanding, but extremely gratifying, CRA career path.

Author's Story

I thoroughly enjoyed working as a regional CRA. I consider myself fortunate to be able to count the number of travel debacles on one hand, with countless outstanding travel experiences as the "norm." However, the savvy regional CRA recognizes that extremely negative/inconvenient travel experiences are the exception and are best endured with patience and humor.

One of the most frustrating travel experiences of my monitoring career resulted in the cancellation of two monitoring visits, getting a collective five hours of sleep in three days and a thirteen-hour travel day home with nothing to show for my efforts.

I was scheduled to conduct two monitoring visits in Northeast Canada: One site was in Montreal and the other was in Newfoundland, a beautiful northern island in Canada that I had always wanted to visit. The first night of my journey I never made it out of the U.S. due to lightning storms in Minneapolis. After a three-hour delay, the airline ultimately rescheduled the flight to the next morning, so I had to reschedule the first monitoring visit. After spending an hour on the phone with the airline representative rebooking my flight to go directly to Newfoundland, I found last-minute accommodations at an airport hotel but had only two hours of sleep due to the early flight the next day. I traveled most of the next day to Ontario and then took the final flight to Newfoundland.

As we approached Newfoundland, we were unexpectedly diverted to Nova Scotia due to high winds. After sitting in the Nova Scotia airport for what seemed an eternity, I made the decision to reschedule the second monitoring visit, as I had a sinking feeling that we were never going to get to Newfoundland. I found another airport hotel and implored the kind-hearted front desk clerk for the most meager accommodation. I spent an additional two hours on the phone with the airline representative, and they finally rebooked my journey home, Nova Scotia to Calgary to Seattle to San Diego. This was a thirteen-hour travel journey.

The result of my exhausting travel experience? Zero monitoring visits conducted and almost five hours speaking to hotel and airline representatives on the telephone.

One of my most outstanding travel experiences as a monitor was when I went to New York City the evening before Halloween for a monitoring visit on the holiday itself. I was upgraded to first class on every flight. Upon my arrival in the city, I was upgraded to a five-room suite at a beautiful hotel, which included a spectacular view of the Hudson River and the city skyline. The pre-study monitoring visit was for a retrospective data collection study that was simple in design; the meeting at the site took two hours and after I finished my remaining work, I spent the rest of the afternoon sight-seeing and enjoying the outrageous Halloween display by New Yorkers.

What a way to work!

–Elizabeth

Career Preparation

How does someone prepare for this complex, challenging career? Today, most CRAs have a bachelor's degree in nursing or in one of the health, natural or medical sciences. Many universities offer postgraduate courses in clinical research (some web-based). There are courses taught by professional societies, such as the Drug Information Association (DIA) and the Association of Clinical Research Professionals (ACRP).

The ratio of open CRA positions vs. CRAs available to fill them ebbs and flows with the economic climate, disease treatment trends and other critical factors. The COVID-19 pandemic created a new therapeutic area for study conduct, COVID vaccines and treatments. These new COVID studies, in addition to established therapeutic area clinical trials starting or ongoing regularly, have created an immediate, critical need for CRAs with the rising study workload. This need has eliminated the previous requirement for clinical research staff to have two years of monitoring experience before transitioning to a CRA role. The industry now views the clinical research experience many investigational site staff have gained as transferrable. Recruiters and hiring managers have had to become open-minded when considering overall clinical research experience to meet the incredible need for CRAs. This has enabled hard-working, motivated and intelligent site personnel to achieve long-held career aspirations.

There are many more CRA training programs and development opportunities in existence as a result of the wave of new clinical researchers entering the industry. Virtual classroom and online clinical research courses taught by industry professionals (study coordinators, CRAs, project managers, etc.) teach the fundamentals of the noted roles and sometimes provide internships and job placement assistance for a nominal fee.

More pharmaceutical and CRO companies are recruiting for new CRAs at universities and offer college internships with prospective positioning for qualified candidates.

Almost every major CRO offers a CRA training program. These are targeted to individuals with clinical research experience looking to transition to the CRA role: experienced study coordinators, data managers, project assistants, investigational pharmacy personnel, etc. After the training, the CRO hires the individual as an entry-level CRA.

Another option is to take an entry-level position at a CRO or pharmaceutical company as a project or clinical trials assistant and work toward a CRA position. This is a longer route that requires willingness to take a pay cut and a proverbial step backward to ultimately move forward, but it does work. Generally speaking, CROs tend to hire more first-timers than large pharmaceutical companies. However, don't exclude the pharmaceutical companies from your list when sending out resumés. Once you get your first CRA position, give it everything you have. A good track record is the greatest asset to furthering your career.

There are CRA coaches for hire who will help those interested in becoming CRAs develop their interviewing and networking skills and update their resumes and social media profiles to help land an interview and CRA position. These individuals are not recruiters but provide a fully dimensional CRA grooming process.

Individuals looking to learn about the CRA role need look no further than social media for content and educational tutorials. Clinical research authors, speakers and influencers post videos and educational content on LinkedIn, Tik Tok, Instagram and other online platforms.

Most sponsor companies have two to four levels of available CRA positions. The differences are primarily related to experience. One key difference is the CRA's ability to evaluate a potential study site and determine whether that site has the expertise, experience, resources and patients to do a particular study well. A CRA who can consistently find good investigators and who can generate accurate, timely data with a minimum of enrollment problems is a valuable asset to a sponsor company or CRO.

As noted earlier in this chapter, the impact of technology on clinical trials requires CRAs to be computer and platform savvy with such programs as EDC, cloud-based trial platforms/systems and clinical trial management systems, among others, used to review and manage data, queries, enrollment, adverse events and protocol deviations. As a result of internet-driven data analysis/collection, remote monitoring is now an essential element of site management. CRAs must also be familiar with systems that manage time entry, expense reports and training within their own organizations.

Experienced CRAs should have a good understanding of the scientific method, which enables them to recognize actions and procedures that could bias a study and invalidate the data. Expertise in these key areas is developed only over time, which is why experience and proven performance are of such high value. Generic job descriptions for two levels of CRAs, plus a job summary comparing tasks for entry level and advanced CRAs, are included in Appendix D.

Once on the job, knowledge, networking and common sense are your best weapons. You never outgrow your need to learn. Be prepared to read quite a bit. At the top of your reading list should be the federal regulations that govern the conduct of clinical research. All CRAs should read the regulations periodically and be aware of possible regulatory updates. Don't rely too heavily on the advice of colleagues because they may not have read the regulations recently. The ICH Guidelines and the Belmont Report should also be on your list of required reading.

CRAs must constantly educate themselves on different diseases and medical conditions and on new drugs and devices. You need to have enough of an understanding to be able to recognize things that are problematic as you monitor sites. You won't be offering medical opinions or advice, but knowledge of basic information in each therapeutic area you monitor is necessary.

SOPs are an important tool for CRAs and should be used to help manage work and as an overall guidance. This means the CRA does not always have to rely on intuition or ethical standards; SOPs will provide a basic level from which to approach tasks and problems. Sponsors and CROs should have a complete set of SOPs to govern monitoring activities, including:

- Investigator selection.
- Risk-based monitoring.
- Onboarding and training of new CRAs.
- Clinical trial agreement.
- Collection and maintenance of study documents.
- Evaluation and selection of investigational sites.
- Initiation of a clinical trial.
- Routine monitoring of a clinical trial.
- Remote monitoring of a clinical trial.
- Source data verification/source data review.
- Investigational product handling and accountability.
- Site visit monitoring reports.
- Reporting noncompliance.
- Study closeout.
- Audits of clinical sites.
- SAE reporting.
- Protocol deviation reporting.

CROs and pharmaceutical companies rely on quality assurance measures to ensure the integrity and accuracy of data collected, and this extends to monitoring proficiency and accuracy of the CRAs they employ. CRAs are evaluated on the onsite conduct of all monitoring visit types (evaluation, initiation, interim monitoring and closeout visits) at periodic intervals by qualified clinical management/senior CRA staff to ensure regulatory and study compliance. This evaluation by the individual assessing the CRA includes specific assessment of all elements of each visit type. Specific interim monitoring visit evaluations include additional review of source/CRF data, drug accountability logs and regulatory documents by the CRA evaluator to ensure the accuracy of data previously reviewed by the CRA currently being assessed. The individual evaluating the CRA will also observe site staff relations and investigator discussions to ensure professionalism and diligence.

The CRA should develop a large network of colleagues. One of the best ways to do this is through membership in professional associations. ACRP (acrpnet.org), the Society of Clinical Research Associates (SOCRA) (socra.org) and DIA (diaglobal.org) are three of the largest associations. It's a good idea to join at least one of these groups. All above noted associations have journals, provide training and offer information and sponsor meetings and workshops. Each also has an annual conference, with continuing education sessions, panels on industry trends and issues and opening sessions with well-known industry influencers/speakers. Try to attend at least one professional meeting each year, as these are great learning opportunities as well as perfect networking events. There are also speaking opportunities for CRAs at these conferences; they require abstract submission and acceptance on the proposed speaking topic but help develop critical speaking and leadership skills important to the CRA role. Check out their websites and talk with current members to get a feel for which organization best meets your particular needs.

There are clinical research education and networking groups, such as GCP Café (gcpcafe.com), and clinical research podcasts that provide clips, blogs and interviews about the industry and relevant CRA training items as a means of educating CRAs/clinical researchers.

Finally, rely on your common sense as well as your business sense. The people participating in your studies are your customers; without them you are out of work. Treat them accordingly. Be polite, courteous and kind. Return calls and emails promptly. Before visiting a site, contact the staff and tell them what you will be doing during the visit, who you wish to have available and how long you plan to be there. A detailed discussion of the business approach to monitoring is covered in the chapter on monitoring.

In the Future

What's coming in the future?

The more movement there is within a job category, the more opportunity it brings. The CRA job has always had a high turnover rate, primarily because it involves a lot of travel and many people reach a point at which their family responsibilities limit their travel availabilities. CRAs who are well-versed in their jobs and complete their responsibilities in a professional manner should have no trouble finding and maintaining good positions.

As the CRA role evolves, so do those of some other closely aligned positions in clinical research, primarily the data manager and the project manager. Since these positions need to work closely together for successful research projects, people holding these positions tend to become knowledgeable about each of them. Frequently, the project manager position is a step up for a CRA, especially when the CRA may reach the time when significant travel becomes problematic. The CRA job, on the other hand, is often seen as a step up the career ladder for a data manager. As people become more experienced and more familiar with the details of how research projects function, they are more apt to obtain new positions that might integrate all three of these functions.

Another role gaining traction in clinical research is that of the clinical trial educator (CTE) or site engagement specialist. The need for CTEs has increased exponentially in the highly competitive research landscape, which is focusing more on investigator, staff and sponsor collaboration, study training, and education and patient-centric clinical trials. The CTE has the therapeutic expertise to better train and facilitate investigational staff understanding of protocol design, endpoints, eligibility criteria and investigational product modalities. There is a science to patient recruitment that involves strategic collaboration between investigators, study staff and physician/facility referrals, as well as a specific understanding to successfully utilize electronic medical records and laboratory databases in the search for potential research subjects.

The CTE is a strategic role with therapeutic and clinical operations expertise to bridge the gap between site/patient education/awareness of clinical studies and patient recruitment. The CTE can ease the investigational site burden by answering site questions, proposing recruitment strategies and serving as a reminder of study importance to investigational sites with frequent communication and support techniques. The CTE builds investigator networks that identify study sites and solicit interest from physicians in study conduct. They have even employed compliance and retention training to study patients.

CTEs are most often RNs, but the position can also be fulfilled by other clinical specialists with expertise in a specific therapeutic area (respiratory therapists, dieticians, pharmacists).

There is a trend toward certification for CRAs—certification will be helpful for differentiating yourself professionally. Currently, both ACRP and SOCRA offer certification programs for CRAs. Both programs require previous experience and passing a written examination. Although it is not necessary at this point for a CRA to be certified, it does add to a person's credentials and credibility. At some point in his or her career, the CRA should investigate and work toward achieving certification. A certified CRA may have an edge when it comes to being hired or promoted. In the future, it may well become standard practice for CRAs to be certified.

Ambition is integral for career progression and to prevent career stagnation. As a CRA grows within their position, so does the desire for increased responsibilities and commensurate pay. Some CRAs feel they can advance internally and will work with their line managers for a promotion/pay increase, while others feel they need to move to another company for a dramatic increase in salary/position. The prospect of a promotion and change in climate that accompany a move is appealing; however, there are also benefits to staying and growing with a company, such as consistent work history on a CV. Recruiters expect some degree of "jumping" from position to position, but a CV with inconsistent or historically short work histories is a red flag to hiring managers. Unfortunately, new CRAs sometimes feel that the only way they can move to the next level in their CRA career is by changing companies. Sometimes a new CRA only has to have a year or more of CRA experience to move to a CRA 2 position and a significant salary increase. This sometimes happens after employers have previously been too slow to promote new employees and increase salaries. This has prompted organizations to provide CRAs an accelerated promotion path and larger salary increases to stay competitive and retain employees.

There are many opportunities for successful CRAs to expand their careers into new, yet related, areas. Be ready and prepared for change, as change always occurs over time.

Your Value

The importance of the CRA role in clinical research cannot be over-emphasized. CRAs are on the front line and play a major role in study conduct and quality. Bad studies are not usually the fault of site personnel; they result from poor planning and study design and from improper selection, preparation and training of the study staff. A CRA may not be involved in planning and study design; but selection, preparation and training are usually CRA responsibilities. Few people on the drug development team have as much direct impact on study quality and timeliness as the CRA.

The CRA also has an influence on the bottom line for a drug program as the main defense against data errors during clinical trials, which can cost millions of dollars to correct. The CRA also as a major impact on the timely completion of trials, assuring that company development timelines are realistic and are met or exceeded. It's not hard to understand the value of a good CRA in terms of program quality and cost.

Key Takeaways

- CRAs are paramedical personnel who perform a variety of clinical research monitoring activities in support of a drug development program.
- CRAs must be self-starters with excellent interpersonal relationship skills, detail-orientation and excellent written and oral communication skills.
- CRAs must possess a breadth of clinical knowledge enabling them to provide investigative site personnel with the information they need to perform good clinical trials.
- CRAs need to be adaptable and be able to work under a wide variety of conditions.
- CRAs should stay abreast of technology and innovations that impact clinical trials and the monitoring role.
- CRAs should develop a large network of peers and colleagues.

- CRAs play a major role in the conduct, quality and timeliness of clinical trials.
- Industry trends and technology serve as the impetus for new CRA/education positions.

CHAPTER 2

The History Behind the Regulations

Good Clinical Practice (GCP) is the internationally recognized ethical and scientific-quality standard for designing, conducting, recording and reporting trials that involve the participation of human subjects. Compliance with this standard provides public assurance that the rights, safety and well-being of trial subjects are protected, consistent with the principles that have their origin in the Declaration of Helsinki and that the clinical trial data are credible.

GCPs are derived from federal regulations, ethical codes, ICH guidelines and official guidance documents. They evolved because of concerns about the treatment of human research subjects around the world and about the reliability of the data and conclusions from trials. Concern about data and conclusions goes beyond the need to protect subjects in clinical trials, extending to the greater goal of protecting all patients who use pharmaceutical products. There are serious consequences for not following the GCPs, including loss of revenue and loss of reputation. Also, not following GCPs can expose sponsors and investigative sites to legal liability, not only from study subjects, but also from future users of a medication (class action suits, for example).

Understanding why the regulations were developed and some of the factors that will undoubtedly lead to additional regulations in the future will help you become a better CRA.

Over the course of the past few years, several large institutional review boards (IRB) have had their activities curtailed by the Food and Drug Administration (FDA) and the Office for Human Research Protection (OHRP) because of serious problems and deficiencies found during inspections. Because of these findings, clinical trials at some of these institutions had enrollment halted or were closed completely. Sponsor companies suffered because they were counting on the data to support their new drug applications (NDA), and the respective institutions suffered because of the loss of study revenues and the intangible loss of their status in the clinical trials community. The discovery of serious problems at a handful of IRBs has already resulted in increased government surveillance, primarily by increasing the number of IRB inspections, and a reorganization within the U.S. Department of Health and Human Services (HHS) to better handle this increased surveillance.

There have also been concerns raised about potential problems inherent in genomics research, both from an ethical viewpoint and because genomics involves new and untried research techniques. It is likely that changes in federal regulations will further tighten research requirements. CRAs should be aware of these changes and be prepared to make appropriate adjustments in the way they work with investigative sites and clinical trials. It is wise to be aware of the current research environment and be prepared for impending changes. You will be a better CRA if you know why the pharmaceutical industry is so highly regulated and why the primary vehicles for human subject protection—IRBs and informed consent—are so important.

Crisis is an impetus for change. Crises breed controversy, which leads to the involvement of Congress, which then enacts legislation. Some of the major milestones in regulations and in human subject protection, and the crises that spurred them, where appropriate, are discussed below.

Regulation and Human Subject Protection Milestones

1848: Drug Importation Act

The first regulatory action regarding drugs came in 1848, when Congress enacted a law that required the U.S. Customs Service to stop the import of adulterated drugs.

1862: Bureau of Chemistry

In 1862, President Abraham Lincoln appointed Dr. Charles M. Wetherill, a chemist, to serve in the new U.S. Department of Agriculture (USDA). This was the beginning of the Bureau of Chemistry, which in 1927 became the Food, Drug and Insecticide Administration. The name was changed to the Food and Drug Administration (FDA) in 1930.

1906: Food and Drugs Act

Until the Food and Drugs Act was signed by President Theodore Roosevelt in 1906, there was no comprehensive statute regulating drugs. Before this, standard medical practice consisted of activities such as purges and bloodletting. There were very few effective drugs on the market. All products could be freely advertised and sold and were readily available without a prescription. Then came Harvey W. Wiley.

Wiley was the chief chemist at the USDA from 1883 to 1912. He had a driving interest in the adulteration of food and drugs and set up a plan to investigate food preservatives. In 1902, Wiley set up his "poison squad"—a group of young, unmarried men who had volunteered to test foods Wiley thought might contain unhealthy preservatives or coloring agents. The squad lunched together, trying the various substances Dr. Wiley wanted to test. Judgment on the degree of harm the substances caused was based on how sick the men got after eating them. The experiments were carried out over the course of five years, and proved conclusively that many preservatives found in food were harmful.

It was, at least in part, because of Wiley's work that Congress passed the 1906 Pure Food and Drugs Act, which prohibited the interstate transportation of adulterated and misbranded foods, drinks and drugs. It didn't limit companies from producing the items, but it cut down on their ability to widely market them, as these items could not be taken across state lines.

1938: Food, Drug and Cosmetic Act

The next major crisis was precipitated by the use of Elixir of Sulfanilamide. Sulfanilamide was a tablet—a very large tablet—used to treat infections. The manufacturer wanted to market it for children, but the tablet was too big for them to swallow. The company decided to make it into a liquid by adding diethylene glycol, the principal ingredient in antifreeze. The company was able to get a liquid form and tested it for flavor—it tasted just fine. Unfortunately, the company never tested the resulting elixir for toxicity. It was very toxic, causing the deaths of more than a hundred people, many of them children.

The FDA had no authority to withdraw the product from the market for safety reasons, because there were no regulations regarding safety. The agency could, however, remove it for mislabeling. It was called an elixir, and elixirs had to contain alcohol, which Elixir of Sulfanilamide did not. Based solely on this finding, the FDA was able to have the unsafe product removed from the market.

As a direct result of this tragedy, Congress passed the 1938 Food, Drug and Cosmetic Act. For the first time, a premarket approval of "new drugs" was required for safety. "New drugs" meant new chemical entities or combinations. Drugs marketed prior to 1938 were specifically exempted (grandfathered in) as long as their labeling didn't change. There was no definition of safety in the act; however, the general understanding was that the benefits must outweigh the risk. The act also did not require active approval by the FDA. Unless the FDA objected within 60 days of the new drug application NDA being filed, the manufacturer could automatically begin marketing. No proof of efficacy was required. Between 1938 and 1962, most NDAs that were filed were essentially just testimonials from physicians.

1947: Nuremberg Code

After the Nuremberg Trials of Nazi leaders during 1945-1946, a series of supplemental trials were held. One trial, officially known as United States v. Karl Brandt et al. and commonly referred to as The Nazi Doctors Trial, was held from Dec. 9, 1946 to July 19, 1947. The judges and prosecutors in this court trial were all from the U.S. The 23 defendants (including 20 physicians)—all members of the Nazi Party—were charged with murder, torture and other atrocities committed in the name of medical science.

When the final judgment in the Nazi Doctors Trial was delivered on July 19, 1947, 15 of the 23 defendants were found guilty. Seven were sentenced to death. Four presiding American judges issued a 10-point code that described basic principles of ethical behavior in the conduct of human experimentation. This 10-point code is known as the Nuremberg Code. Although the Code focuses on the ethical treatment of humans in non-therapeutic research (research not intended to result in a cure for a condition), the elements described formed the cornerstone for the guidelines and regulations we have today and reflect that:

- Informed consent should be obtained without coercion.
- The experiment should be useful and necessary.
- Human experiments should be based on previous experiments with animals.
- Physical and mental suffering should be avoided.

- Death and disability should not be expected outcomes of an experiment.
- The degree of risk taken should not exceed the humanitarian importance of solving the problem.
- Human subjects should be protected against even remote possibilities of harm.
- Only qualified scientists should conduct medical research.
- Human subjects should be free to end an experiment at any time.
- The scientist in charge must be prepared to end an experiment at any stage.

1962: Kefauver-Harris Amendments (Drug Amendments of 1962)

In the late 1950s, thalidomide was being tested extensively in Europe, and to some degree in the U.S. It was a sleeping pill, and pregnant women were included in the testing groups. Unfortunately, it had a terrible effect on the fetus when taken during the first trimester, and many children born to women who had taken thalidomide suffered from phocomelia, a shortening of the limbs which resulted in arms that looked like flippers. Dr. Francis Kelsey at the FDA was responsible for much of the research that defined the link between phocomelia and thalidomide use in pregnancy.

The Kefauver-Harris amendments, passed in part due to the outcry and public support for stronger drug regulation because of the thalidomide tragedy, formed the basis of the current Investigational New Drug (IND) application regulations. For the first time, drugs were required to have proven efficacy, as well as safety. Also for the first time, an active FDA approval was required, beyond the review and 60-day waiting time. In addition, this law required mandated reporting of adverse events and disclosure of risks in advertisements.

Much to the chagrin of pharmaceutical manufacturers, as part of this regulation the FDA also had to re-review all the NDAs submitted between 1938 and 1962 to see if products met the new efficacy standard. There were numerous lawsuits over the definition of substantial evidence of efficacy, including the Pharmaceutical Manufacturers Association vs. the FDA, and suits by almost all major pharmaceutical manufacturers. This controversy led to the definition of the "adequate and well-controlled" clinical investigations required today.

1964: Declaration of Helsinki

The World Health Organization (WHO) spent more than 10 years working on the statement of ethical principles that became known as the Declaration of Helsinki. This document defined rules for therapeutic and non-therapeutic research. It repeated the Nuremberg Code requirement for consent for non-therapeutic research but allowed for enrolling certain patients in therapeutic research without consent. The Declaration of Helsinki also allowed legal guardians to grant permission to enroll subjects in research, both therapeutic and non-therapeutic, and recommended written consent—an issue not addressed in the Nuremberg Code. In addition, the Declaration of Helsinki required review and prior approval of a protocol by an IRB. Several revisions have been made to this document, including a Clarification.

1979: The Belmont Report

The National Research Act, passed by Congress in 1974, created the National Commission for the Protection of Human Subjects of Biomedical and Behavioral Research. This commission wrote a document entitled Ethical Principles and Guidelines for the Protection of Human Subjects of Research, which became known as the Belmont Report when it was published in 1979. The three basic principles of the Belmont Report are respect for persons, beneficence and justice.

1. Respect for persons is manifested by the informed consent process, as well as in safeguards for vulnerable populations such as children, pregnant women, mentally disabled adults and prisoners. Other important concerns of respect for persons include privacy and confidentiality.
2. Beneficence has two general characteristics: do no harm and maximize benefit while minimizing risk. Beneficence is manifested in the use of good research design, competent investigators and a favorable risk/benefit ratio.
3. Justice implies fairness and is manifested in the equitable selection of subjects for research, ensuring that no group of people is "selected in" or "selected out" unfairly based on factors unrelated to the research. This means that there must be appropriate inclusion/exclusion criteria and a fair system of recruitment.

The Belmont Report formed the cornerstone for the ethical treatment of human subjects in research.

1987: IND Rewrite Regulations

Additional regulations were enacted after three extreme examples of abuse illustrated the need for further protection of human subjects.

Tuskegee Syphilis Study

In this study, which began in 1932 and extended for more than 40 years, several hundred black males with syphilis were enrolled. They were not informed about the purpose of the study, but were told that government doctors were examining people for "bad blood." Even after penicillin became available and was known to be effective for syphilis (1943), the males in this study were not treated with it. This study was not stopped until 1973, when treatment was given as needed. In 1997, President Clinton made a formal apology to study subjects and their families.

Jewish Chronic Disease Hospital Study

In 1963, physicians at this hospital were interested in studying the nature of human transplant rejection. To do this, they injected live cancer cells into indigent, elderly patients suffering from a variety of chronic debilitating diseases, without their consent. The subjects were not told about the live cancer cells because the physicians thought the cells would be rejected anyway, and they didn't want to alarm the subjects.

Acres of Skin

This book, by Allen M. Hornblum, revealed some of the abuses of testing in the Holmesburg Prison in Philadelphia, where subjects underwent extensive and painful testing of numerous chemicals to see their effect on the skin. Paying the prisoners $100 to be in a study, compared to the 10 cents a day they were paid for prison jobs, undoubtedly influenced their willingness to participate in these trials.

These studies were carried out from the mid-1950s through the mid-1970s. There were three principal objectives of the 1987 IND Rewrite Regulations: protecting the safety of subjects in clinical trials; ensuring the adequacy of clinical trial designs to support marketing approvals; and assuring the quality, integrity and validity of the data that form the bases of FDA approval decisions. Not only was patient/subject safety covered by aspects of these regulations, but the regulations were the impetus for greatly expanded statistical sections in protocols. From relatively short, basic descriptions of the analyses to be done, they became full-blown, detailed plans. For the first time, the FDA became a real partner in ensuring both adequate trial design and the generation of data that would stand rigorous inspection.

1988: Expedited NDA Approval Process for Life-Threatening Illnesses

Primarily as a result of the AIDS crisis, Congress enacted the 1988 Expedited NDA regulations. The purpose of these regulations was to establish procedures to expedite the development, evaluation and marketing of new therapies intended to treat people with life-threatening and severely debilitating illnesses, especially where no satisfactory alternative therapy existed. These regulations provide for consultation with the FDA early in the development process to review and agree on the design of non-clinical and clinical studies. They also provide for treatment protocols under which an investigational drug can be provided to patients throughout the clinical development program and review period, prior to marketing. (These studies are known as expanded access or named patient trials.) Because nothing else is available to treat these illnesses and people are dying from them, the risk/benefit assessment is more lenient than for other investigational drugs.

In consultation with the FDA, companies may be allowed to collapse phase 2 and 3 studies together (see Chapter 5 for an explanation of the phases of drug testing); however, in this case, phase 4 post-marketing surveillance studies are often a condition of approval. If post-marketing studies are required, the company is given a time period (usually two to three years) within which the studies must be completed, and these studies must be submitted, reviewed and approved or marketing approval may be withdrawn.

1992: Prescription Drug User Fee Act

In the years preceding the Prescription Drug User Fee Act (PDUFA), the FDA was under fire because it took so much longer to review and approve drugs in the U.S. than it did in Europe. Congress asked why. The FDA replied that the agency didn't have enough people available to do the job any faster. In response, Congress enacted PDUFA in 1992, which provided the FDA with more people to review human drug applications. The funds for acquiring additional review staff came from fees collected from the firms developing drugs and biologics. The goal was to reduce the time required to review and evaluate certain drug applications without compromising the quality of the review.

The industry was, and is, willing to pay. The fees associated with this program have sped up the review time for NDAs. For 2023, the fee a sponsor had to pay for submitting an application requiring clinical data was $3,242,026 while the fee for an application not requiring clinical data, or for a supplement requiring clinical data, was $1,621,013.

These fees are actually a small price to pay for accelerating NDA approval, when you consider that every day saved is worth about $1.4 million (based on a good, but average, drug that brings in about $500 million in annual sales.)

1993: NIH Revitalization of Act of 1993

This was signed into law to establish guidelines for the inclusion of women and persons from racial and ethnic minority populations in clinical research. The goal of this law, and other guidelines, is to ensure that research findings are generalizable to the entire population.

1997: FDA Modernization Act

PDUFA was considered a success. The problem with PDUFA, however, was that the period for collecting fees expired after five years. In 1997, Congress reauthorized PDUFA for an additional five years by enacting the FDA Modernization Act (FDAMA). Not only did this act extend PDUFA, it also increased patient access to investigational drugs and mandated an expanded database on clinical trials that was accessible to patients. It also accelerated the review of important new drugs, like those used to treat conditions with high morbidity and mortality where no treatment already existed, in part by allowing one pivotal trial rather than two in certain circumstances. FDAMA also requires child testing in certain categories of drugs for which pediatric use is expected. FDAMA mandates the most wide-ranging agency reforms since 1938, including not only the provisions listed above but also others designed to accelerate the review of devices, regulate advertising of unapproved uses for approved drugs and devices, and regulate health claims for foods.

2022-Food and Drug Omnibus Reform Act

The Food and Drug Omnibus Reform Act (FDAMA) signed into law in December 2022 includes funding for clinical trial diversity legislation such as the Diverse and Equitable Participation in Clinical Trials (DEPICT) Act and the Diversifying Investigations Via Equitable Research Studies for Everyone (DIVERSE) Trials Act.

DEPICT directs the FDA to issue regulations requiring sponsors to develop a diversity plan for clinical trials and gives the agency the authority to mandate post-approval studies or post-marketing surveillance if the clinical trials conducted to support a drug application did not meet the enrollment targets.

Under the new omnibus legislation, pharmaceutical and biotech companies are now required to submit diversity action plans for phase 3 or pivotal trials. These plans should include specific enrollment goals and supporting rationale. Per the legislation, plans "shall apply only with respect to clinical investigations for which enrollment commences after the date that is 180 days after publication of final guidance required under this section."

The FDA will be tasked with analyzing the plans provided by sponsors and publishing annual aggregate reports for approved therapies. These reports have to be submitted to Congress. The FDA is also required to conduct one or more public meetings to solicit input from all stakeholders on ways to increase clinical trial diversity.

It is important to note that the legislation failed to include proposed provisions to give the FDA the authority to mandate postmarketing studies for companies that do not meet their diversity plan goals.

Summary

The regulations and the ethics documents are in place to ensure the safety and well-being of human subjects involved in research. The government has made tremendous strides to ensure not only that subject protections are in place, but also that safe drugs reach the market. A list of readings is included in the appendices, in case you'd like more history and background about why the business of clinical trials is as regulated as it is today.

Key Takeaways

- Regulations are often a response to abuse of human research subjects and to concerns about the validity of data and conclusions from clinical trials.
- The primary vehicles for human subject protection are IRBs and informed consent.
- The Declaration of Helsinki and the Belmont Report are critical documents for the protection of human subjects in research.
- The FDA, by means of PDUFA and FDAMA, has made significant gains in accelerating the process of making new drugs available for patients who need them.
- Problems with clinical trials and trial oversights may well lead to increased regulation.
- Requirements for diversity in clinical trials enacted into law.

CHAPTER 3

Regulations and GCPs

This chapter discusses the regulations and guidelines a CRA must be familiar with and understand.

An informal survey of a few large investigative sites showed that many CRAs exhibit a lack of knowledge of the regulations. This is especially true of those new to the business. Unfortunately, many of these same CRAs think they have a good working knowledge of the regulations. How can this happen? Very easily. Instead of reading the regulations for themselves, too many people rely on information by asking someone else who may not have actually read them either. This leads to misinformation, self-perpetuating myths and misinformation.

It is a good practice for CRAs to carry pocket-sized copies of the FDA regulations and ICH/GCP guidelines or bookmark links to FDA regulations (ecfr.gov/current/title-21) and ICH E6(R2) (database.ich.org/sites/default/files/E6_R2_Addendum.pdf) and the FDA website (FDA.gov) for reference during monitoring visits and discussions with study staff to explain or support a questioned directive.

FDA Regulations for Clinical Trials

As a CRA, you will want to make sure you have a thorough understanding of the regulations. This will help to keep your sites in compliance. The regulations CRAs should be familiar with are:

- 21 CFR Part 11—Electronic Records and Electronic Signatures.
- 21 CFR Part 50—Protection of Human Subjects.
- 21 CFR Part 54—Financial Disclosure by Clinical Investigators.
- 21 CFR Part 56—Institutional Review Boards.

- 21 CFR Part 312—Investigational New Drug Application.
- 21 CFR Part 314—Applications for FDA Approval to Market a New Drug.

If you are working with devices, you should be familiar with:

- 21 CFR Part 812—Investigational Device Exemptions.
- 21 CFR Part 814—Premarket Approval of Medical Devices.

If you are working with biologics, you also want to be familiar with:

- 21 CFR Part 600—Biological Products; General.
- 21 CFR Part 601—Biologics-Licensing.
- 21 CFR Part 610—General Biological Products Standards.

The first six parts listed above encompass the Good Clinical Practice (GCP) sections of the Code of Federal Regulations, and they form the basis of the regulations pertinent to conducting clinical trials in the U.S.

Since the job of a CRA is to monitor clinical trials, it follows that the CRA must have a good working knowledge of these regulations. The regulations tell us what is actually required by the FDA when involved in conducting clinical studies. They cover the responsibilities of sponsors, investigators and IRBs for conducting trials involving human subjects.

Exploring the FDA's website, www.fda.gov, is a great way to find all kinds of information about conducting trials. Taking some time to look around and delve into different topics on the web will be time well spent for a CRA. From this site, you can branch off into information about drugs, biologics and devices.

ICH Guidelines for Good Clinical Practice

In addition to FDA regulations, CRAs must be familiar with the ICH Guideline for Good Clinical Practice. Although not yet required by regulation in the U.S., ICH E6(R2) has been adopted by the FDA as an official guidance. Many sponsor companies require their studies to follow ICH E6(R2), as well as FDA regulations.

The ICH was organized to provide opportunities for standardized regulatory initiatives to be developed with input from both governmental bodies and industry representatives. ICH is comprised of 14 member nations and several industry organizations. The ICH guideline from 1997 defines Good Clinical Practice and provides a unified standard for designing, conducting, recording and reporting on clinical trials involving human subjects. Compliance with good clinical practice ensures that the rights, well-being and confidentiality of human subjects are protected and that trial data are credible.

FDA Guidances and Information Sheets

The FDA also publishes a number of guidances and information sheets that are very useful in the conduct of clinical trials. These give further explanation to the regulations, including current interpretations and thought processes of the FDA. They often include questions and answers for items that are of particular interest. Although the guidances do not carry the weight of regulations, it is highly recommended that they be followed, as they explain the FDA's expectations for the conduct of trials.

Links to specific guidances and information sheets can be found on the FDA website. Some of the more useful guidances are:

- Information Sheet Guidance for Sponsors, Clinical Investigators, and IRBs, Frequently Asked Questions, Statement of Investigator, (Form FDA 1572) (Revision 1), Draft Guidance, May 2021.
- Conduct of Clinical Trials of Medical Products During the COVID-19 Public Health Emergency, Guidance for Industry, Investigators, and Institutional Review Boards, March 2020, Updated Aug. 30, 2021.
- A Risk-Based Approach to Monitoring of Clinical Investigations, Questions and Answers, Guidance for Industry, April 2023.
- Informed Consent, Draft Guidance for IRBs, Clinical Investigators, and Sponsor, July 2014.
- Use of Electronic Informed Consent in Clinical Investigations—Questions and Answers, Guidance for Institutional Review Boards, Investigators, and Sponsors, December 2016.
- Exception from Informed Consent Requirements for Emergency Research, Guidance for IRBs, Clinical Investigators and Sponsors, April 2013.

- Recruiting Study Subjects, Guidance for Institutional Review Boards and Clinical Investigators, January 1998.
- Disqualified/Restricted/Assurance List for Clinical Investigators.
- Using a Centralized IRB Review Process in Multicenter Clinical Trials, Guidance for Industry, March, 2006.
- FDA Inspections of Clinical Investigators, Guidance for IRBs, Clinical Investigators and Sponsors, June 2010.
- Investigator Responsibilities—Protecting the Rights, Safety and Welfare of Study Subjects.
- Waiver of IRB Requirements for Drug and Biological Product Studies—Information Sheet, 2017.
- Content of Human Factors Information in Medical Device Marketing Submissions, Draft Guidance for Industry, December 2022.
- Guidance for Industry and Investigators Safety Reporting Requirements for INDs and BA/BE Studies, December 2012.
- Electronic Source Data in Clinical Investigations, Guidance for Industry, 2013.
- Payment and Reimbursement to Research Subjects—Information Sheet, January, 2018.
- Diversity Plans to Improve Enrollment of Participants from Underrepresented Racial and Ethnic Populations in Clinical Trials, Draft Guidance for Industry, April 2022.

CRAs should familiarize themselves with these guidances as well as with the regulations. Exceptions from informed consent are discussed in detail in Chapter 9. Risk-based monitoring practices are detailed in Chapter 14.

FDA Compliance Program Guidance Manuals

There are also a number of FDA Compliance Program Guidance Manuals (CPGM) that can be helpful to a CRA. These are the manuals FDA personnel use when they conduct inspections of clinical investigators, sponsors or IRBs.

All of these manuals can be found on the FDA website. Those of particular interest include:

- CPGM for Clinical Investigators and Sponsor-Investigators (7348.811).
- CPGM for Sponsors and Contract Research Organizations (7348.810).
- CPGM for IRBs (7348.809).

These manuals will tell you exactly what the FDA will focus on during inspections.

NIH-Regulated Research

CRAs were not generally involved in monitoring trials conducted under the auspices of HHS until the COVID pandemic. Sponsors ran joint trials during the pandemic in the quest to develop a COVID vaccine. For example, the National Institute of Allergy and Infectious Diseases (NIAID), part of the National Institutes of Health (NIH), provided trial funding and development with a known sponsor for COVID study conduct.

There are other occasions, however, when a sponsor may run a joint trial with an NIH group, such as the National Cancer Institute (NCI). In this case, the trial must be conducted by HHS regulations, which differ somewhat from FDA regulations. For example, HHS regulations contain specific sections on working with vulnerable subjects, such as pregnant women, children and prisoners, which are not found in FDA regulations. The FDA and HHS have developed a comparison of their respective regulations on human subject protections (https://www.fda.gov/science-research/good-clinical-practice-educational-materials/comparison-fda-and-hhs-human-subject-protection-regulations).

FDA Bioresearch Monitoring Program

The FDA requires that the biomedical research it regulates conform to GCP standards as found in FDA regulations. To help ensure that GCP standards are followed, the agency inspects clinical trials. (Note that what the FDA calls inspections are commonly called audits by others.) The FDA's program of inspections/audits is called the Bioresearch Monitoring (BIMO) program and covers all of the parties involved in regulated clinical trials, including clinical investigators, IRBs, sponsors, monitors and CROs. FDA audits are covered in Chapter 19.

Good Clinical Practice

Good Clinical Practice (GCP) is not a single document that can be referenced, printed or read. The phrase Good Clinical Practice was, in fact, coined by the industry and is a standard for the design, conduct, performance, monitoring, recording, analysis and reporting of clinical trials. The purpose of GCP is to protect human subjects in trials, as well as the general population who will use the products being tested once they are available on the market. GCPs comprise the FDA regulations and guidance documents, the ICH guidelines for good clinical practice and codes of ethical conduct, such as the Declaration of Helsinki and the Belmont Report. They are recognized as overall standard operating procedures for the conduct of clinical research and encompass the informed consent process, accurate collection of data, maintaining audit trails, reporting adverse events, investigator oversight and record retention. All of these items are covered in this book. Compliance with GCPs ensures not only that the rights and safety of study subjects are not compromised, but that the integrity of the data collected is maintained.

Common Rule Updates

A major component of GCP in the U.S. is the Federal Policy for the Protection of Human Research Subjects, which is enforced by a number of federal agencies that support clinical research. Known as the Common Rule, the policy puts forth requirements for informed consent and IRB review, among other issues.

The Common Rule, established in 1991, applies any time human subjects research is conducted using federal funding; therefore, federal agencies, academic institutions and healthcare research institutes are among the top qualifying institutions. The rule grew out of prior HHS regulations as well as a number of international developments in bioethics, including the Nuremberg Code, the Declaration of Helsinki and the Belmont Report. In 2011, the federal agencies began a regulatory overhaul of the rule to bring it up to date with current research practices and issues.

The revised rule, implemented in January 2019, includes new requirements for informed consent, the delineation of several new and expanded exempt categories of research, the creation of a new classification of "broad consent," the introduction of limited IRB review, the discontinuation of IRB continuing review and an update to the description of vulnerable populations.

The touchstone of the requirements is new language that states that informed consent must begin with "a concise and focused presentation of the key information that is most likely to assist a prospective subject or legally authorized representative in understanding why one might or might not want to participate in the research." This statement, according to the revised language, must be "organized and presented in a way that facilitates comprehension." The informed consent document should be readable, engaging and clear. Patients also must be given the chance to ask questions and discuss anything they might not understand.

The revised Common Rule suggests that prospective study subjects be provided a description of five "factors" at the beginning of the informed consent process, as well as at the beginning of the informed consent form:

- Consent is being sought and participation is voluntary.
- The purposes of the research, expected duration of participation and procedures to be followed.
- The reasonably foreseeable risks and discomforts.
- The benefits to the prospective subjects, or others, that may reasonably be expected from the research.
- Appropriate alternative procedures or courses of treatment that may be advantageous to the prospective subject.
- The rule also requires that informed consent forms be published online—to a federal website—within 60 days of the close of enrollment of the clinical study. Most likely that posting will be done by the sponsor.

Contacting the FDA

The FDA invites contact from sponsors, investigators and IRBs with respect to questions about proper procedures or interpretation of regulations. Most companies have a specific procedure to follow for calling the FDA. If a CRA has a question for the FDA, he or she should check with the sponsor company's regulatory department to be sure that it is acceptable to call. Company procedures may require that the regulatory department make all FDA contact. Contact numbers for all FDA offices are available on the FDA website.

In conclusion, there are many sources of information available to CRAs that will help them ensure compliance when working with investigative sites on clinical trials. CRAs should utilize these resources when doing their jobs.

Key Takeaways

- The FDA regulations pertaining to clinical trials are found in 21 CFR Parts 11, 50, 54, 56, 312 and 314.
- The ICH GCP guidelines should be followed in clinical trials.
- The FDA publishes many guidelines and information sheets pertaining to the appropriate conduct of clinical trials.
- Good clinical practices are the ethical and clinical standard for designing, conducting, analyzing, monitoring and reporting on clinical trials.
- There are differences between FDA and HHS rules for doing research in human subjects.
- CRAs should read and be familiar with the regulations that pertain to clinical trials and the ICH guidelines.

CHAPTER 4

Roles and Responsibilities in Clinical Trials

A clinical trial is a study done in human subjects to investigate a potential new drug, device or biologic product. There are three primary groups involved in the conduct of clinical trials: sponsors, clinical investigators and IRBs. This chapter looks at the specific regulatory responsibilities each of these three has when it comes to conducting clinical trials. Also involved are regulatory agencies (FDA, HHS) and the human subjects who participate in trials. Although many of these responsibilities are discussed in more detail in other chapters, this chapter will give you a summary of responsibilities as they appear in FDA regulations.

Sponsors

FDA regulations at 21 CFR 312.3(b) define a sponsor as "a person who takes responsibility for and initiates a clinical investigation. The sponsor may be an individual or a pharmaceutical company." For this book, a sponsor is the pharmaceutical or device company that initiates a clinical trial for one of its products. The regulatory responsibilities of sponsors are found primarily in 21 CFR 312, Subpart D - Responsibilities of Sponsors and Investigators.

Sponsors are responsible for:

- Selecting qualified investigators.
- Providing investigators with the information they need to conduct an investigation properly.
- Ensuring proper monitoring of the investigation.
- Ensuring that the investigation is conducted in accordance with the general investigational plan and protocols contained in the IND.
- Maintaining an effective IND with respect to the investigations.

- Ensuring that the FDA and all participating investigators are promptly informed of significant new adverse effects or risks with respect to the drug.
- Additional specific responsibilities of sponsors are:
- Selecting only investigators who are qualified by training and experience as experts to investigate the drug.
- Shipping investigational new drugs only to investigators who are participating in the investigation.
- Obtaining appropriate information from the investigator, including a curriculum vitae, Form 1572—Statement of Investigator, financial disclosure, outline of the study protocol for phase 2, 3 or a general outline of the planned investigation for phase 1.
- Selecting monitors who are qualified by training and experience to monitor the progress of the investigation.
- Monitoring the progress of all investigations involving an exception from informed consent.
- Giving each participating clinical investigator an investigator brochure.
- Keeping each participating investigator informed of new observations discovered by or reported to the sponsor on the drug, particularly with respect to adverse effects and safe use.
- Monitoring the progress of all clinical investigations being conducted under the sponsor's IND.
- Upon discovering that an investigator is not complying with the Form FDA-1572, the general investigational plan or the regulations, promptly securing compliance or discontinuing shipments of the investigational new drug to the investigator and ending the investigator's participation in the investigation.
- Reviewing and evaluating the evidence relating to the safety and effectiveness of the drug as it is obtained from the investigator. If determining that its investigational drug presents an unreasonable and significant risk to subjects, the sponsor will discontinue those investigations that present the risk. The FDA, all institutional review boards and all investigators who have at any time participated in the investigation of the discontinuance must be notified.

- Maintaining and retaining adequate records and reports.
- Permitting the FDA to inspect records and reports relating to clinical investigations.
- Maintaining written records of the disposition of the investigational drug.
- Retaining reserve samples of any test article and reference standard identified in and used in any of the bioequivalence or bioavailability studies described in the regulations at 21 CFR 320.38 and 21 CFR 320.63 and releasing the reserve samples to the FDA upon request in accordance with and for the period specified in 21 CFR 320.38.

This means that the sponsor is essentially responsible for all operational aspects of the clinical trials it sponsors.

Sponsor Delegation of Duties to a Contract Research Organization (CRO)

ICH defines a CRO as "a person or an organization (commercial, academic or other) contracted by the sponsor to perform one or more of a sponsor's trial-related duties and functions."

In many instances, the sponsor will delegate a portion of clinical trial-related responsibilities to a CRO. This is dependent on sponsor capabilities, logistics, location, finances, company size and personnel. Some CROs are delegated a small portion of responsibilities such as central lab, or monitoring responsibilities. Other CROs serve as a "one stop shop" and provide a variety of services such as central lab, Interactive Voice Response Systems (IVRS), study supplies and study supplies shipment, project management, data management, safety, medical writing, investigator selection, study startup and monitoring responsibilities for a study.

The regulations describe the transfer of responsibilities in detail:

Section. 312.52—Transfer of obligations to a contract research organization:

(a) A sponsor may transfer responsibility for any or all of the obligations set forth in this part to a CRO. Any such transfer shall be described in writing. If not all obligations are transferred, the writing is required to describe each of the obligations being assumed by the CRO. If all obligations are transferred, a general statement that all obligations have been transferred is acceptable. Any obligation not covered by the written description shall be deemed not to have been transferred.

(b) A CRO that assumes any obligation of a sponsor shall comply with the specific regulations in this chapter applicable to this obligation and shall be subject to the same regulatory action as a sponsor for failure to comply with any obligation assumed under these regulations. Thus, all references to "sponsor" in this part apply to a CRO to the extent that it assumes one or more obligations of the sponsor.

Institutional Review Boards (IRBs)

In the regulations at 21 CFR 56.102(g), an IRB is defined as "any board, committee or other group formally designated by an institution to review, approve the initiation of and conduct periodic review of biomedical research involving human subjects. The primary purpose of such review is to assure the protection of the rights and welfare of the human subjects." As a side note, institution means any public or private entity or agency (including federal, state and other agencies), to include hospitals, universities, private medical clinics and so forth.

For our purposes, an IRB is a committee that formally reviews and approves a trial before it can start with the primary goal of protecting human subjects of research. There is an entire chapter devoted to IRBs in this book, but their responsibilities will be summarized here in order to compare and contrast them with those of sponsors and investigators.

The regulatory responsibilities of IRBs are found primarily at 21 CFR 56—Institutional Review Boards, which requires that IRBs follow regulations regarding IRB organizations and personnel and follow written procedures, including those for:

- Conducting initial and continuing review of research and reporting those findings to the investigators.
- Determining which projects require review more than once annually.
- Ensuring prompt reporting to the IRB of changes in the research.

- Ensuring that changes are not implemented before IRB review, except where necessary to eliminate apparent immediate hazards to human subjects.
- Promptly reporting to the IRB, institution and the FDA any unanticipated problems involving risk to human subjects, any instance of serious or continuing noncompliance with regulations or IRB requirements and any suspension or termination of IRB approval.
- Reviewing proposed research at convened meetings with a majority of members present, including at least one member whose primary concerns are non-scientific.
- Requiring that information given to subjects as part of informed consent meets the regulations.
- Notifying investigators in writing of its decision to approve or disapprove the proposed research, or of any modifications required to secure approval.
- Conducting continuing review of the research at least annually, or more often, depending on the degree of risk.

The IRB is primarily responsible for the ethical aspects of the clinical trial.

Clinical Investigator

In the regulations at 21 CFR 312.3(b), an investigator is defined as "an individual who actually conducts a clinical investigation (i.e., under whose immediate direction the drug is administered or dispensed to a subject). In the event the investigation is conducted by a team of individuals, the investigator is the responsible leader of the team. "Sub-Investigator" includes any other individual member of that team. Investigators are discussed in detail in another chapter of this book.

The regulatory responsibilities of investigators are found primarily at 21 CFR 312, Subpart D - Responsibilities of Sponsors and Investigators. Under 21 CFR 312.60, an investigator is responsible for:

- Ensuring that an investigation is conducted according to the signed investigator statement (Form FDA 1572), the investigational plan (protocol) and the applicable regulations.
- Protecting the rights, safety and welfare of subjects under his or her care (including obtaining informed consent for each human subject to whom the drug is administered, except for exceptions noted in the regulations).
- Controlling the drugs under investigation.

In addition, for FDA-regulated drug studies, the investigator must sign a Form 1572. By signing this form, the investigator agrees to:

- Conduct the study in accordance with the protocol.
- Personally conduct or supervise the investigation.
- Inform study subjects that the study drugs are being used for investigational purposes.
- Ensure that the requirements for obtaining informed consent (21 CFR 50) and for obtaining IRB review (21 CFR 56) are met.
- Report adverse experiences that occur during the course of the investigation to the sponsor, in accordance with 21 CFR 312.64.
- Read and understand the material in the investigator's brochure, including the potential risks and side effects of the drug.
- Ensure that all associates, colleagues and employees assisting in the conduct of the study are informed about their obligations.
- Maintain adequate and accurate records as per 21 CFR 312.62 and make those records available for inspection in accordance with 21 CFR 312.68.

The investigators must also ensure that an IRB compliant with 21 CFR 56 will be responsible for the initial and continuing review and approval of the clinical investigation, and will:

- Promptly report all changes in research activity to the IRB.
- Promptly report all unanticipated problems involving risk to human subjects or others.

- Will not make changes to the research without IRB approval, except where necessary to eliminate apparent immediate hazards to human subjects.
- Additional investigator responsibilities under 21 CFR 312.60 include:
- Maintaining adequate records of drug disposition.
- Preparing and maintaining accurate subject case histories that record all observations and other data pertinent to the investigation, including case report forms, signed and dated consent forms, medical records, progress notes, etc.
- Retaining all records appropriately and for the required time periods.
- Furnishing progress, safety and final reports to the sponsor.
- Providing financial disclosure information to the sponsor as required.
- Providing assurance of IRB review.
- Allowing FDA inspections of records and reports.

The investigator, then, is primarily responsible for the conduct of the trial.

Other Research Partners

The FDA, HHS and regulatory agencies around the world also have a major role in clinical research. These agencies regulate clinical research conducted in their countries by maintaining and enforcing the regulations covering research, and issuing guidance and other documents detailing acceptable research practices. They interact with sponsors throughout a sponsor's development program, dispensing advice and working with the sponsor on the initiation and continuation of the program. The FDA also performs inspections of sponsors, investigative sites and IRBs to ensure both the safety and well-being of study subjects and the integrity of the data. When the research program is complete, the FDA reviews the studies and the data and makes a decision about whether the sponsor can proceed with marketing of the new product. In effect, regulatory agencies act as overseers to ensure clinical research is done properly and new medications are safe and effective to be used in the general population.

There is one more major contributor to the research process—the subjects who actually volunteer and participate in research studies. They are the unsung heroes without whom new drugs and devices could not be tested and brought to market. Study subjects deserve a big round of applause from all of us.

Occasionally, there is also a role for an institution in clinical research. This often occurs in large teaching hospitals, for example, where a separate department within the institution handles some matters, such as grants and contracts, for all investigators affiliated with the institution.

The diagram below shows the interactions between the different entities involved in clinical trials. The solid lines designate primary interactions, while the dotted lines show secondary interactions.

The sponsor interacts primarily with investigators (sites) and the FDA. In the past, sponsors rarely had contact with IRBs. This has changed somewhat with multi-center trials, as sponsors often submit the protocol and consent to a central IRB that will review the study for all, or most, of the individual sites. In this case, however, the sites still communicate directly with the IRB with regard to other documentation that is site specific.

The clinical investigators are the primary link to both the IRB and, of course, the study subjects. It is rare for anyone other than the investigator and his or her staff to interact with study subjects, although upon occasion, a subject may contact an IRB with concerns about the study. If an institution is involved, there will be interactions between the appropriate institution departments and the investigators involved in research at the institution.

The FDA, although interacting primarily with the sponsor, may also interact with sites (and the institution) and conducts inspections of sponsors, investigative sites and IRBs.

Managing Relationships

With so many groups involved in a clinical trial, there are a lot of relationships to manage. Not only are there relationships between the groups mentioned above, but there are those within each group to think about as well. Many of these associations appear in other chapters.

As with all relationships, respect for the other people and their problems and situations can go a long way to smoothing out a rocky relationship. Think about "working with people" rather than "working for me." If you can maintain this attitude, it will go a long way toward ensuring a good relationship.

Key Takeaways

- Regulations contain the key responsibilities for the primary groups involved in clinical trials.
- In general, the sponsor is responsible for the operational aspects of the clinical trials it sponsors. The sponsor can choose to delegate a few or all of these responsibilities to a CRO.
- The IRB is primarily responsible for the ethical aspects of the clinical trial.
- The investigator is primarily responsible for the conduct of the trial.
- Other research partners are the study subjects and regulatory agencies.
- Maintaining good relationships among study partners is critical to a successful clinical trial.

CHAPTER 5

The Research Process

This chapter presents an overview of the research process for new pharmaceutical compounds, looking first at preclinical work, then at clinical development. Also briefly discussed are the two main documents that must be filed with the FDA. One of these is the Investigational New Drug (IND) application, which is filed before studies can begin in humans. The other is the New Drug Application (NDA), which is the formal request for permission to market a new product. It is important that CRAs comprehend the entire drug development process, even though they will not be involved in every step. This will help the CRA understand why things happen as they do and to participate knowledgeably in the process.

Figure 1. FDA drug development process

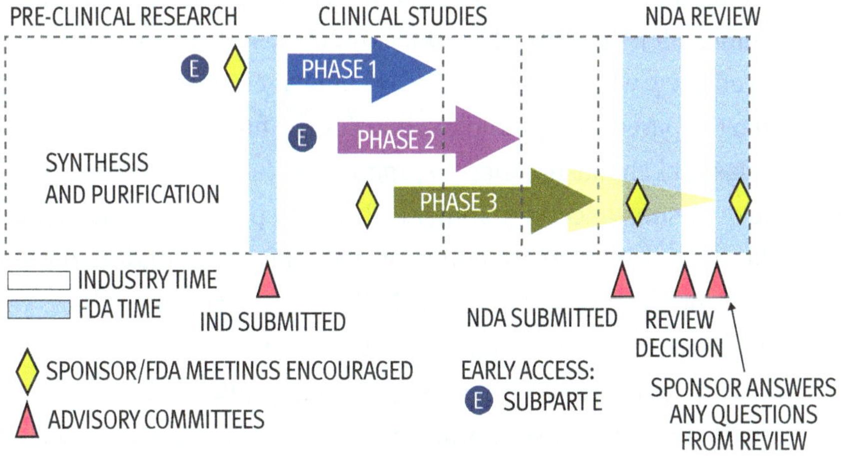

Source: FDA

Preclinical Research

This section looks at drug discovery and the preclinical work that must be done before phase 1 studies in humans can begin. Preclinical refers to studies that do not involve human subjects. Clinical studies are studies conducted with human subjects. Note that sometimes people refer to research as preclinical, even though non-human work can continue after clinical studies have begun. Also, the terms preclinical and nonclinical can be used interchangeably.

The purpose of preclinical studies is to provide information on safety and, if possible, efficacy, in order to begin conducting clinical studies in humans. The information gathered from preclinical studies provides the pharmaceutical company, the FDA and the IRB with enough evidence to make reasonable decisions about exposing humans to the compound. The information from preclinical studies includes data on acute toxicity, the kinetics and metabolism of the drug and organ sensitivity. Most importantly, these studies determine a starting dose with an acceptable margin of safety so that there is minimal chance of endangerment to human study subjects.

Drug Discovery/Development

The discovery of new substances, which subsequently become marketed drugs or biologics, occurs in a number of ways. There is direct research, during which medicinal chemists create compounds with structures likely to evoke the kind of physiological effect they are looking for. Another approach is to change the molecular structure of known compounds in the hope of improving safety or efficacy, while creating a new chemical entity that is sufficiently different from the parent compound to allow for the filing of a new patent. In addition to classical chemistry, there are many new laboratory tools for developing viable drug substances. Computer technology provides many methods for molecular structuring and screening for potential compounds to develop. Other methods include research using artificial intelligence algorithms, gene sequencing, gene vector delivery and recombinant DNA.

Biological products are a well-known category of drug study/discovery. According to the FDA's glossary of drug terms, biological products "include a wide range of products such as vaccines, blood and blood components, allergenics, somatic cells, gene therapy, tissues and recombinant therapeutic proteins. Biologics can be composed of sugars, proteins, nucleic acids or complex combinations of these substances, or may be living entities such as cells and tissues. Biologics are isolated from a variety of natural sources—human, animal or microorganism—and may be produced by biotechnology methods and other cutting-edge technologies. Gene-based and cellular biologics, for example, often are at the forefront of biomedical research and may be used to treat a variety of medical conditions for which no other treatments are available."

Naturally occurring compounds are another source of potential pharmaceuticals. A number of drugs originated from soil samples (antibiotics), plants (digitalis) and other natural materials, such as coral (prostaglandins). Michael Kopcha, director of the FDA's Office of Pharmaceutical Quality explained the term "naturally derived drug" in a WebMD Magazine article titled "A Closer Look at Naturally Derived Drugs." Prior to the creation of the first drug made using chemistry "nearly all drugs came from natural sources such as plants, animals, and fungi. Even today, drug manufacturers isolate many ingredients in drug products from natural sources," Kopcha wrote. "One interesting example is cannabidiol, the active ingredient in an FDA-approved seizure drug. The drugmaker isolates cannabidiol (CBD) from the Cannabis sativa plant, more commonly known as marijuana. CBD does not cause the 'high' associated with marijuana."

Asked how the FDA assures the quality of naturally derived drugs, Kopcha explained that, like all drugs, "they must be made so that they are consistently safe and able to provide their intended benefit. To do this, drug manufacturers must meet quality standards that ensure every dose of a drug is of the appropriate strength and free of contamination and defects. The FDA has a dedicated botanical team to address unique considerations for developing complex drugs derived from plants. This helps the FDA assure that manufacturers of plant-derived drugs are capable of meeting quality standards prior to approval. This is another reason why you can have confidence in your next dose of medicine, no matter the source." In fact, the article says, 6 percent of FDA-approved drugs are natural products.

Serendipity plays a role in any research program. Some exciting compounds have been discovered by accident. Many drugs are marketed for an indication that was discovered by accident during studies for the primary indication. One example is Rogaine. This compound, minoxidil, was originally developed as an antihypertensive (Loniten). Its hair-growing capability wasn't known until subjects enrolled in the hypertension studies began exhibiting accelerated hair growth—in all the wrong places. Women weren't thrilled with new mustaches and bushy eyebrows. Based on this unwanted side effect, the company eventually developed a topical formulation of minoxidil as a hair-growth product.

Once researchers identify a promising compound for development, they conduct experiments to gather information on:

- How it is absorbed, distributed, metabolized and excreted.
- Its potential benefits and mechanisms of action.
- The best dosage.
- The best way to give the drug (such as by mouth or injection).
- Side effects or adverse events, often referred to as toxicity.
- How it affects different groups of people (such as by gender, race or ethnicity) differently.
- How it interacts with other drugs and treatments.
- Its effectiveness as compared with similar drugs.

Preclinical Studies of Product Candidates

Once a compound appears to be a viable product candidate, it must be determined if the compound is reasonably safe for initial testing in humans and exhibits pharmacological activity that might justify developing it commercially. The preclinical work will focus on collecting data and information to establish that humans will not be exposed to unreasonable risks in early-phase clinical studies. This evidence will be presented to the FDA in an IND application.

The first step is to determine the basic physical, chemical and biological characteristics of a new compound with the following actions:

- Preliminary analytical methods and release criteria must be defined prior to beginning toxicology studies. Methodology and release criteria will change and become better defined as more work is completed and additional information becomes available.
- Data must be developed that will provide evidence of the stability of the compound for the duration of the toxicology studies and clinical trials.

- A formulation of the compound for use in animals and humans must be developed.
- Bioavailability studies must be done to demonstrate equivalence each time the formulation is changed.
- For biologics (monoclonal antibodies, vaccines, etc.), steps such as the identification of adventitious agents and the characterization of cell lines must be completed. (Adventitious agents are impurities or contaminates; for example, all vaccines that are bovine-based must now be checked for mad cow disease.)

The outcomes for these parameters change as the preclinical studies progress. They may even change as phase 1 and phase 2 studies in humans are carried out. This ongoing process will result in a final formulation by the time phase 3 studies begin.

There will be a final collection of analytical methods, release criteria and formulation prior to beginning phase 3 studies, and all excipients must be identified both quantitatively and qualitatively. (An excipient is an inert substance that forms part of the vehicle for delivering a drug (e.g., gum arabic or starch.)

Once a compound is characterized and satisfactory stability data are in hand, preclinical studies can be initiated. The type of studies and their design will vary depending on the intended use of the drug or biologic being developed. The purpose of preclinical studies is to characterize the toxic effects of the compound with respect to target organs, dose dependence and relationship to exposure. The studies must normally be conducted using two routes of administration: the route intended for human administration—oral, nasal, topical, etc.—and intravenous (IV). If the IV route will solely be used in humans, then no other route needs to be studied in preclinical investigations.

These preclinical studies will establish a number of different things, including:

- The highest dose of the compound that can be tolerated, as well as a low dose that evokes no overt toxicity, in order to determine initial dosing in humans and to characterize potential organ-specific adverse events.
- Proposed dosing, route of administration and duration of treatment for phase 1 studies.

- Whether the observed adverse effects are reversible.

The recommended preclinical safety studies necessary to obtain marketing approval for a pharmaceutical include: genotoxicity studies, single and multiple (repeated) dose toxicology studies, local tolerance studies and teratology or reproductive studies.

Other preclinical studies that must be completed are pharmacology studies for safety and pharmacokinetic studies that identify absorption, distribution, metabolism and excretion (ADME) of the compound—known as ADME studies.

These studies are all conducted in compliance with regulatory guidelines, which are typically harmonized between the U.S., Europe and Japan, thus accepted globally. In addition, Good Laboratory Practices (GLPs) are strictly followed for documentation and to ensure the integrity of the data. The GLPs are the toxicology counterpart to the GCPs.

To ensure the ethical treatment of animals during these studies and to guarantee that the animals do not suffer any unnecessary pain or distress, there is an independent group called the Institutional Animal Care and Use Committee (IACUC), which must review and approve all animal studies before they begin. It also monitors the progress of these studies through real-time reporting from the attending veterinarian. The IACUC reports directly to the highest official at the facility and is independent from any scientific or management influence. Guidelines for animal studies are covered under the Animal Welfare Act, which is law; infractions are punishable by fine and/or imprisonment.

The IND Application

The FDA becomes involved in a drug development program when the sponsor has completed enough preclinical work with the compound to determine it is safe enough to begin human trials and has filed an IND with the FDA. This is when the compound changes in legal status under the Federal Food, Drug and Cosmetic Act. It becomes an investigational drug and is subject to specific regulatory requirements.

Approval of INDs is passive. The sponsor may begin clinical trials 30 days after submission of the IND unless the FDA indicates there is a problem. Most companies will contact the FDA a few days prior to the 30-day expiration period just to be sure they will be able to proceed with the trials.

The IND contains all known information about the compound. In general, the IND includes:

1. Animal pharmacology and toxicology studies. These are the preclinical data that allow the FDA to make an assessment about whether the compound is reasonably safe for initial testing in humans.
2. Any previous experience with the compound in humans from non-U.S. studies.
3. Chemistry, Manufacturing and Control information.
4. The protocol and investigator information. This includes a complete protocol so the FDA can assess whether the risk for the initial trials (phase 1) is acceptable as well as information about the qualifications of the investigator(s).
5. Assurance that a duly-formed IRB will be responsible for initial and continuing review of the trial.
6. If involved, the responsibilities that have been delegated to the CRO.
7. The general development plan for the drug.

The IND must be updated on an annual basis. In the update, the sponsor includes any new information about the drug, as well as the results of any studies that are still active or were completed during the year. This information will include current enrollment numbers, adverse events information and the overall study status. The update also includes the clinical plan for the next year. This information keeps the FDA abreast of what is happening with the compound over time. Amendments to the IND may be filed at any time.

Amendments are filed for any changes in protocols, medicine strength, investigators or the development program. The regulations pertaining to INDs are found in 21 CFR 312.

A CRA will rarely have any involvement with the IND; however, when it is time for the annual update, the CRA may be asked to contact sites for current information needed for the update. When this happens, there are often critical timelines involved, so the CRA will need to collect the information in a timely manner.

Clinical Trials

In this section we will discuss the clinical development of a compound. The term clinical implies human studies, as opposed to animal studies. Clinical trials are research studies that involve the active participation of people (trial subjects) to test the safety and efficacy of new medical treatments. Clinical studies are not begun until a reasonable amount of preclinical work has been completed and there is evidence that the compound is potentially safe for use in humans.

Clinical trials are divided into phases: 1, 2, 3 and 4. Many companies also use the designation of phase 3b, which will also be defined in this chapter. (Note that you may also see the phases numbered using Roman numerals I, II, III and IV.) The phases simply serve as markers or milestones in the drug development process and are not necessarily distinct, consecutive periods. For example, in some cases phases 2 and 3 can be combined, and phase 2 may start before phase 1 is complete. However, each phase does have distinct characteristics and purposes, and each is important to the development program.

Phase 1 Clinical Trials

During phase 1, the investigational drug or biologic is given to humans for the first time.

Phase 1 studies, frequently referred to as safety studies, enroll a small number of subjects. The total number of subjects in phase 1 is usually between 20 and 100. Subjects are usually healthy volunteers although, in some cases, patients with the target disease are studied. The type of subject depends on the nature of the disease and the expected toxicity of the investigational drug. It would not be ethical, for example, to give healthy subjects a toxic investigational drug meant to treat one of the cancers.

The purpose of phase 1 studies is to determine the metabolic and pharmacologic action of the investigational drug in humans; assess the adverse effects associated with different doses; and, perhaps, get an indication of whether or not there is any evidence of efficacy. Subjects are usually given increasing doses of the test product until the side effects reach the point that they are no longer tolerable; this is part of establishing the maximum dose that can be used in humans. Because of the lack of knowledge about the drug, phase 1 studies include special testing (serial lab tests, timed pharmacokinetic (PK) tests, safety testing like ECGs). Since this is the first time humans are exposed to the investigational drug, these studies are very closely monitored by medical personnel. Phase 1 studies are often done in special testing facilities designed for this work—phase 1 units/facilities. Frequently, subjects may be required to stay several nights, or more, so phase 1 facilities are set up with sleeping, dining and recreational facilities.

Some investigational sites/investigators specialize in phase 1 research only and have large, state of the art phase 1 units. Some investigators/investigational sites include phase 1 capabilities in their portfolio and some larger CROs own phase 1 units in the U.S.

Essentially, phase 1 should provide the researcher with sufficient information about the investigational drug's pharmacokinetics and pharmacological effects (safe dose range and adverse effects) to permit designing safe, well-controlled, scientifically sound phase 2 studies. The primary concern of phase I is subject safety.

A lot of preclinical work must be done before phase 1 studies can begin. The types of phase 1 study designs include single ascending and multiple ascending dose studies, studies with different patient cohorts for dosing to determine recommended phase 2 dose, food effect studies, drug-drug interaction studies, bioavailability and bioequivalence studies.

Phase 2 Clinical Trials

When the appropriate phase 1 studies have been completed and sufficient safety data are in hand, phase 2 studies are initiated. Phase 2 studies are rigid, well-controlled studies in a relatively small homogeneous patient population, usually no more than a few hundred subjects in total. These subjects have the target disease, but no other confounding illnesses. Phase 2 usually consists of double-blind, well-controlled studies using a placebo or comparator drug, or both. Their purpose is to determine whether or not the investigational drug demonstrates efficacy for the proposed indication within the safe dose range established in phase 1. Short-term adverse effects and risks are also assessed. While the focus of phase 2 studies is primarily efficacy, they also assess safety. Dose-range finding (e.g., establishing a minimum and maximum effective dose) and PK data correlating blood levels of the investigational drug with pharmacological effect (also known as the pharmacokinetic/pharmacodynamic relationship) are also studied during phase 2.

Near the end of phase 2, most sponsors will meet with the FDA to review the results obtained to date and present their plans for phase 3. This is called the end-of-phase 2 meeting. The FDA views these meetings as being of considerable assistance (to both the FDA and the sponsor) for planning later studies of the compound. Pursuant to the provisions of PDUFA, agreements reached at these meetings are binding on the FDA and the sponsor.

Remember, there are preclinical studies that may have been active during phase 1 but must be completed before phase 2 can start.

Phase 3 Clinical Trials

Phase 3 studies are initiated only if the data generated in phases 1 and 2 have a satisfactory safety profile and there is sufficient evidence of efficacy. The purpose of phase 3 studies is to demonstrate the safety and efficacy needed to assess the risk/benefit relationship for the intended use of the investigational drug and to provide adequate data for the product package insert.

Phase 3 studies are expanded, controlled studies in large patient populations (often thousands of patients) that represent the types of patients the compound is intended to treat after it is marketed. They may extend over several years. The development plan for the compound usually includes many different studies, including more than one multicenter study using the same or similar protocols. Multicenter studies are those for which multiple investigative sites all follow the same protocol and for which the data are pooled together in one group for analysis.

The FDA requirement for registration of a drug is two "adequate and well-controlled" (primary efficacy) studies. However, under the FDAMA legislation of 1997, the FDA may allow one study instead of two for a product for which it is determined (by the FDA) that "data from one adequate and well-controlled clinical investigation and confirmatory evidence (obtained prior to or after such investigation) are sufficient to establish effectiveness." The decision to do one, rather than two, adequate and well-controlled studies is not one that a sponsor will make on its own. This decision will be made after consultation with and support of the FDA.

As is the case for phases 1 and 2, there are a number of preclinical studies that must be completed before or during the phase 3 program. The completion of these studies is required before a sponsor can file the NDA with the FDA.

Notes on studies in women and children

Recently there has been a greater emphasis on studying new compounds in women and children. These populations were previously understudied and many compounds do not work the same way in women or children as they do in men. Consequently, the FDA determined that studies should include women and children if the compounds would be used to treat them after marketing. The rationale is that it is preferable to determine the effects of the compound under the controlled conditions in clinical trials as opposed to uncontrolled use of the drug after marketing.

CRAs should have basic knowledge about the testing of compounds in women of childbearing potential, pregnant women and children.

Women of childbearing potential are a major concern in clinical trials because of the possibility of unintentional exposure of an embryo/fetus before data are available relative to potential risk. Some teratology work (segments I and II testing) is usually done before entering women of childbearing potential into a clinical trial, although this is not essential.

In the U.S., women of childbearing potential may be included in early studies prior to completion of reproductive toxicology studies, providing that the studies are carefully monitored and all precautions are taken to minimize exposure in utero. This generally involves pregnancy testing and establishment of highly effective methods of birth control. Monitoring and testing should continue throughout the trial to ensure compliance with all measures intended to prevent pregnancy.

If women of childbearing potential participate in a clinical trial prior to completion of the teratology studies, the informed consent process should clearly indicate the possible risk associated with taking the investigational drug since effects on the embryo/fetus are unknown. If pregnant women are to be enrolled in clinical trials, all reproductive toxicity studies and genotoxicity tests must be completed. Data from any previous experience in humans will also be needed.

If children are to be included in clinical trials, repeated-dose toxicity studies and all reproductive toxicity and genotoxicity studies should have been completed. In addition, safety data from previous studies in human adult populations should be available.

The New Drug Application

The NDA is a formal request to be allowed to market a drug. The sponsor submits the NDA to the FDA at the time the primary efficacy studies (phase 3) are complete. The company is essentially telling the FDA that it has completed the necessary safety and efficacy requirements needed for approval. This signals the end of phase 3, although there are likely to be some studies still in progress.

In the NDA, as in the IND, the sponsor is informing the FDA of everything that is known about the drug to date. This includes copies of all protocols and case report forms from studies. These applications can be enormous. The regulations for NDAs are found in 21 CFR 314. They delineate the particular information that must be included.

Field-based CRAs are unlikely to be involved in helping put together an NDA submission. However, CRAs who are based in-house may well be involved in helping to assemble the clinical section. Often CRAs are involved in a last-minute push to retrieve and/or clean up data needed for the NDA. CRAs also may be asked to re-verify information from sites when questions arise during the NDA writing process.

Part of the NDA is the proposed package insert that the sponsor would like to use with the drug. This is the information that goes with the drug that tells physicians about the drug and how it should be used. The package insert negotiations between the sponsor and the FDA can be extensive.

There is an active approval process for an NDA (as opposed to the passive 30-day wait for an IND). The sponsor must receive a formal approval letter from the FDA before marketing of the drug can begin.

Phase 3b Clinical Studies

A sponsor will frequently have some studies that are still active at the time it files the NDA for a new compound. There are also studies that may be initiated and conducted while the NDA is pending approval. These studies are known as phase 3b studies. The purpose of these studies may be to gather additional safety data, to gather information on additional indications for the drug or to assess its use in special patient populations such as geriatric patients.

Phase 4 Clinical Studies

Phase 4 studies are those conducted after the approval of the NDA, often to determine additional information about the safety or efficacy profile of the compound. They consist of studies:

- Required as a condition of approval by the FDA.
- Required as long-term safety studies by the FDA.
- Conducted to study the compound in comparison with other marketed products.

- Designed to familiarize physicians with the compound.

If the sponsor was allowed to file the NDA with one, rather than two, adequate and well-controlled studies, the FDA may require that one or more additional confirmatory studies be completed within a certain time period of the approval. This is a condition of the approval; if it is not met, the approval may be withdrawn.

The FDA may also require that a sponsor do a long-term safety study as a condition of approval. These studies are often referred to as epidemiologic or post-marketing surveillance studies. These may be required because the FDA has seen problems with similar compounds or because the compound is novel and the FDA thinks additional safety information will be beneficial.

During the development time for the compound, other drugs may have been approved by the FDA and become the new standard of care for the disease or condition. In this case, the sponsor may want to do additional studies comparing its drug to these new compounds. The sponsor may also wish to look at different formulations, dosages, durations of treatments or medical interactions with other compounds commonly used by people with the disease targeted by the drug. Note that if the sponsor wants to evaluate the compound for a new (additional) indication, a new NDA will need to be filed for the new indication(s), but it will not require repeating studies. Studies designed to familiarize physicians with the new drug are sometimes referred to as marketing studies. Physicians may be given a relatively small amount of the new drug to use in an open-label manner with appropriate patients and will be required to collect some data, usually only safety data, on these patients. The goal of the sponsor of these studies is to have the physician become familiar with the product.

There are other types of "studies" that do not actively involve treating patients with investigational devices or products, such as "registry studies" and "retrospective chart review" studies.

According to the Virginia Commonwealth University Office of Research and Innovation, "A registry is an organized system that uses observational study methods to collect uniform data (clinical and other) to evaluate specified outcomes for a population defined by a particular disease, condition or exposure and that serves one or more predetermined scientific, clinical or policy purposes."

Data tokenization in clinical research studies

Data "tokenization" replaces some sensitive data element with a substitute known as a token—a randomized number with no actual meaning. There is growing interest in the use of tokenization in clinical research studies because it protects sensitive information while enabling the sharing of data and long-term tracking of individuals.

Enthusiasm is building for the tokenization of clinical research participants to link information from trials to real-world data (RWD) on the same patients. Unique, anonymized identifiers, or tokens, have been used for many years to link different sources of patient-level RWD while protecting patient privacy, according to Tim Riely, vice president of clinical data analytics at IQVIA. Processes and systems are in place to do the same on the clinical research side and join the two to find the overlap, Riely says.

Tokenization is a means to "future-proof" studies and entire research programs, according to Sandy Leonard, senior vice president of partnerships and RWD at HealthVerity. When done on the front end, the process can help study sponsors nimbly respond to the evidence requirements for regulatory approvals.

Submission of real-world evidence as a complement to trial data can reduce if not remove postmarket commitments, says Kathleen Mandziuk, vice president of real-world solutions and tokenization at ICON. If companies already have a cohort of patients exposed to a drug, tokenization can also be useful for product positioning in the market.

Tokens provide a way to stitch together data fragments from trials and the real world, potentially in lieu of a phase 4 or long-term follow-up study, said Vera Mucaj, chief scientific officer at Datavant.

Retrospective chart review studies involve review/analysis of pre-existing data, such as based on data already collected in a medical record.

Key Takeaways

Preclinical

- Preclinical trials do not involve human subjects.
- Clinical trials involve human subjects.
- Before clinical trials begin, the sponsor must file an IND with the FDA.
- The IND must include results from the preclinical studies.

- Animal studies are monitored to ensure ethical treatment.
- The IND is filed after significant preclinical testing has been done on a compound and it appears to be reasonably safe for use in humans.
- There is no formal FDA approval for an IND. A sponsor must wait 30 days after filing the IND before starting studies in humans.
- INDs must be updated annually. The update contains what was learned about the compound during the year and the clinical plan for the following year.

Clinical

- Phase 1 studies are small safety studies usually done in healthy volunteers.
- Phase 2 studies are usually the first studies in patients with the disease or condition of interest.
- Phase 3 studies are large, comprehensive safety and efficacy studies.
- Phase 3b studies are those being conducted during the time the compound is in the FDA review cycle.
- Phase 4 studies are conducted after approval of the compound.
- There is an increased emphasis on conducting studies in women and children.

NDA

- The NDA is the sponsor's formal application to market a new drug.
- The NDA is filed when the primary safety and efficacy studies are complete.
- The FDA must formally approve a drug before it can be marketed.

CHAPTER 6

Devices and Biologics

The FDA is responsible for protecting public health by assuring the safety and effectiveness of a variety of medical products, including drugs, devices and biological products. It also has responsibility for advancing public health by helping to speed innovations that make treatments more effective, safer and more affordable. Although much of the information in this book is geared toward the study of drugs, many CRAs will also be involved in clinical trials of devices and biological products. The precepts of conducting good research (GCPs, etc.) are the same in any clinical trial, but there are some differences in the regulations when the potential product is a device. This section discusses some of the differences.

The FDA's Center for Devices and Radiological Health (CDRH) is responsible for both the premarket and postmarket regulation of medical devices. The CDRH page can be found on the FDA website. A medical device is a product used for diagnosis, therapy or surgery purposes in patients and that acts by physical, mechanical or physico-chemical (drug/device combination) means. Medical devices include a wide range of products that vary in complexity from tongue depressors to artificial hearts and X-ray machines.

The FDA recognizes different classes of medical devices, based on their design's complexity, their use characteristics and their potential for harm if misused. "Class" refers to the level of regulatory control attached to the device. The definitions pertaining to the classification of devices are found in 21 CFR 860 (Medical Device Classification Procedures).

Class I devices are subject only to the general controls authorized by or under sections 501 (adulteration), 502 (misbranding), 510 (registration), 516 (banned devices), 518 (notification and other remedies), 519 (records and reports) and 520 (general provisions) of 21 CFR 860. A device is in Class I if these general controls are sufficient to provide reasonable assurance of the safety and effectiveness of the device, if the device is not life-supporting or life-sustaining, its use is not of substantial importance in preventing impairment of human health, and it does not present a potential unreasonable risk of illness or injury. Examples of Class I devices are examination gloves and elastic bandages.

Class II devices are subject to special controls because general controls alone are insufficient to provide reasonable assurance of its safety and effectiveness. Special controls can include the need for performance standards, post-market surveillance, patient registries, the development and dissemination of guidance documents and other appropriate actions that the FDA deems necessary to provide this assurance. Examples of Class II devices are powered wheelchairs and infusion pumps.

Class III devices, which are usually novel devices, require the submission of a premarket approval application (PMA). These devices tend to have a higher risk or raise new safety and effectiveness questions that must be answered before they are approved for marketing. Data in a PMA application must demonstrate a "reasonable assurance" of safety and effectiveness. Examples of Class III devices include implantable pacemakers and automated external defibrillators.

There are several types of marketing applications a medical device manufacturer may submit to CDRH. The most common types of premarket submissions include:

- **Premarket Notification (510k)**—Some Class I and most Class II devices require a 510(k) premarket notification to the FDA. In a 510(k), the sponsor must demonstrate that the new device is "substantially equivalent" to a predicate device in terms of intended use, technological characteristics and performance testing, as needed. Data in a 510(k) submission must demonstrate that the new device is substantially equivalent in safety and effectiveness to a Class II device already on the market. Some Class I and Class II devices are exempt from the 510(k) notification requirement. For example, an elastic bandage classified under 21 CFR 880.5075 is exempt from premarket notification provided that it does not exceed the exemption limitations stated in 21 CFR 880.9.
- **Premarket Approval (PMA)**—Class III (high-risk) devices require a PMA application. A PMA is the most stringent type of premarket submission. Before the FDA approves a PMA, the sponsor must provide

valid scientific evidence demonstrating reasonable assurances of safety and effectiveness for the device's intended use.

- **De Novo Classification Request**—The De Novo process provides a pathway to classify novel medical devices for which general controls alone, or general and special controls, provide reasonable assurance of safety and effectiveness for the intended use but for which there is no legally marketed predicate device.
- **Humanitarian Device Exemption (HDE)**—HDE provides a regulatory pathway for Class III devices that are intended to benefit patients with rare diseases or conditions. In order for a device to be eligible for an HDE, a sponsor must first obtain designation as a Humanitarian Use Device, which is granted through an application to FDA's Office of Orphan Products Development.

Most device applications cleared under the 510(k) program are based on nonclinical testing with no clinical data, while the majority of PMA applications contain clinical data.

Many devices are designed and developed as tools to accomplish a specific task that is already an established practice, so the intended patient population and anticipated effects of the device are known before testing begins. This is different from the drug development process, where a new molecular entity may be identified before determining any potential clinical applications.

Another major difference between device and drug development is the interpretation of safety events seen in a clinical trial. A control group is almost always necessary to interpret safety information from a drug trial, while a control group may not be needed to identify adverse events related to the use of a device.

Premarket trials tend to be simpler than drug trials when demonstrating safety with regard to intended use, and compliance is usually easier to measure in device trials. There are a number of other differences between device and drug trials. For example, it may not be possible to "blind" the device, so many device trials are done with the investigator and subject both being aware of the device being used. It also may not be possible to have a direct comparison with a competitor device, either because there may not be a comparable device or because of the logistics involved.

When studying a drug, the dosage may be an issue; with a device, the size of the device may be an issue, especially in implantable devices. Implanting a device may carry a greater risk than prescribing a drug, especially in later-phase trials when more is known about a drug. Depending on the device, there may be more precise endpoint determination (especially when there is electronic information storage on the device). Many endpoints in drug trials, on the other hand, are quite subjective (think of a depression rating scale versus a "hard" measurement such as blood pressure).

There are also some differences in the collection and reporting of medical events between device and drug trials. These are discussed in more detail in the adverse events chapter.

If you will be monitoring device trials, it is recommended that you read the device regulations found in 21 CFR Part 812 (Investigational Device Exemptions) and 21 CFR Part 814 (Premarket Approval of Medical Devices). 21 CFR Part 860 (Medical Device Classification Procedures) and 21 CFR Part 803 (Medical Device Reporting), which covers adverse event reporting, will also be helpful.

Biologics and Vaccines

The Center for Biologics Evaluation and Research (CBER) is the organization within the FDA responsible for ensuring the safety and efficacy of vaccines; blood and blood products; xenotransplantation; and cell, tissue and gene therapies designed for the prevention, diagnosis and treatment of human diseases, conditions or injury. The CBER page can be found on the FDA website.

A Biologics License Application (BLA) is a request for permission to introduce a biologic product into interstate commerce (21 CFR 601.2). This means approval for marketing. The BLA is regulated under 21 CFR 600-680. The application, which shows the clinical efficacy and safety of a biologic product in humans and requests marketing approval in the U.S., is usually submitted to the FDA after completion of phase 3 trials.

The regulations that apply to drugs also apply to biologics. In addition to these, the regulations in the preceding paragraph regulate the BLA.

Vaccine clinical development follows the same general pathway as drugs and other biologics. A sponsor that wishes to begin clinical trials with a vaccine must submit an IND to the FDA. The IND describes the vaccine, its method of manufacture and quality-control tests for release. Also included is information about the vaccine's safety and ability to elicit a protective immune response (immunogenicity) in animal testing, as well as the proposed clinical protocol for studies in humans.

The NIH has guidelines for "Research Involving Recombinant or Synthetic Nucleic Acid Molecules," that state:

> **Section I-A-1-a.** For experiments involving the deliberate transfer of recombinant or synthetic nucleic acid molecules or DNA or RNA derived from recombinant or synthetic nucleic acid molecules into human research participants (human gene transfer), no human gene transfer experiment shall be initiated (see definition of initiation in Section I-E-4) until Institutional Biosafety Committee (IBC) approval (from the clinical trial site) has been obtained and all applicable regulatory authorization(s) and approvals have been obtained.
>
> **Section I-B. Definition of Recombinant and Synthetic Nucleic Acid Molecules**
>
> In the context of the NIH Guidelines, recombinant and synthetic nucleic acids are defined as:
>
> (i) molecules that a) are constructed by joining nucleic acid molecules and b) that can replicate in a living cell, i.e., recombinant nucleic acids;
>
> (ii) nucleic acid molecules that are chemically or by other means synthesized or amplified, including those that are chemically or otherwise modified but can base pair with naturally occurring nucleic acid molecules, i.e., synthetic nucleic acids; or
>
> (iii) molecules that result from the replication of those described in (i) or (ii) above.

Institutional Biosafety Committees (IBC) are "the cornerstone of institutional oversight of recombinant DNA research," according to the HHS website.

It is important for CRAs to be aware that institutions that conduct this type of research (including some investigational vaccine treatments) are subject to additional oversight by IBCs. The IBC oversight includes additional requirements for drug containment, storage, preparation and dispensation practices at the institution performing the research, among many other things. There are specific IBC requirements that institutions have to meet before they can conduct these types of trials. CRAs need to ensure they are aware of IBC oversight and institutional requirements for trial conduct when monitoring these types of studies at their investigational sites.

Clinical trials for vaccines are typically done in three phases, just like for drugs and biologics. Initial human studies, referred to as phase 1, are safety and immunogenicity studies performed in a small number of closely monitored subjects. Phase 2 studies are dose-ranging studies and may enroll hundreds of subjects. Protection from the specific pathogen starts to be reviewed in this phase. Finally, phase 3 trials typically enroll thousands of individuals and provide the proof of effectiveness and safety required for licensing.

After the successful completion of all three phases of clinical development, the sponsor can submit a BLA. To be considered, the application must provide the FDA review team (medical officers, microbiologists, chemists, biostatisticians, etc.) with the efficacy and safety information necessary to make a risk/benefit assessment and to recommend or oppose approval of the vaccine.

As is the case for drugs, vaccine approval also requires the provision of adequate product labeling to allow healthcare providers to understand the vaccine's proper use, including its potential benefits and risks, to be able to communicate with patients (and parents if the vaccine is for use in children) and to safely deliver the vaccine to the public. The FDA continues to oversee production of vaccines after the vaccine and the manufacturing processes are approved in order to ensure continuing safety.

Until a vaccine is given to the general population, all potential adverse events cannot be anticipated. Thus, many vaccines are required to undergo phase 4 studies after they are on the market. There is also a Vaccine Adverse Event Reporting System (VAERS) to help identify any problems with a vaccine after marketing begins.

Many large pharmaceutical companies are adding vaccines to their portfolios because of growth opportunities. Vaccine area growth means that more CRAs will have the opportunity to work on vaccine trials. Although vaccines and drugs fall under the same regulations, there are some significant differences in vaccine trials. One fundamental difference in the trials is that vaccines are typically given to healthy individuals in the hope that the vaccine will keep them from contracting the disease of interest (e.g., flu). Since these trials take healthy people and expose them to an investigational product (the vaccine), there is very little tolerance for risk.

Vaccine trials tend to be extremely large, and recruiting large numbers of healthy people can be very resource-intensive. There is also an issue of retaining subjects for the duration of the trial, as the site does not normally see the subjects again after the administration of the vaccine until the very end of the trial. Enrollment time also may be very short, especially if you need to "catch the season," as with the flu. When a new strain of flu is expected to become endemic, for example, studies on a vaccine to prevent it must be done before the flu season commences.

COVID Vaccine Development

In December 2020, the FDA granted Emergency Use Authorization (EUA) for COVID-19 vaccines developed by Pfizer/BioNTech and Moderna. Vaccines typically take from 10 to 15 years to develop, but these two messenger RNA (mRNA) vaccines were developed in record time—less than one year—because of the public health emergency.

In a phase 3 study with 30,000 participants, including groups at higher risk of COVID-19 (those over age 65 and individuals with underlying health conditions), Moderna's vaccine was 94.1 percent effective in protecting against COVID-19 disease and 100 percent effective in protecting against severe COVID-19 infection, defined as requiring hospitalization or supplemental oxygen support. The Pfizer/BioNTech vaccine demonstrated similar efficacy in multiple studies. However, the efficacy of both vaccines declined over time and the original vaccines were less effective against new strains of the SARS-CoV-2 virus that caused COVID infections, leading to a need for new vaccines that targeted the emerging strains.

Since the initial EUAs were granted, the development of COVID vaccines, boosters and treatments has grown. Trials are still underway for bivalent COVID vaccines and the mRNA technology is now also being applied to other therapeutic areas.

This presents a new opportunity for CRAs. If you will be working with biologics, including vaccines, you may want to become familiar with 21 CFR Part 600 (Biological Products: General), 21 CFR 601 (Licensing) 21 CFR Part

610 (General Biological Products Standards) and NIH Guidelines for Research Involving Recombinant or Synthetic Nucleic Acid Molecules.

Key Takeaways

- CDRH is responsible for both the premarket and post-market regulation of medical devices.
- There are a number of differences between device and drug trials.
- CBER is responsible for vaccines; blood and blood products; xenotransplantation; and cell, tissue and gene therapies.
- The regulations that apply to drugs also apply to biologics and vaccines.
- There are other regulations and institutional requirements that apply specifically to devices and to biologics.
- One of the main differences in vaccine studies is that the vaccines are normally given to healthy study subjects.
- The vaccine area is growing very rapidly.

CHAPTER 7

Globalization of Clinical Trials

Many diseases, such as diabetes, hypertension and HIV/AIDS, have now become global in scope. Instead of being confined to a small geographic area or one group of people, diseases have become more prevalent among many different cultural groups. Newer global markets have sponsors conducting clinical trials in countries that would hardly have been considered in the past, for many reasons. Some populations around the world have used considerably fewer medications than in more developed countries, making it easier to assess the effects of a study medication. Also, some diseases have an extremely low incidence in developed countries (e.g., malaria), but there is still a need for new medications; these medications could not be developed without conducting trials in countries where the disease is still prevalent. Another reason for the increase in the number of global trials is that some developing nations require local clinical trial data for product registration (e.g., India and China).

There has been a large increase in the number of clinical trials conducted in countries outside the U.S. over the past decade, especially in later-phase studies that enroll large numbers of subjects and have higher per-subject costs. In fact, many multicenter trials currently being conducted have a mixture of both U.S. and non-U.S. sites. By 2009, the average phase 3 trial was taking place in 34 countries.

According to ClinicalTrials.gov, of 452,005 trials listed in the database (as of May 2023), only 31 percent were conducted in the U.S., while 53 percent were based in other countries. Five percent of trials operated in both the U.S. and other countries; 11 percent did not specify.

Using sites in emerging markets such as Central and Eastern Europe, China, India and Latin America in later-stage trials often enables sponsors to increase subject recruitment and cut costs while establishing a presence in these emerging markets. With the huge increase in global trials, sponsors have had to broaden their procedures and processes to handle the varying regulato-

Figure 1. Percentage of registered studies by location

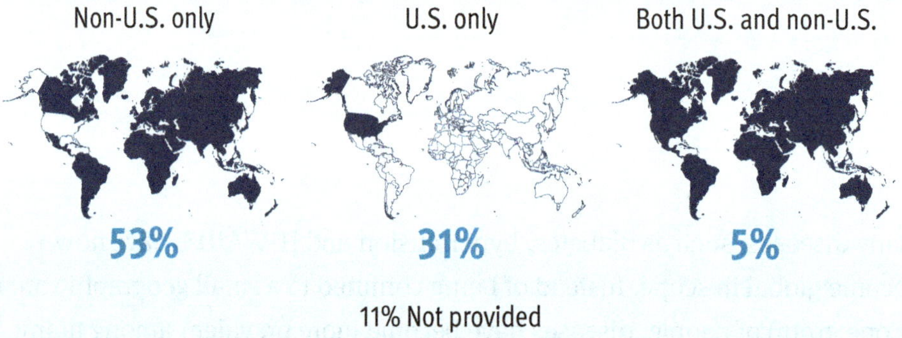

Source: ClinicalTrials.gov

ry and cultural requirements of many counties. Note that if these trials are to be used for registration in the U.S., they must follow FDA regulations, as well as those of the country that is conducting the trial.

Completing trials in other countries may help the sponsor register the product more quickly in these countries and in the U.S., as well as reduce its overall development time and cost. Cutting costs has become a critical aspect of research and development programs; so as long as costs continue to be lower in emerging markets, the trend toward conducting studies in these areas of the world will undoubtedly continue to rise.

Another reason emerging markets are becoming more enticing locations for clinical research is that there is a growing middle class in many of these countries, such as China, India and Indonesia, with increasing spending on public healthcare by governments and by individuals.

Managing Multinational Trials

Many CRAs are working on trials in which some, if not all, of the investigative sites are in other countries. Some CRAs actually travel to other countries to monitor non-U.S. sites. Even if the CRA is not actually monitoring non-U.S. sites, activities often involve the U.S.

There are some inherent difficulties when studies involve sites in different countries. Language, cultural differences and time zone differences can make working together a challenge. Translating study materials into other languages can be expensive and time consuming. Working with a translator makes meetings awkward, and misunderstanding cultural differences can cause embarrassment. Differences in standard medical practice are important to recognize, as are differing attitudes toward medical care. For example, in some countries patients would never think to complain about an issue that would be seen in the U.S. as an adverse event. Projects can go awry simply because of misunderstandings and difficult personal interactions due to cultural differences.

The distribution and storage of study products can be difficult in terms of time, cost, the environment and accountability. Storage can be an issue, especially if the product needs to be temperature controlled, refrigerated or frozen. Conditions can vary considerably in some countries, especially where basic utility services are not available on a regular basis.

It can also be difficult to transfer data from the site to the sponsor in a timely manner. If electronic data transfers are being used, the required connections may not always be reliable or available. If relying on mail services, it may take a much longer time for the transfer. These issues need to be recognized and addressed before the trial begins.

Global trials should be conducted with the same ethical principles as trials run in the U.S. They should follow all national and international regulatory requirements, as well as ICH guidelines. There are certainly some ethical issues to consider. For example, in Europe as well as other non-U.S. countries, there is a bias against using placebo controls in clinical trials. It is felt that it is not ethical to withhold active medication from someone suffering from a medical condition that could be treated. Informed consent may not mean the same thing in another country that it does in the U.S. Written consent may not be possible, so one might have to work with a witness who can explain and interpret what will happen in the study. Payments to subjects and to investigators can be an issue and should be appropriate to the local economy.

These issues need to be considered and managed. To help with ethical issues, some companies have an IRB in the U.S. review the study and related issues, as well as a local IRB in the trial country.

If a sponsor is large, more resources may be available to facilitate global trials. Many large sponsors have offices in multiple countries, so people are available who speak both English and the local language, understand the cultural climate and can assist colleagues coming from the U.S. to work at investigative sites. Some sponsors also use CROs based in foreign countries to monitor trials, which is another good resource. Even when an in-country CRO is used, however, it is likely that sponsor personnel from the U.S. will need to visit non-U.S. sites periodically.

As a CRA, if you have involvement with non-U.S. sites, there are some basic things you will want to keep in mind that will make for smoother interactions when working with them:

- Time differences are significant. You may need to adjust your working hours to be available earlier or later in the day to talk to your non-U.S. colleagues. You cannot expect others to always adhere to your most convenient times. This is especially true when contacting study site personnel, who are not sponsor employees.
- Although many other people around the world speak English, it is often not their first language. You may need to speak more slowly to be understood. Try not to use slang, abbreviations, colloquialisms, etc. that may not be familiar to others. Check to be sure what you said is clear to the other person. If you are speaking in person, watch the other person's body language for clues. It's easier to confirm that everyone is on the same page than it is to fix misunderstandings later.
- In email and instant message communications, be mindful that your colleagues may not have English as their first language and that grammar, punctation, spelling and word use may be a little different, with some errors. Be patient and read things slowly and carefully to ensure correct interpretation.
- Cultural differences can be landmines. We've all heard stories about gaffes made because of these differences, from using the wrong word in a situation to making a gesture that has a completely different meaning to giving an inappropriate gift. Go slowly, ask people with more experience, watch others—be aware. The internet has scores of references about appropriate etiquette in other countries, as do libraries and bookstores.
- When in large meetings or teleconferences with non-U.S. investigational or sponsor personnel, be sure to avoid uncomfortable or controversial topics such as politics, religion or world events. Individuals on the same study team may hold dramatically different views on these topics.

Discussing them can be unprofessional and cause discord within a study team.

- Remember that some people are better with spoken English than written English or vice-versa. Think as much about what you write as what you say.
- Ensure that your passport is renewed and current, as you may have to travel internationally at the last minute.
- Large meetings, such as investigator or study startup meetings, with many speakers and long sessions are tiring, especially when English is not your first language. Take time at these meetings to speak individually with people to see if they have questions. Note: It is important to build in more breaks—longer breaks—into meetings with participants from multiple countries or who speak multiple languages.
- Allow more time for monitoring visits. You may need extra time to develop trust and cooperative relationships, as well as for study-related activities that need to be carried out. When you are traveling long distances, it would be counterproductive to cut your visit short without accomplishing everything that needs to be done.
- Be nice. Be pleasant. Be friendly. This will go a long way toward good, professional working relationships.

If you are lucky enough to be involved in non-U.S. studies, enjoy the opportunities afforded by travel to other countries and working with people from other cultures; you may never have this wonderful good fortune again.

Key Takeaways

- Many multicenter trials being conducted today have a mixture of both U.S. and non-U.S. sites:
- Working with multinational sites presents numerous challenges, including logistical problems due to travel and different time zones.
- Cultural and language differences need to be carefully considered when working in other countries.

- Global trials should be conducted with the same ethical principles as trials run in the U.S.

CHAPTER 8

Institutional Review Boards and Data Safety Monitoring Boards

When conducting clinical trials, the safety of human subjects comes first. The two main safeguards for human subjects are Institutional Review Boards (IRB) and the informed consent process. This chapter covers IRBs—what they are, their purpose and how they function. Another entity frequently used to enhance safety/review safety data in clinical trials is a Data Safety Monitoring Board (DSMB), which will also be discussed later in this chapter.

The regulatory definition of an IRB is "any board, committee or group formally designated by an institution to review, approve the initiation of and conduct periodic review of biomedical research involving human subjects. The primary purpose of such review is to assure the protection of the rights and welfare of the human subjects." Notice that an IRB must approve a study before it can start. All research done in humans in the U.S. must be approved by an IRB. (21 CFR Part 56 contains the regulations that pertain to IRBs.)

Since many companies do research globally, a CRA should be aware that ethical reviews of protocols are conducted outside the U.S. The Independent Ethics Committee (IEC) is the body analogous to an IRB in countries outside the U.S. The IEC is an independent body, the responsibility of which is to ensure the protection of the rights, safety and well-being of human subjects involved in a trial by reviewing and approving/providing a favorable opinion on the trial protocol and informed consent. Both IRBs and IECs have one fundamental purpose: to protect the rights, safety and welfare of human subjects in research. In general, IECs give a favorable opinion about the research, rather than an actual approval; this difference in wording is the main difference between the two groups. For all purposes, the favorable opinion of an IEC carries the same weight and is just as binding as the approval of an IRB; it is especially viewed as such for any studies that will be submitted to the FDA for registration purposes.

Our discussion, however, will focus on IRBs and the U.S. regulations for IRBs and investigators. An investigator who is planning to conduct a trial must contact an IRB, submit the appropriate materials, including the proposed protocol and consent form, investigator's brochure, any study manuals, any recruitment materials and patient-facing materials, etc. and wait for formal approval from the IRB before initiating the trial. Interacting with and asking an IRB for approval are the responsibilities of the clinical investigator, not the pharmaceutical company sponsoring the research. (Note: Occasionally a sponsor may submit documents to the IRB on behalf of investigators.) However, the CRA will verify the investigator's IRB approval for the sponsor.

Types of IRBs

There are two types of IRBs: those that are affiliated with an institution and those that are not. Unaffiliated IRBs are called independent, central/commercial or national IRBs. They can be used by any researcher who is not constrained by institutional policy to the use of a particular institutional review board.

Here are the most common scenarios for the use of a local vs. a central/commercial IRB. If an investigator is affiliated with an institution (hospital or university, etc.) that has an IRB and if that investigator is conducting the trial or any part of the trial at the institution, then he or she would normally use the institution's IRB (also known as the local IRB). If the trial is being conducted at an investigator's private practice or dedicated research site and the investigator and site are independent from an institution with an IRB, then the investigator would use the central/commercial IRB. There are situations in which an investigator has institutional affiliation but would still use a central/commercial IRB. Some investigators serve as professors at large academic institutions but maintain a private medical practice where clinical trials are also conducted. In this case, despite the professorship at the academic institution, if the investigator is only conducting study activities at his/her private practice and the practice is independent from and not affiliated in any way with the academic institution/IRB, then the central/commercial IRB could in most cases be used. However, each situation is unique and governed differently.

Independent IRBs (also known as commercial, or central IRBs), those not affiliated with a particular institution, are available to any investigator who is not constrained by institutional affiliation that requires him or her to conduct clinical trials at the institution or affiliate locations and to use the institutional IRB. Independent IRBs are available to independent investigators with private practices, dedicated research sites/networks and institutions that lack an institutional IRB. Independent IRBs are frequently used for multi-center studies in non-hospitalized patients.

Study sponsors prefer to use independent IRBs when possible because, in general, they tend to review studies more quickly (turnaround time). The IRBs at some teaching hospitals, for example, can take three to six months to review a protocol, while most independent IRBs have a review time of less than one month. Sometimes sponsors or investigators may express concerns about having research reviewed by an IRB that is not local and may not be as familiar with the investigative site, the investigator or the community. To counteract concerns, the better independent IRBs visit investigative sites and have methods of determining community attitudes and other local issues in order to appropriately approve or disapprove research.

A more common trend to mitigate the long approval timeframes of large institutional/academic health site IRBs is the practice of deferring the local IRB responsibilities to a central IRB. These large institutions enlist the assistance of well-established central IRBs to complete study review and approval; they essentially delegate the institutional IRB responsibility to a central IRB (the central IRB will essentially serve as the local IRB). The basic process is that the institutional IRB will complete review of the study and accompanying materials and, if contingently approving the study, will send the study materials on to the central IRB for final verification and approval. This is usually done in cases where the institutional local IRB is backlogged with internal study review or is experiencing extremely long review timeframes. Delegating study review responsibilities to a central IRB expedites the study submission and approval process, which allows institutions to stay competitive with their counterpart institutions, as well as with local private physicians and research sites that use central IRBs. Another term for this is when a local IRB has a reliance agreement with a central IRB for review/approval of studies at their institution.

If an investigator is conducting a study at more than one institution (e.g., two hospitals), IRB approval is required from each institution where the study will be conducted.

IRB Responsibilities

Whether or not the IRB is affiliated with a particular institution, its primary responsibility is to protect the rights and welfare of human subjects participating in clinical research. To fulfill this responsibility, the IRB must answer two basic questions:

1. Should the study be done at all? Do the benefits outweigh the risks?
2. If so, what constitutes adequate informed consent?

Should the Study be Done at All? (Benefit vs. Risk Assessments)

When determining whether or not the study should be conducted, the IRB must consider several items. The IRB members must have assurance that the study is scientifically valid; in other words, that there is a properly designed protocol. However, it is not the responsibility of an IRB to judge the scientific merit or worth of the trial. For example, it is not the function of an IRB to decide whether we need another drug for hypertension but rather to determine if the research methods being used to study that potential antihypertensive are valid.

Risks to the subjects must be minimized, so the IRB will look for a sound research design that does not expose human subjects to unnecessary risk. It will also ascertain if the protocol uses procedures that would be performed on these patients, both diagnostically and treatment-wise, even if they were not in the study, when appropriate.

The IRB must determine whether the anticipated benefit to subjects and the overall knowledge to be gained from the research compare favorably to the risks. In this evaluation, the IRB considers only those risks and benefits that may result directly from the research, excluding the risks and benefits the subjects would have encountered even if they had not been involved in the research (just in the standard treatment for the condition). Remember, there are always risks involved in doing research. The IRB will also want to know what the subject selection process is, in order to ensure that the selection is equitable and that no groups of potential subjects are routinely excluded or included based on non-study related characteristics. Depending on the particular study, some of these characteristics might include sex, race, ethnic background, weight, smoking, educational background, etc. In making this assessment, the IRB will consider the particular setting in which the research will be conducted, as well as the purposes of the research.

What Constitutes Adequate Informed Consent?

If the IRB determines that the answer to the first question (Do the benefits outweigh the risks?) is yes, then it will consider the consent form submitted by the investigator. It is a regulatory requirement that informed consent is sought from each subject or the subject's legally authorized representative before that person may be enrolled in the research project. By regulation, informed consent must be documented, which is usually done by having the subject sign a written copy of the consent document. (Consents are discussed in detail in the next chapter.)

There is a specific process to the development and finalization of the informed consent form for a study, relative to the sponsor and the institutional and independent IRBs used by sites. The sponsor/CRO is responsible for developing an appropriate informed consent form template. It is submitted to the independent IRB for review/approval. The investigative sites using institutional IRBs have to change sponsor language and or/include specific institutional language into the informed consent templates, which are then submitted to their respective institutional IRBs for review/approval. The sponsor also has to approve the informed consent template changes made by sites using institutional IRBs. The back-and-forth review process of the informed consent template between sites and sponsors can extensively delay site activation if the parties cannot agree in a timely manner.

Along with written consent, there must be provisions in the research plan for ongoing safety monitoring of the data with the goal of ensuring the safety of subjects during the research. It's not sufficient, for example, to have all adverse event data reviewed only at the completion of a trial—data must be regularly reviewed throughout the study period in case problems arise as more is learned about the drug, device or procedure under investigation.

The IRB will also determine whether or not there are adequate provisions in the research to protect the privacy of the research subjects, as well as to maintain the confidentiality of the data, where appropriate.

Payments to study patients and advertising are considered by the FDA and IRBs as part of the consent process, as both might encourage a subject to enroll in a trial. If subjects are to be paid for their participation in the research, the IRB will review the planned compensation to ensure that it does not constitute an undue influence or coercion, which could influence the subject's decision to participate. Ideally, subjects would not take the risks involved in study participation simply because of compensation. The IRB's decision will be based not only on the amount subjects may receive for being in the study but also on the setting in which the study will take place. An amount that may be coercive in one setting may not be in another. Due to the patient's stipend listed in the informed consent form, sites often require the draft or final budget around the time of the IRB study submission as the stipend is an element of their budget.

The IRB will also review any proposed advertising to ensure it does not make misleading or untruthful claims and does not constitute undue influence. Glowing claims of success for a new treatment, for example, can also influence subjects to participate in a trial they might otherwise not want to be involved in. (See Chapter 16 for more on advertising.)

Vulnerable Subjects

Sometimes special, vulnerable populations are studied in research trials. Vulnerable subjects include children, pregnant women, prisoners, people with physical or mental disabilities, people with acute or severe mental illness and people who are economically or educationally disadvantaged. If any of these categories of people are going to be included in the research, the IRB needs to determine whether or not there are sufficient additional safeguards to protect them from coercion or undue influence. There are a number of NIH regulations (45 CFR 46) regarding research in various vulnerable populations. IRB members, investigators and others involved in these types of research, including CRAs, should familiarize themselves with this information.

California's bill of rights for study subjects

California's Experimental Subject's Bill of Rights states that any person who is requested to consent to participate as a subject in a research study involving a medical experiment or who is requested to consent on behalf of another has the right to:

- Be informed of the nature and purpose of the experiment.
- Be given an explanation of the procedures to be followed in the medical experiment and of any drug or device to be used.
- Be given a description of any attendant discomforts and risks reasonably to be expected from the experiment, if applicable.
- Be given an explanation of any benefits to the subject reasonably to be expected from the experiment, if applicable.
- Be given a disclosure of any appropriate alternative procedures, drugs or devices that might be advantageous to the subject and their relative risks and benefits
- Be informed of the avenues of medical treatment, if any, available to the subject after the experiment or if complications should arise.
- Be given an opportunity to ask any questions concerning the experiment or other procedures involved.
- Be instructed that consent to participate in the medical experiment maybe withdrawn at any time and that the subject may discontinue in the medical experiment without prejudice.
- Be given a copy of a signed and dated written informed consent form when one is required.
- Be given the opportunity to decide to consent or not to consent to a medical experiment without the intervention of any element of force, fraud, deceit, duress, coercion or undue influence on the subject's decision.

State and Local Regulations

The IRB must determine that the research does not violate any existing state or local laws or regulations or any applicable institutional policies or practices. Some states, for example, California and Massachusetts, have regulations that may exceed federal regulations. People working in these states and others should be familiar with their state requirements for conducting research.

As an example, California requires that an experimental subject's bill of rights be provided to every study subject in a trial. For an example of a subject's bill of rights based on California's experimental subject's bill of rights, see below. In another example, in 2015 Alabama lowered the age of consent to

18 years old (previously 19 years) for IRB-approved research conducted by an accredited college or university.

IRB Review of Proposed Research

An IRB considers each research project submitted for review separately. In order to determine if the research meets all the criteria discussed above. The IRB will review:

- Investigator qualifications.
- Study protocol and supporting documents.
- Proposed consent form.
- Subject compensation, if applicable.
- Advertising, if applicable.

Materials Submitted to the IRB by an Investigator

To ensure an adequate review, the investigator submits a number of materials to the IRB for review, including the following:

- A current curriculum vitae (CV) that includes his or her qualifications for conducting the research, including education, training and experience.
- The study protocol, which includes or addresses the following items, as applicable:
  - Title of the study.
  - Purpose of the study, including any expected benefits.
  - Sponsor of the study.
  - Results from previous related research.
  - Subject inclusion/exclusion criteria.
  - Study design, including a discussion of the appropriateness of the research methods.
  - Description and schedule of the procedures to be performed.
  - Provisions for managing adverse events.

  - Payment to subjects for their participation.
  - Compensation for injuries to research subjects.
  - Provisions for protecting subject privacy.
  - Extra costs to subjects for participation in the study, if applicable.
  - Extra costs to third-party payers because of a subject's participation, if applicable.
- The investigator brochure or package insert, if applicable.
- The proposed informed consent document, containing all appropriate elements.
- All subject advertisements and recruitment procedures. In general, advertising includes anything that is directed toward potential research subjects and is designed for recruitment.
- Statement of Investigator (Form 1572), if applicable. This form is required for all FDA-regulated studies conducted under an IND. (Some IRBs do not require this, but many do.)
- Grant application for federally-funded research, if applicable.
- Any other specific forms or materials required by the IRB, such as an application form.

For investigators who use the sponsor-designated central IRB for the study, often the sponsor/CRO will submit regulatory documents to the central IRB on their behalf. Investigators/sites still have to send the necessary site regulatory documents to the sponsor/CRO regulatory staff tasked with central IRB submissions, but the overall IRB submissions are completed by the sponsor/CRO.

Most IRBs (local and central) use online, electronic systems to support IRB submissions. Essential and regulatory documents are electronically uploaded/submitted into the IRB system by institutional or CRO regulatory staff making the submission and the submissions are routed to the IRB board reviewing the study. In the past, IRB submissions consisted of multiple copies of regulatory documents for each IRB member reviewing the study, sent via interoffice delivery systems at institutions, with hours spent at copy machines, requiring mountains of paper.

IRB Deliberations

After documents are received from an investigator, an IRB will schedule the protocol review. For the initial review of a protocol, the committee will meet to decide whether or not to approve the proposed research. In order to make this decision, the group will review all the submitted materials and discuss the proposed research, followed by a vote. The IRB may approve the project or request changes or additional information in order to approve it or disapprove it. Please note that an investigator can sit on an IRB, but he or she cannot participate in the discussion leading to the vote or the voting for his or her own research, as this would constitute a conflict of interest. The IRB will usually provide documentation of the investigator's abstinence from voting on the study in which he or she is participating. This is usually documented in IRB meeting minutes, the IRB membership roster for the committee that reviewed the trial, the IRB approval letter or separate IRB documentation. This does not solely involve investigators. Site research pharmacists, study coordinators (i.e., any investigative research staff that sit on the IRB) must abstain from voting on the study in which he or she may be involved. It is not only the responsibility of the CRA to ask the critical question when conducting the site evaluation visit, it is just as much the responsibility of the investigational site staff to disclose which site members sit on the IRB during the initial study discussions/site evaluation visits. CRAs are also obligated to collect a copy of the documentation verifying that the investigator and/or staff in question did abstain from voting on the study for the internal study file.

The IRB must notify the investigator in writing that the study is approved. If a study is rejected, the IRB will also notify the investigator in writing of its action and must allow the investigator to address the IRB concerning the decision either in writing or in person.

Any planned advertising must be approved before use, although this does not have to be approved before the study begins. It depends on whether the sponsor anticipates the need for recruitment advertisement when a study first starts or later on "just in case." A robust advertising campaign and IRB approval happens before study start, so it can be used by sites immediately when activated. This happens if a study has an enormous enrollment requirement, if a study is for a rare disease or has difficult eligibility criteria. If the study is in a common therapeutic area, not difficult to enroll, and research sites/investigators already have access to the population in their database, then advertising may come after study initiation. Advertising also starts after the fact when subject recruitment has been slower than expected. However, IRB approval of the study and the consent form must be obtained prior to patient enrollment.

As detailed throughout this book, CRAs must be diligent and proactive in the conduct of their job responsibilities and with the many tasks that require collaboration with sites to complete. I once had a CRA friend who was assigned to a site with an overworked but well-meaning study coordinator. The site was close to activation. All that was pending was the IRB approval letter, which the study coordinator had not gotten around to requesting. The CRA did not want to miss the Site Initiation Visit (SIV) schedule deadline and took it upon herself to contact the IRB and request the letter. She obtained the approval letter almost immediately and sent it to the harried SC, who appreciated the gesture and the thoughtfulness of the CRA.

Investigator Reporting Responsibilities

Throughout the study, the investigator must report any protocol changes or amendments to the IRB. Any change that would increase risk to subjects must be approved by the IRB prior to implementation. Protocol amendments and changes can also be submitted by CRO/sponsor staff to the central IRB for those applicable sites. The only exception to this is when the change is necessary to eliminate an apparent immediate hazard to the safety and well-being of the subjects, in which case it should be implemented immediately, followed by a timely notification and submission to the IRB. For example, if it is determined during a trial that taking a particular concomitant medication is unsafe, investigative sites would be notified by the sponsor to immediately stop giving that particular medication to study patients. Sites would do this immediately, then notify their IRBs. These exceptions are quite rare.

The investigator must also promptly report "immediately reportable" adverse events to the IRB. These usually include deaths and other serious adverse events that are unexpected during the study. Each IRB has their own reporting requirements for adverse events reporting and what is deemed reportable. Occasionally deaths may be the expected outcome in a study; in this case, the reporting rules may change, and deaths will not be reported as immediately reportable adverse events. This exception is also quite rare. (Adverse event reporting is discussed in detail in Chapter 15.)

The investigator must promptly report any unanticipated problems that arise during the research that involve risk to the study subjects or others to the IRB.

The investigator is required to submit periodic reports to the IRB detailing the progress of the study. This will be submitted at least annually and may be required on a more frequent basis.

The investigator must also report a change in location/facilities or a change in investigator status, for example, if the Principal Investigator retires, or transitions to a Sub Investigator role and a new Principal Investigator assumes study responsibility. This includes updated paperwork such as a Form 1572, CV, financial disclosure, new informed consent documents, etc.

Continuing Review of a Research Study

The IRB will review each research project at least annually, although the IRB may require updates on a more frequent basis, such as quarterly, based on the degree of risk to which subjects are exposed. At the continuing review, the IRB will ensure that the risk/benefit relationship remains acceptable, that the consent and study documents being used are still appropriate and that the selection of subjects has been equitable.

To help make these determinations, most IRBs will require the investigator to submit an IRB-specific form about the progress of the study, including enrollment figures, withdrawals, adverse events and unanticipated problems, protocol violations, etc. at each review period. The IRB will also want to see a copy of the consent form currently in use, advertising and any other appropriate documents. The IRB will ask for any protocol amendments that were made during the time period, especially if they were not previously reviewed by the IRB. This information allows the IRB to determine whether or not the research can continue.

All research must be reapproved at least annually. The investigator will receive written notification of each formal reapproval. Rereview and reapproval continue throughout the entire research project, until such time as all subjects have completed their participation and the project is closed.

If an investigator is not submitting the required study updates to the IRB for review, the IRB has several options. The IRB may send the investigator a reminder that he or she is required to submit the update, with a deadline for receipt of the requested materials. If the reminder does not work, the IRB may put enrollment on hold until the updates are received and reviewed. In the worst-case scenario, the IRB may withdraw approval of the study. It is important to remember that each approval is good only for a specified time period. If reapproval is not received prior to the expiration date of the previous approval, the study is out of compliance with the regulations.

Expedited Review

Upon occasion, an IRB may utilize an expedited review process for minor changes in previously approved research; this may be done only during the time period for which the approval was authorized. Expedited review may be done by the IRB chairperson or by experienced members who are designated as expedited reviewers. Items may be approved by expedited review, but they cannot be rejected. If the expedited reviewer(s) thinks something should be rejected, it must go to the full board for review. The board also must be made aware of all expedited review decisions, which is usually done at the first regular meeting following the review.

Expedited review is never used in circumstances in which the risk to human subjects increases. It cannot, in general, be used for the initial review of a research study. There are a few exceptions by which initial review of a project can be done using expedited review, but these are not the kinds of studies in which CRAs would normally be involved; these exceptions are published in the Federal Register. If you are interested in reading more about this, there is an FDA guidance document called Categories of Research That May Be Reviewed by the Institutional Review Board (IRB) Through an Expedited Review Procedure.

IRB Membership

An IRB must have at least five members, a quorum. IRB membership should be selected to assure appropriate diversity, including representation by multiple professions, multiple ethnic backgrounds and both genders, and must include both scientific and non-scientific members. The members must possess the appropriate professional competence to review the diverse types of protocols received. Most IRBs also have alternate members to ensure a quorum if a regular member is unable to be present.

There must be at least one member who is not affiliated with the institution (and who has no immediate family member affiliated with the institution) other than his or her IRB membership. There must also be one member whose interests and background are non-scientific (lay person). It is acceptable for one IRB member to fulfill both of these criteria. In addition, an IRB that reviews FDA-regulated products (drugs, biologics and devices) should have at least one member who is a physician.

IRB Operations

IRBs are required by regulation to follow written procedures. IRBs are audited by regulatory authorities, and they will be held responsible for having the appropriate written procedures and for following them. They must also carefully document their decisions and retain this documentation appropriately.

Conflict of Interest

No IRB member may participate in the initial or continuing review of any project in which he or she has a conflicting interest in the research. A person whose research is being reviewed may be present at the IRB meeting to answer questions and provide information about the project, but he or she should not be present for the discussion leading to the vote or during actual voting. The minutes of the meeting or IRB documentation need to reflect that the person was not present to alleviate any claim of conflict of interest.

IRB Registration

In 2009, the FDA began requiring the registration of IRBs that review FDA-regulated studies. Registration gives the FDA more complete information about the IRBs that review these studies and will:

- Facilitate sharing educational and other information with the IRBs.
- Assist the FDA in scheduling and conducting IRB inspections.

- Help the FDA prioritize IRB inspections.

Once registered, IRBs are required to review and submit current information every three years, although some information, such as a change in the IRB chairperson, is required to be submitted within a certain amount of time after the change occurs.

IRB registration is not accreditation or certification by the FDA, nor does it address issues of the IRB's competence, expertise or ability to conduct reviews.

FDA Guidance Documents for IRBs

There are a number of FDA guidance documents that discuss topics relevant to IRBs. Some of the more useful ones include:

- Institutional Review Board (IRB) Written Procedures Guidance for Institutions and IRBs, May 2018.
- FDA Institutional Review Board Inspections, April 2018.
- Institutional Review Board (IRB) Review of Individual Patient Expanded Access Requests for Investigational Drugs and Biological Products During the COVID-19 Public Health Emergency Guidance for IRBs and Clinical Investigators, June 2020.
- Considerations When Transferring Clinical Investigation Oversight to Another IRB, Guidance for IRBs, Clinical Investigators, and Sponsors, May 2014.
- IRB Responsibilities for Reviewing the Qualifications of Investigators, Adequacy of Research Sites, and the Determination of Whether an IND/IDE is Needed, Guidance for IRBs, Clinical Investigators, and Sponsors, august 2013.
- Sponsor - Investigator - IRB Interrelationship, January 1998.

Scientific Review Committee

Some medical and academic institutions have an additional scientific panel or committee, known as a "scientific review committee," which is required to review and approve a potential study, in addition to IRB review. This is usually to confirm study science or medical merit or design and represents an additional layer of institutional oversight of potential studies. Therapeutic indications that usually require additional scientific review include oncology studies, pediatric studies and radiology studies; some institutions require scientific review for every study proposed. Institutional requirements for scientific review committees vary.

Scientific review is usually completed in conjunction with IRB review. However, some institutions require scientific review committee approval of a study before it can be submitted to the IRB. This can add additional time to the submission and approval process for the study and needs to be considered when evaluating sites for studies.

Additional Review Committees

Some institutions also have a feasibility committee, which reviews the study prior to a scientific review or IRB review. This is a group of site representatives from each department that review the study for capability, labor, time, etc. Some institutions also have radiology review committees for studies with imaging requirements more than standard of care.

Data Safety Monitoring Boards

A Data Safety Monitoring Board (DSMB), sometimes known as a Data Safety Monitoring Committee (DSMC) or Data Monitoring Committee (DMC), is a group of expert advisors, usually appointed by a sponsor, to periodically review the accumulating data from a clinical trial, primarily to assess the continuing safety of trial subjects. The purpose of this committee is to advise the sponsor, after review of the data to date, whether or not the trial should continue in its present form, be modified or perhaps even be discontinued.

DSMBs were used in some clinical trials as early as the 1960s, mainly in large, randomized multi-center trials sponsored by the NIH and the Department of Veterans Affairs (VA), in which mortality and morbidity were the primary outcome measures. The establishment of these committees was based not only on the premise that monitoring of the accumulating study data is essential to ensure the ongoing safety of trial subjects but also on the premise that sponsor representatives closely involved in the design and conduct of a trial might not be fully objective in reviewing the interim data for any emerging concerns.

FDA regulations do not require the use of DSMBs in trials except under 21 CFR 50.24(a)(7)(iv) for research studies in emergency settings in which the informed consent requirement is excepted.

A DSMB consists of people who are external to the trial organizers, sponsors and investigators in order to minimize bias. They must have the appropriate expertise to evaluate the data, and members usually include one or more medical people, a statistician and others, as appropriate. They may meet on a regular schedule based on time, such as every six months, or they may meet based on enrollment (e.g., after every increment of 50 enrolled subjects) or on some other "trigger" appropriate for the trial. The DSMB will receive the data from the study up to the cut-off date for that review.

During its review, it will look at the data, have the DSMB statistician run some appropriate programs for looking at aggregate data, discuss the findings and inform the sponsor of its recommendation. This review usually results in one of three possible recommendations: Continue the trial as is, continue with modifications (or more frequent DSMB review) or stop the trial because of safety concerns. Although the DSMB recommendation is not binding, sponsors take these recommendations very seriously and usually abide by them.

All clinical trials require safety monitoring, but not all trials require monitoring by a DSMB. DSMBs have usually been used for large, randomized, multi-center studies that evaluate treatments intended to prolong life or reduce risk of a major adverse health outcome, such as cancer or cardiovascular events. They are recommended in controlled trials in which mortality or major morbidity is the outcome measured or in trials that have a high risk of severe outcomes. They are not usually needed for trials looking at less serious outcomes or for early-stage trials.

Adding a DSMB to a trial adds cost and resources, as well as additional administrative complexity, so the FDA does not recommend using a DSMB unless the trial meets particular criteria related to safety, practicality and scientific validity. The FDA has a guidance document Guidance for Clinical Trial Sponsors: Establishment and Operation of Clinical Trial Data Monitoring Committees, which provides additional information and the FDA's current thinking on the use of DSMBs, as well as practical information relating to the establishment and function of such groups.

A CRA usually will not have any reason to interact with a DSMB. However, there can be situations in which an upcoming DSMB review will necessitate the rapid collection and cleaning of data from study sites. In this case, the CRA may be expected to retrieve data for the subjects included in the DSMB review without regard to the normal monitoring schedule. The CRA may need to spend significant time on the phone with study coordinators or may have to make additional monitoring visits to ensure that the necessary information is available for the DSMB.

Applicable early phase studies will use a safety committee to review available safety and dosing data to determine if dose escalation is safe or if the current dose needs extra evaluation with additional subjects or if a stop is required due to dose-limiting toxicities. This can also help determine a recommended phase 2 dose.

Some studies may involve committees to assure appropriate study oversight, as well as committees for the adjudication of specific medical events.

Key Takeaways

IRBs

- IRBs are one of the primary safeguards for the protection of human subjects in research.
- CFR Part 56 contains the regulations that pertain to IRBs.
- An IRB must approve a study and the informed consent document before the study can begin.
- There are two types of IRBs: those that are affiliated with an institution and those that are independent (i.e., not affiliated with an institution).
- The IRB must make a risk/benefit assessment for each proposed project.
- There are special regulations concerning research in vulnerable subjects (children, pregnant women, prisoners, etc.).

- State and local research regulations must be followed.
- IRBs must approve advertising and subject compensation.
- An investigator must report adverse events and study progress to the IRB at least annually.
- Continuing review of a study must be done at least annually.
- Expedited review may not be used for the initial review of a project, except in particular instances published in the Federal Register.
- IRB members may not vote if they have a conflict of interest.
- IRBs reviewing FDA-regulated research must register with the FDA.

DSMBs

- DSMBs are appointed by the sponsor to review study safety on a periodic basis.
- DSMBs are used primarily for clinical trials in which high morbidity or mortality is anticipated.
- FDA regulations do not require the use of a DSMB except for research studies in emergency settings in which informed consent is accepted.
- After review, a DSMB makes a recommendation to the sponsor concerning whether the study should continue as it is, continue with modifications or be discontinued.

CHAPTER 9

Informed Consent

One of the main safeguards for the protection of human subjects in research is informed consent. This chapter discusses informed consent, including governing regulations, how a consent form is written, CRA review and administration, and the emergence of electronic informed consent.

The decision whether or not to participate in a study is not an easy one. There is the hope of help and the desire to please the physician investigator, as well as apprehension and fear of the unknown. To help a potential subject make a decision that is not based purely on emotions such as fear and hope, everything possible must be done to provide complete information in a format that is readily accessible and easy to read, along with sufficient time to make an informed decision and the freedom to discuss this decision with family, friends and their personal physician, if desired.

Informed Consent is defined by the ICH E6(R2)—Guidelines for Good Clinical Practice as:

> A process by which a subject voluntarily confirms his or her willingness to participate in a particular trial, after having been informed of all aspects of the trial that are relevant to the subject's decision to participate. Informed consent is documented by means of a written, signed and dated informed consent form.

The two key words in this definition are "voluntarily" and "informed." These words form the cornerstone of ethical conduct in clinical research and are in place to protect the rights and safety of the subjects who participate in research. Potential subjects of clinical research must understand what they are getting into and must be free to decline to participate. The freedom to say "no" with a clear conscience and no fear of repercussion is an aspect of the consent process that must be considered. Many people have a certain reverence for their personal physicians; they want to please their physicians and will do as they direct. This carries over into the informed consent process and needs to be understood by physicians involved in research. CRAs should advise investigators to be conscious of this phenomenon. Investigators must make every effort to help potential study subjects understand that it is entirely acceptable if they choose not to participate. It is also important for subjects to understand that during a trial, as per ICH E6(R2) 4.8.10(m), "the subject's participation in the trial is voluntary and the subject may refuse to participate or withdraw from the trial at any time, without penalty or loss of benefits to which the subject is otherwise entitled."

Author's Story

I once visited two large academic health centers in the same week; one was in Canada and one was in a large East Coast city in the U.S. Though the academic institutions had similar services for patients and similarities in research infrastructure and personnel (including extensive SOPs to support research conduct and experienced and educated staff acting as study coordinators), one dramatic difference lay in by whom and how informed consent was obtained. Both processes followed by each institution were ethical and had the subject's best interest as the highest priority. The institution in Canada had the study coordinators obtain consent to prevent bias and ensure the subjects did not feel coerced or pressured to participate in the study because their personal physician was the investigator. The U.S. institution had only physician investigators obtaining consent to ensure the study patient was adequately informed about all aspects of study participation. They felt physician investigators were the most qualified to do this.

–Elizabeth

Monitoring Informed Consent

Informed consent should be one of the primary areas of concentration during a CRA's monitoring visits, both because it is so important ethically and because it is a frequent deficiency found during clinical investigator inspections conducted by the FDA. The problem is not that the consent process is not being done, but that it is not being done correctly. Common problems are:

The timing of the administration of consent may not be correct, meaning that the consent is not always obtained before any study-related procedures take place.

- Proper signatures are not always obtained.
- The consent form is poorly written.
- There are missing required elements.
- The amended informed consent is not signed.
- Re-consenting of study subjects with an amended informed consent does not occur in a timely manner.
- Inappropriate staff (not medically trained or qualified) are conducting the informed consent process/obtaining informed consent.

The first step in monitoring informed consent is to be familiar with the requirements, both for the document itself and the process. There are three basic requirements that a consent form must meet:

- It must completely and accurately describe all of the activities required by the protocol and what the subject's participation will involve.
- It must be able to be read and understood by the study subjects.
- It must contain all the elements required by regulation (21 CFR Part 50).

In other words, consents must inform, be comprehensible and comply with regulations. Here is a closer look at each of these requirements.

Activities and Participation

Potential study subjects need to be told about the study and their involvement in detail to be able to make an informed decision regarding their participation. Subjects need to know they will be participating in research, what is required of them, their rights as research subjects, and the potential benefits and risks they will face. The required elements of consent will be discussed later in this chapter. All the requirements (tests, procedures, activities, etc.) of the protocol must be described, including how these various activities will have an impact on the subjects, both in terms of personal discomfort and any lifestyle changes. Subjects also need to know when each activity must be done and how long it will take for each activity and study visit.

Readability and Comprehension

It is difficult to adequately inform potential subjects about a study without overwhelming them. A consent form may contain a very detailed description of protocol activities and consequences, but if it is a long, multiple-page document, a subject may not have a good feel for what will happen because the document is simply too long and presents too much information to comprehend. Writing a consent that properly informs without overwhelming is mostly the result of common sense and experience. It is important to keep this balance in mind if you are writing or reviewing a consent form.

Writing a comprehensible consent is as difficult as making it informative without being overwhelming. The consent form needs to be technically correct, yet intelligible for non-medical people. Consent forms should be written at approximately the fifth- to eighth-grade levels. This is a challenge in an industry filled with jargon, acronyms, medical terminology and highly educated people.

In general, the shorter the sentences and the fewer syllables per word in the text, the easier it will be to understand. Make a conscious effort to use terminology such as "teaspoons" instead of "cubic centimeters" and "milliliters" or "high blood pressure" instead of "hypertension." There is no substitute for experience; after you have written a few consent forms, it becomes easier. There are formulas that will give you a good estimate of the grade level of your document. For example, Microsoft Word includes the Flesch-Kincaid Grade Level tester, which pops up after spelling and grammar checks have been done on a document.

Elements

The last of the three requirements for a proper consent form is to make it compliant with federal regulations. 21 CFR part 50.25, which contains the elements of informed consent, is one of the more straightforward regulations. It clearly lists the elements that must be present in a consent form (basic elements) and those that are optional (additional elements).

Basic Elements of Consent

Part 50.25 lists the basic and additional elements of consent must be present in all consent forms. They are:

(1) A statement that the study involves research, an explanation of the purposes of the research and the expected duration of the subject's participation, a description of the procedures to be followed and identification of any procedures which are experimental.

(2) A description of any reasonably foreseeable risks or discomforts to the subject.

(3) A description of any benefits to the subject or to others which may reasonably be expected from the research.

(4) A disclosure of appropriate alternative procedures or courses of treatment, if any, that might be advantageous to the subject.

(5) A statement describing the extent, if any, to which confidentiality of records identifying the subject will be maintained and that notes the possibility that the Food and Drug Administration may inspect the records.

(6) For research involving more than minimal risk, an explanation as to whether any compensation and an explanation as to whether any medical treatments are available if injury occurs; and, if so, what they consist of or where further information may be obtained.

(7) An explanation of whom to contact for answers to pertinent questions about the research and research subjects' rights, and whom to contact in the event of a research-related injury to the subject.

(8) A statement that participation is voluntary, that refusal to participate will involve no penalty or loss of benefits to which the subject is otherwise entitled, and that the subject may discontinue participation at any time without penalty or loss of benefits to which the subject is otherwise entitled.

Additional Elements of Consent

Part 50.25 also lists the additional elements of consent, which should be included, as appropriate, are:

(1) A statement that the particular treatment or procedure may involve risks to the subject (or to the embryo or fetus, if the subject is or may become pregnant) which are currently unforeseeable.

(2) Anticipated circumstances under which the subject's participation may be terminated by the investigator without regard to the subject's consent.

(3) Any additional costs to the subject that may result from participation in the research.

(4) The consequences of a subject's decision to withdraw from the research and procedures for orderly termination of participation by the subject.

(5) A statement that significant new findings developed during the course of the research which may relate to the subject's willingness to continue participation will be provided to the subject.

(6) The approximate number of subjects involved in the study.

Since ICH guidelines mandate the inclusion of these additional elements, they usually appear in most informed consent forms, if appropriate.

One way to ensure that all elements are present in a consent form is to have an explicit heading for subsections that address each element. In any case, it must be clear that each of the elements is addressed in the form so subjects are properly informed and that the form will not be found deficient in a regulatory review.

Some states and institutions also have requirements that may have an impact on the content form. California, for example, requires that an Experimental Research Subject's Bill of Rights be attached to all consent forms.

In addition, the final Health Insurance Portability and Accountability Act (HIPAA) rule was published on Aug. 14, 2002, which allows the authorization form for all uses and disclosures of a patient's protected health information to be combined with the informed consent form. This authorization form can also be signed separately. The choice is up to the individual investigative site.

Tips for Effective Informed Consent Form Review During Monitoring Visits:

- Review the IRB approval letter to determine that the correct or latest version of the Informed Consent Form (ICF) was signed by the subject and/or guardian.
- There may be more than one signed ICF per subject depending upon whether the ICF was revised—confirm this.
- Know the IRB-approved current ICF version date, if there is more than one version that requires signature for all Consents/Assents/PK/Tissue Sampling/Pharmacogenetics/Partner Consents.
- Confirm that all sequential pages of the ICF are present, in chronological order, and there are none missing.
- Confirm that all pages have been initialed and dated by the subject and/or guardian as required.
- Determine if the HIPAA document is separate or incorporated into the ICF.
- Confirm that the HIPAA has been signed and/or checked "yes" by the subject and/or guardian to allow for records review.
- Does this study involve pediatrics? If the answer is yes, assess for pediatric assents in addition to parent/guardian consent.
- Check to ensure that the individual obtaining consent has the knowledge, experience and training to appropriately obtain consent and that they have been appropriately delegated this responsibility per the delegation of authority log.
- Cross-check staff signatures on the delegation of authority log with the informed consent form to ensure accuracy and legitimacy.
- Ensure that the subject and/or guardian signed and dated the ICF prior to research procedures. This can be accomplished a variety of ways, such as, if the informed consent form has a space for the time consent was obtained, it can be compared to the time study procedures were completed, if that is documented. Sometimes the timing of procedures is required to be documented in the source/CRF, if it is dependent upon

dose time or serial assessments, etc. There are ways to confirm time of procedures relative to time of consent.

- Confirm that the subject printed his or her own name and date on the ICF in addition to signing own his or her own name. (Check delegation log and compare signatures of staff.)
- Confirm that the person obtaining consent signed and dated the document on the same day as the subject and within a reasonable timeframe. Some consent forms have "time" requirements on the signature page and this sheds light on such things as when the investigator signed the consent compared to when the patient signed the consent, etc.
- Confirm that the Witness and/or Legal Guardian signature line was completed appropriately.
- Ensure that the amendments/revisions to the ICF contain appropriate safety or amendment updates per Investigator Brochure changes or protocol amendment release.
- Confirm that the PI's address and contact information is in the ICF, including an emergency or after-hours phone number.
- Confirm that the ICF process is documented in the subject's source and includes such important points as: confirmation that the informed consent was obtained prior to study procedures, that the subject was given appropriate time to review the consent and ask questions, that the investigator was available for questions, the ICF date, time and version, and that the subject was given a signed copy. Some sites use a checklist to document this, or document a paragraph attesting to this in the source document or electronic medical record (EMR).
- Confirm that the investigator also obtained and/or signed the informed consent as appropriate per institutional or IRB signature requirements.
- If reconsenting of the subject was required, ensure that the subject's re-consenting was conducted appropriately, and that this was updated in the subject's source.
- Ensure that a subject reconsented in a timely manner relative to the amended consent approval date. For example, if a site received the approved amended consent in January, and the subject's next visit

was in February, but they were not reconsented until March, there is a problem.

Obtaining Informed Consent

Informed consent must be obtained from subjects at the proper time and in the proper manner. The first thing to remember is that no person may be involved as a research subject unless the person or the person's legally acceptable representative (LAR) has given consent. According to ICH E6(R2), an LAR is an individual, juridical or other body authorized under applicable law to consent on behalf of a prospective subject to the subject's participation in the clinical trial. Secondly, a subject's consent must be obtained before the subject is involved in any study-related activity. A CRA should always check a consent and when it was signed during the study enrollment period. The time of consent versus when the subject started the study is almost always checked during FDA inspections of investigative sites.

There are two types of consent forms: short form and long form. Both must be approved by an IRB before use.

The Short Form Consent

The short form consent may be used in circumstances when, in the best judgment of the investigator, it would be the most appropriate way for the subject to comprehend and give informed consent. This form supplements and documents an oral presentation of the information provided to the study subject as part of the consent process. If this method is used (21CFR 50.27-Documentation of Informed Consent):

- The form must state that all elements of consent required by regulation have been presented orally to the subject or subject's legally-appointed representative.
- There must be a witness to the oral presentation.
- The IRB must approve a written summary of what is to be said to the subject or his or her representative.
- Only the short form itself is to be signed by the subject or his or her representative.

- The witness will sign both the short form and a copy of the written summary.
- The person obtaining the consent will sign a written copy of the summary.
- A copy of the short form and the summary will be given to the subject or his or her representative.

The Long Form Consent

This is the standard consent form and process and is the consent method of choice whenever possible. The main difference between the two forms is that the long form spells out in writing everything that is presented orally when the short form is used. Consequently, no summary is needed. The subject signs and dates two copies, one to keep and one for the investigator.

Author's Story

After years of reviewing informed consent forms at different investigational sites, you become familiar with different IRB signature requirements for obtaining informed consent. Some IRBs allow a person different from the investigator to perform the consent discussion, obtain consent from subjects and sign the consent form, as long as they are appropriately trained, delegated and experienced. This is evidenced by the signature line "signature of individual obtaining consent" or "signature of researcher" on the consent form. Other IRBs require the investigator to sign the consent form, either as the "investigator obtaining consent" or in addition to the individual obtaining consent as "signature of the investigator."

Several years ago, I was monitoring a skin infection study at an investigational site. They were a high-enrolling medical practice and had enrolled 15 patients in the study. It was my first monitoring visit to the site and I was reviewing all the current and new subject informed consent forms for accuracy and completeness.

The IRB managing the study had very specific informed consent signature requirements; the investigator and the individual conducting the informed consent discussion were both required to sign the consent. The study coordinator was new to research and had obtained and signed consent for all of the study patients. I was concerned that her inexperience would affect her ability to effectively obtain consent from a study patient.

In reviewing each consent form, I noticed that the study coordinator had signed each consent form correctly on the "signature of individual obtaining consent" line. However, the investigator had not signed one consent form; the signature line on the last page of each consent form was blank where "investigator signature" was required. Some of these study subjects had been consented three-to-four months ago. I informed the investigator of this oversight, advised the investigator to retrain the study coordinator and advised that the investigator inform the IRB of these deviations immediately so the IRB could advise on their specific corrective action. It served as a crucial reminder of the importance of delegating an appropriately trained and experienced individual the task of obtaining consent for study patients.

–Elizabeth

The Consent Process

As a CRA, you will not be involved in the actual consent process. However, since it is a CRA's responsibility to ensure that investigative sites conduct their studies in accordance with GCPs, the CRA should be able to advise investigators and their staff on consent activities.

It is a best practice for investigational sites to have an informed consent standard operating procedure, guideline or documented process to ensure consistency and accuracy of staff conducting/signing/documenting the informed consent process.

It is also recommended that investigators directly participate in training staff on appropriate conduct of the informed consent process and/or obtaining informed consent, to demonstrate investigator oversight of staff training and procedures that involve patient safety. Best training practices include:

- Have staff observe the investigator conducting several different informed consent discussions on several different types of patients (adults, children) to have a fully dimensional exposure to the informed consent process.

- Have the investigator observe the conduct of several informed consent discussions with subjects by the site staff member being trained to ensure the appropriate process and information provision.
- Have the staff member review several informed consent forms completed by other staff members to ensure proper signatures, dates and content and to ensure that all safety information and informed consent elements are present.

Here are some suggestions that can be discussed with investigators and study coordinators regarding the informed consent process; these may be particularly helpful for those at the site who are inexperienced with the consent process:

- Provide the subject with a quiet place to review the consent form; ensure they spend an appropriate amount on this review.
- Ensure the subject is given the opportunity to take the ICF home, if desired, to review with his or her personal physician, family or whomever they desire to assist them in making an informed decision.
- Ensure that an appropriately trained, experienced and delegated member of the investigational staff or an investigator reads the consent form while the subject follows along. This usually improves comprehension and is helpful for subjects who may not read well.
- Have the presenter summarize what was read, emphasizing the important points of the consent and the procedures the subject will need to perform.
- Always ask the subject if there are any questions. Answer them completely and truthfully.
- Ensure that the investigator is on site during the consent process to provide oversight and answer questions.
- Never try to convince a subject to participate.
- Ask the subject some questions about the consent material to determine how well the subject understood what was presented. This will often generate additional questions from the subject.
- A video presentation of the consent form can be an effective tool. If the investigative site has someone who is a particularly good presenter,

this person could describe the study in the video. In addition to ensuring that all subjects hear the same thing, the video documents what was said. Videos, however, should never be used in lieu of the involvement of the investigator, who should always be present to talk with subjects and to answer questions. All patient-facing materials must be IRB-approved.

- The consent process should not be rushed. Subjects must be given ample time to assess, evaluate and discuss the information they have been given before having to make a decision. Some investigational sites take over an hour to conduct an entire informed consent process.
- The investigator or investigational site staff member obtaining consent should document the informed consent process in a progress note or similar format, detailing that consent was given, no study-related procedures were done prior to signing the informed consent and a copy of the informed consent document, both signed and dated, was given to the subject.

Author's Story

I was once monitoring ICFs with a colleague at a large academic health center that had a main site and a number of network satellite sites. The main site and network satellite sites had different informed consent forms. The investigator's brochure had just been revised to reflect updated study drug safety information and the informed consent forms for the main and satellite sites were likewise updated with the applicable safety language. My colleague and I were reviewing the ICFs of reconsented subjects, when she noticed a difference in the content of the main site ICF vs. the network site ICFs. She had previously worked as a study coordinator and was trained to automatically review ICF content as well as signature requirements (in her review of the ICFs during monitoring visits). The ICF version for the satellite sites was missing a paragraph from the updated safety information, that was present in the main site consent. It had inadvertently been omitted, and a number of subjects at the satellite sites had been reconsented with the incorrect ICF version. Thanks to my colleague's "eagle eye," we were able to help the site correct a major protocol violation. This example speaks volumes of the critical need for CRAs to be aware of ICF content, and not just signature requirements, of the sites they monitor.

— Elizabeth

Exceptions to Consent

Exceptions to consent may be made in two situations for patients using investigational products. The first situation is for research involving the single emergency use of a test article in a single individual, as provided for in 21 CFR 50.23. The second involves entire studies in which, because of the expected circumstances, it is not generally feasible to obtain consent before patients must be treated (21 CFR 50.24). Both of these situations are discussed below.

Individual Exceptions

Occasionally, a circumstance will arise in which an investigator feels there is a subject who would benefit from the use of an investigational product, but who is not in a study or who would not qualify for the study. For example, there may be a patient who is near death from a severe infection and all suitable marketed antibiotics have been tried, but the infective bacteria are resistant to all of these drugs. The patient does not qualify for any ongoing study. Under this exemption, this patient may be treated with one of the new, powerful antibiotics that might cure his infection. Although a physician may treat a patient with an investigational product in a case like this, he must follow the regulations discussed.

According to the regulations, obtaining informed consent is feasible unless, before the use of the investigational product, both the investigator and a physician who is not otherwise participating in the clinical investigation certify, in writing, all of the following:

- The human subject is confronted by a life-threatening situation necessitating the use of the test article.
- Informed consent cannot be obtained from the subject because of an inability to communicate with, or obtain a legally effective consent from, the subject.

- Time is not sufficient to obtain consent from the subject's legal representative.
- There is no alternative method available of approved or generally recognized therapy that provides an equal or greater likelihood of saving the life of the subject.

The exception is if immediate use of the test article is, in the investigator's opinion, required to preserve the life of the subject and time is not sufficient to obtain the independent determination in advance of using the test article. In this case, the determination of the clinical investigator shall be made and within five working days after use of the article be reviewed and evaluated in writing by a physician who is not participating in the clinical investigation.

The documentation required must be submitted to the investigator's IRB within five working days after the use of the test article. If the investigator wants to be able to use the product for this type of patient more than just the one time, the necessary documentation must be submitted to the IRB and approved, as for any study.

Exception to Informed Consent Requirements for Emergency Research Studies

In some types of studies, obtaining informed consent from study subjects prior to their participation may not be possible. Examples of these studies are those in which the subject is in a life-threatening trauma situation, such as a head injury or heart attack. Not only are the subjects in these studies not able to give consent prior to being treated, but there may not be time to identify and locate a subject's legally authorized representative before treatment must begin. Frequently, these studies have a relatively short window of opportunity for treatment (e.g., treatment must commence within two hours of the injury).

Exceptions or waivers from consent must be approved in advance of the study by the IRB. It is not the investigator or the sponsor who makes the determination of whether or not the exception is allowed. It must be approved by an IRB, with the concurrence of a licensed physician (who may or may not be a member of the IRB) who is not associated with the research project. In order for the IRB to make this determination, the following must be documented:

- The subject is in a life-threatening situation, available treatments are unproven or unsatisfactory and the collection of valid scientific evidence is necessary to determine the safety and effectiveness of the particular intervention.

- Informed consent is not feasible because:
  - The subject will not be able to give consent because of his or her medical condition.
  - The intervention under investigation must be administered before consent can be obtained from the subject's LAR.
  - There is no way to identify the individuals likely to become eligible for participation in the study.
- Participation in the research may have a direct benefit to the subject because:
  - The subject is in a life-threatening situation that necessitates intervention.
  - Previous research, both preclinical and/or clinical, provides supporting evidence of the potential for the intervention to provide a direct benefit to the subject.
  - Risks associated with the intervention are reasonable in relation to what is known about the medical condition of the potential class of subjects, the risks and benefits of standard therapy and what is known, if anything, about the risks and benefits of the experimental treatment or intervention.
- The clinical investigation could not practically be carried out without the waiver.
- The protocol defines the length of the therapeutic window based on scientific evidence, and the investigator commits to attempt to contact the subject's LAR or family member within that window of opportunity and ask for consent, if feasible, rather than proceeding without consent. The investigator will summarize efforts to contact legal representatives and provide this information to the IRB.
- The IRB has approved the consent form and the process to be used when informing the subject, when possible, or the subject's LAR or a family member.

- Additional protection of the rights and welfare of subjects will be provided to include:
  - Consultation with the community in which the study will be conducted and the subjects selected.
  - Public disclosure in the community in which the study is to be conducted prior to initiation of the study of plans for the study and the risks and benefits associated with it.
  - Public disclosure following completion of the study of sufficient information to appraise researchers and the community of the study, including demographics of the study population and its results.
  - Establishment of an independent data monitoring committee to exercise oversight of the investigation.

The IRB also has a responsibility to see that the study subject is informed about the nature of the study and his or her involvement in it in as timely a fashion as possible. If the subject remains incapacitated, then the LAR or, if not available, a family member must be updated. The LAR (or family member) should also be told that he or she may request that the subject be removed from the study at any time without penalty or loss of benefit.

Electronic Informed Consent

The integration of the internet and the technology-driven research process has impacted all aspects of clinical research, including the process of informed consent. Researchers now have additional means to communicate study requirements, informed consent content and obtain informed consent from study subjects via audio and video delivery systems, remote conduct of informed consent discussions and utilization of electronic informed consent platforms, computer systems, tablets and devices for this purpose. On December 15, 2016, OHRP and the FDA finalized a guidance on electronic methods of informed consent entitled Use of Electronic Informed Consent, Questions and Answers, Guidance for Institutional Review Boards, Investigators and Sponsors.

The guidance is a recommendation in a question/answer format about the use of electronic informed consent and the impact on the regulated informed consent process. This clarifies the FDA-accepted process and measures for electronic informed consent (eIC)—often called e-consent.

As per the guidance document, page 1, section 1, introduction:

> This guidance provides recommendations on the use of electronic systems and processes that may employ multiple electronic media to obtain informed consent for both HHS-regulated human subject research and FDA-regulated clinical investigations of medical products, including human drug and biological products, medical devices and combinations thereof.

According to the guidance, "electronic informed consent" refers to:

> The use of electronic systems and processes that may employ multiple electronic media, including text, graphics, audio, video, podcasts, passive and interactive websites, biological recognition devices and card readers to convey information related to the study and to obtain and document informed consent.
>
> The guidance also provides recommendations on procedures that may be followed when using an eIC to help:
>
> - Ensure protection of the rights, safety and welfare of human subjects.
> - Facilitate the subject's comprehension of the information presented during the eIC process.
> - Ensure that appropriate documentation of consent is obtained when electronic systems and processes that may employ multiple electronic media are used to obtain informed consent.
> - Ensure the quality and integrity of eIC data included in FDA applications and made available to the FDA during inspections.

Section III, page 7 of the FDA guidance document Instituting an Electronic Informed Consent Process Questions and Answers covers the very important topic of presenting information in the eIC to study subjects as follows:

> **Question: How should information in the eIC be presented to the subject?**

Answer: The eIC must contain all elements of informed consent required by HHS and/or FDA regulations (45 CFR 46.116 and 21 CFR 50.25). The information must be in language understandable to the potential subject or the subject's LAR and conveyed in a manner that minimizes the possibility of coercion or undue influence regarding the subject's decision to participate in a study (45 CFR 46.116 and 21 CFR 50.20). *Understandable* means that the information presented to subjects is in a language and at a level the subject can comprehend, including an explanation of scientific and medical terms. To ensure that the eIC is presented appropriately and that subjects will have enough time to dedicate to the eIC process, the subjects should be informed of approximately how long the process will take and what information will be presented to them.

Any eIC should be easy to navigate, allowing the user to proceed forward or backward within the system and to stop and continue at a later time. Hyperlinks may be provided where helpful. The eIC may also incorporate electronic strategies to encourage subjects to access all of the consent material before documenting their consent.

Electronic informed consent may be used to either supplement or replace paper-based informed consent processes in order to best address the subject's needs throughout the course of the study. For example, some subjects may prefer one method over another. Other subjects may have difficulty navigating or using electronic systems because of, for example, a lack of familiarity with electronic systems, poor eyesight, or impaired motor skills. In such cases, the eIC process may not be appropriate for these subjects.

The FDA guidance also covers the important dynamic of addressing the study subject's questions when utilizing electronic or remote informed consent. Whether the electronic informed consent is obtained from the subject onsite or remotely, the process must allow subjects the opportunity to consider whether or not to participate and to ask questions about the study before signing consent, as well as at any time during the subject's involvement in the research. This may be accomplished by in-person discussions with study personnel or through a combination of electronic messaging, telephone calls, video conferencing or a live chat with a remotely located investigator or study personnel. When live chat or video conferencing is used during the process, investigators and study personnel should remind subjects to conduct the discussion in a private location to help ensure privacy and confidentiality.

Whether following the traditional informed consent process (paper informed consent document and face-to-face discussion with the study patient) or incorporating elements of, or a completely electronic/digital informed consent process, the rules are constant and relevant: the subject's safety and rights must be protected, the subject's right to privacy must be assured and the informed consent must be worded and communicated so that the subject can comprehend and make an informed decision about study participation.

Author's Story

About three years ago, I was evaluating sites for an investigational study that was using an e-consent platform and every site that I evaluated either outright refused to use the e-consent platform or their local IRB did not yet allow the use of electronic informed consent. In speaking with site personnel, it seemed that their resistance to using e-consent was not in the concept but with the platform challenges. E-consent in theory provides a lot of assurance: versioning control, not allowing patients to proceed to the next page of the consent form (on the device or tablet) until they have "checked" the box verifying they have read the page, etc. These site personnel had dealt with e-consent platforms that would freeze or outright crash. Fast forward three years. Many more sites are open to using e-consent, but a number of investigational sites still have reservations. If a study requires the use of e-consent, sponsors have had to make exceptions for investigational sites to be able to print the consent from the device and consent patients by that means. E-consent is still not the accepted standard but is moving in that direction.

–Elizabeth

E-consent Platforms

Common e-consent devices are tablets or touch screen devices. E-consent can involve interactive media as part of the consent process for better patient understanding. E-consent streamlines version control of informed consent forms that has long been a challenge when working with multiple consent versions in a study and tracking what is most current or required for patients. Patients use the device to review the consent pages and verify electronically they have read the content before moving forward to the next screen. E-consent is signed electronically by the study patient. E-consent was widely used during the COVID pandemic.

The FDA issued an August 2021 final guidance document FDA Guidance on Conduct of Clinical Trials of Medical Products During the COVID-19 Public Health Emergency that includes recommendations for obtaining informed consent under specific situations, such as obtaining informed consent from patients in isolation, those unable to travel to the research site, when electronic consent is not available, etc. Page 20 of the appendix includes the following question and answer:

> **Question: How do I obtain informed consent from a patient unable to travel to a clinical trial site where electronic informed consent is not an option?**
>
> Answer: Investigators may also need to obtain informed consent from a potential trial participant or their legally authorized representative when these individuals are unable to travel to the site where the investigator is located due to COVID-19 illness or travel restrictions. When investigators do not have electronic informed consent (eIC) capabilities, methods of obtaining informed consent other than a face-to-face consent interview may still be acceptable if those methods allow for an adequate exchange of information and documentation, and a method to ensure that the signer of the consent form is the person who plans to enroll as a participant in the clinical investigation or is the legally authorized representative of the trial participant. For example, the consent form may be sent to the trial participant or their legally authorized representative by facsimile or email, and the consent interview may then be conducted by telephone when the trial participant or their legally authorized representative can read the consent form during the discussion. After the consent discussion, the trial participant or their legally authorized representative can sign and date the consent form.
>
> Options for returning the document to the clinical investigator may include facsimile, a photographic image sent through electronic means, scanning the consent form and returning it through a secure email account or posting it to a secure Internet address, especially if there are concerns about having

the participant mail a potentially contaminated consent document. Alternatively, the trial participant may bring the signed and dated consent form to his/her next visit to the clinical site, if restrictions on traveling to the clinical trial site are alleviated, or mail it to the clinical investigator. The case history for each trial participant must document that informed consent was obtained prior to participation in the trial. In addition, the person signing the consent form must receive a copy of the consent form.

Although FDA regulations do not require the trial participant's copy to be a signed copy, FDA recommends that a copy of the signed consent form be provided. The trial participant or their legally authorized representative must sign and date the informed consent form before the investigator may conduct any study-related procedures involving the participant. Where it is not feasible for investigators to receive the signed consent form prior to beginning study-related procedures, the investigators should have the prospective trial participant or legally authorized representative confirm verbally during the consent interview that the participant or legally authorized representative has signed and dated the form. In addition, the overseeing IRB must review and approve the planned informed consent process.

Conclusion

A primary safeguard for the rights, safety and well-being of human subjects of research is informed consent. The informed consent process is a complex and important part of conducting clinical research. CRAs must have a working knowledge of consent forms and processes so that deficiencies can be recognized and corrected immediately. It is recommended that CRAs read the regulations governing informed consent (21 CFR part 50). A checklist for reviewing informed consent is found in Appendix C.

There is an updated FDA guidance document on informed consent: A Guide to Informed Consent—Information Sheet, July 12, 2018.

Key Takeaways

- Informed consent is a cornerstone of the ethical conduct of clinical research.
- Informed consent documents must be approved by the IRB before use.
- Informed consent must be obtained before a subject enters a study.
- Informed consent must be documented.
- CRAs must thoroughly assess consent forms to ensure they are correct and that the signatures and dates provided are valid. The proper preparation of forms and conduct of the procedure is vital to truly informed consent.
- Informed consent usually is required for all subjects involved in a research project.
- There are exceptions to the consent process under certain circumstances.
- Electronic informed consent presents an alternative to the traditional face-to-face, paper informed consent process.

CHAPTER 10

Preparing for a Study

Study Design and Statistical Issues

This chapter covers some of the primary activities that must be conducted before starting a study—determining the study design, writing the protocol and developing case report forms. Working with studies, protocols and case report forms are critical parts of a CRA's job, so the CRA must have a good understanding of each of them, even if he or she is not involved in determining study designs, writing protocols or developing case report forms. The chapter begins by discussing some aspects of design, followed by protocols and then case report forms, since this is the usual pattern of their development in a research program.

This chapter is designed to give you basic information. Much of the material that follows is in the form of an annotated outline that gives you the basic considerations for these documents.

Study Design

CRAs should have a basic understanding of the critical aspects of study design. In this section, we will look at some of the terminology that CRAs should be familiar with, as well as a few of the more common study designs. In general, the statistician, in consultation with the medical monitor for a study, will determine which design is appropriate to use. We will also discuss sample size, the controls used in studies and methods for minimizing bias.

Determining Sample Size

There are a number of factors that must be taken into account when determining how many subjects should be entered into a trial. The first of these is the sample size. The sample size for a trial is usually computed by the statistician and is based on three variables:

1. The magnitude of the effect expected between the treatments.
2. The variability of the endpoints to be analyzed.
3. The desired probability of observing the effect with a defined significance. (This is known as the power of the test and is commonly set at least at 80 percent).

The magnitude of the effect is the difference between what you expect to see with your drug and the comparator (placebo or another drug). For example, if you expect your drug to work in 70 percent of the subjects and the drug you are using as a comparator to work in only 50 percent of the subjects, the magnitude of the effect (the effect size) is 20 percent. It is always a bit of a guess to determine the effect size, especially in phase 2 studies with a new compound. This is because you don't have much information about the effect size of your compound until a number of studies have been completed.

In advance of any studies, the effect size is determined by making educated guesses. The problem of approximating the effect size is like the chicken and the egg—you need to know something about the effect size to calculate a sample size, but you can't calculate the sample size without an effect size. Make a guess in the early phase 2 studies, and information gathered from these studies will help determine the effect size. This information is then used to calculate sample sizes for subsequent studies. As the development program progresses and more is known about the investigational drug, the effect size estimates become more accurate and sample sizes become easier to calculate. By the time phase 3 studies are done, the effect size estimates are reasonably accurate.

As the effect size increases, the necessary sample size decreases; that is, it takes fewer subjects to show a statistically significant difference between two treatments when the difference in the effect of the treatments is large.

As for effect size, the estimate of the variability is based primarily on educated guesses in phase 1 and early phase 2 studies, but becomes quite accurate by the time phase 3 studies are done. Variability is also a statistical parameter and will be determined by the statistician, based in part on information from past work and from the clinician involved in the trial.

Given the effect size and the variability, the statistician can construct power curves that will show the sample size needed. These help to ensure that enough subjects are entered into the study to show the treatment effect.

The sample size that results from these calculations tells how many subjects are needed at the end of the trial for valid analyses. However, it is rare for participants to see a trial through to completion; subjects drop out along the way for many reasons. Consequently, you must start with more subjects than you need to compensate for those subjects who do not complete the study. If it is expected that 25 percent of the subjects will drop out along the way, then at least 25 percent more subjects than your sample size calculation must be entered. For example, if the sample size was calculated to be 300 subjects per treatment group, it would need to be increased by at least 75 (25 percent) for a total of 375 subjects per group.

Most of the time a large sample size is better than a small sample size, but both cost control and time become harder to manage as the sample size increases.

Placebo Response versus Placebo Effect

It would be nice to be able to assume that the subjects receiving a placebo treatment during a trial would have no treatment effect at all, but this is far from true. People respond to treatment with placebo, sometimes quite dramatically. For example, in trials for depression or anxiety, it is commonplace to see placebo response rates of 25 percent to 40 percent.

Remember that in clinical trials, subjects get a great deal of care, including frequent visits, lots of medical tests and attention from both the investigator and the study coordinator—all this extra attention could be enough to make them feel better, even if they are being treated only with a placebo.

There have also been numerous studies that show an actual disease state can respond measurably to placebo, including, among others, the lowering of blood pressure, alleviation of post-operative pain and relief of psychiatric conditions such as anxiety, depression, agoraphobia and schizophrenia. Pundits have gone so far as to suggest that placebo might be the next wonder drug. There has been much written about placebo response, but it is outside the scope of this book, so we will not discuss it further. However, you must be aware that it is a real phenomenon and has a significant impact on clinical trials.

Subjects do not have to receive a placebo to benefit from the "placebo effect" while in a trial. Remember that all subjects are receiving the same benefits from the trial—more tests, more visits and more attention. Therefore, subjects receiving the active treatment are as apt to experience a placebo effect as are those subjects being treated with the placebo. Ideally the placebo effect will balance out between groups so that the differences seen can be attributed to the actual drug effect.

Statistical Significance

Statistical significance relates to the probability that an event (such as the difference between two treatments) is due to chance alone. When a sponsor is conducting a study to compare a drug to a placebo or to another active drug, it is hoped there will be a statistically significant difference in favor of the sponsor's drug. The significance level is most commonly set at 5 percent, or $p=0.05$, where p stands for probability.

If the drug appears to be better than placebo in a test at the 0.05 level, it does not prove that the drug is actually better, but it lends a comfort level that there really is a difference in the effect of the two treatments.

Noticing a statistically significant difference does not say anything about the magnitude of the difference or the clinical significance of the difference. Inferences about the actual clinical value of the difference must be made based on the actual value of the variables being studied. For example, let's assume that the final average Hamilton Depression Rating Scale for Depression (HAM-D) total score was 10.6 in the investigational drug group and 13.2 in the placebo group and that the difference (2.6) was statistically significant at $p=0.05$. This means, roughly, that the probability of this difference being due to chance alone is only 5 percent. Whether or not the difference of 2.6 points that separates the two groups is significant clinically would need to be decided by medical personnel.

Control Groups Used in Clinical Trials

What is a control group? Subjects in comparative trials are divided into two (or more) groups: the treatment group and the control group. Subjects in the treatment group receive the investigational drug, while those in the control group receive placebo or an active drug that is already marketed for use. Control groups are used in clinical trials as a baseline against which to compare a new treatment to test that it is both safe and effective. Three main types of control groups—placebo control, active comparator control and historical control—are discussed below.

Placebo Control

Use of a placebo control in a study means that one group is treated with the active drug and another group is treated with a placebo and the results are compared. Use of a placebo helps control for the psychological effect of being in a trial and helps to control for adverse events being attributed to the active drug when in fact they are simply the result of changes in the disease or other outside factors.

In the U.S., placebo-controlled studies are common and accepted, except those for which the use of a placebo would be unethical (such as in an infectious disease known to respond to treatment). In many other countries, the routine use of placebo-controlled studies is less acceptable. However, if a placebo control is not used, it is difficult to tell whether the active medication was really effective, regardless of the size of the effect observed, because the result seen may have been due to the placebo effect rather than to the active treatment.

Active Comparator Control

In cases in which a placebo cannot be ethically used, the investigational drug may be compared to another active compound. The comparator will be an already marketed product; it is frequently an established, standard treatment used for the condition, although it may be the newest and most interesting treatment or the market leader. It is usually the hope of a sponsor that its investigational drug will be shown to be statistically superior to the comparator drug. Remember, though, that the effect seen with one or both of the drugs may be due to the placebo effect, and there is no way to distinguish that in an active comparator trial.

Sometimes both a placebo and active comparator are used in a trial, making three treatment groups. This allows both drugs to be compared to the placebo as well as to each other, eliminating the potential placebo effect problem. In general, it allows for more subjects to receive an active drug rather than placebo. If one-third of the total number of subjects are randomized to each of the three study groups (investigational drug, placebo and active comparator), two-thirds of the subjects will receive an active drug treatment and only one-third will receive placebo treatment. Since most subjects would prefer to receive an active drug, this control scheme often makes a study more appealing.

Historical Control

On occasion, a historical control will be used in a clinical trial. There are two types of historical controls. One is the use of data obtained from the same subjects (on no treatment, the same treatment or a different treatment). Sometimes this is done by a crossover study, which will be discussed later in this chapter.

The other type is a comparison to data obtained from other patients, (again on no treatment, the same treatment or another treatment). This type of trial is seen rather often in the testing of new therapies for cancer, when no other treatment exists. The trial results will be compared to the remission rates or death rates seen in the general population of similar cancer patients when there is no treatment. For example, if the death rate in untreated people with a particular cancer is 35 percent over a particular period of time and if the death rate in study subjects (receiving the treatment) with this same cancer over the same period of time is 25 percent, this might show a significant difference with the use of the investigational drug.

Minimizing Bias

Bias, according to Webster's Dictionary, is "a systematic error introduced into sampling or testing by selection or encouraging one outcome or answer over others." In clinical trials, these systematic errors distort the data, which may lead to an incorrect conclusion.

Bias may be introduced in a clinical trial from anyone who might be able to exert some influence over it, including the sponsor, the investigator, a monitor or study subjects. An investigator could introduce bias by placing subjects in study groups based on how the investigator felt each particular subject would react to one treatment over another. Bias may also be introduced in assessing a subject's response to a medication, based on how well the assessor (investigator, coordinator) thinks the given treatment will work. It is difficult to give an impartial judgment if you have a particular point of view, in this case, the expected result of a treatment.

The two main techniques used in clinical trials to eliminate bias are blinding and randomization.

Blinding

Blinding refers to a lack of knowledge of which treatment is being used with a subject in a clinical trial. The primary people who may be blinded in a trial are the subjects, the investigator (and staff), monitors and statisticians. Blinding is achieved by making the treatments look the same for each treatment group. If it is impossible to make the treatments look the same, blinding can be achieved by having someone who is not otherwise associated with the trial prepare and administer the treatment, while the investigator remains blinded while doing assessments of the subject. The most common blinding schemes are:

- **Triple blind.** The subject, the investigator, the sponsor's monitors and statisticians all do not know which treatment is being received by a particular subject.
- **Double blind.** Neither the subject nor the investigator knows which treatment is being received by a particular subject.
- **Single blind.** The subject does not know which treatment is being received, but the investigator does know.
- **Open label.** No blind is used. Both the investigator and the subject know which treatment the subject is receiving.

Randomization

Randomization is the method by which study subjects are randomly assigned to treatment groups. It is usually done by means of a randomization code scheme, most often generated by a validated computer program. Randomization helps to reduce bias in a trial by ensuring there is no pattern in the way subjects are assigned to the treatment groups. It also allows the blind to be broken for one subject without breaking it for all other subjects at the same time.

If subjects were assigned to treatment groups A and B one after the other as they came in, the investigator would not be blinded, as he or she would always know which treatment group would be assigned next, even if the drug itself is blinded. (See Table 1)

Table 1: Assignment scheme

Subject	1	2	3	4	5	6	7	8	9	10	11	12
Drug	A	B	A	B	A	B	A	B	B	B	A	B

In a randomized assignment, the investigator will not be able to know the pattern because it is random. When blinded study drugs are sent to an investigative site, they are labeled by subject number, Subject #101, Subject #102 ... etc. The investigator and site personnel will know only the subject number, not the underlying treatment or the underlying randomization scheme. A random treatment pattern for the same two treatments, A and B, might look like:

Table 2: Random treatment pattern

Subject	1	2	3	4	5	6	7	8	9	10	11	12
Drug	B	B	A	A	A	B	B	B	A	B	A	A

Note that there are 12 subjects in each randomization scheme and that six subjects receive each treatment in each scheme. In the random scheme, however, it is not easy to predict the next treatment, as there is no particular order to the scheme. Sometimes randomization is done in blocks, in which each block of subjects has the same number of people on each treatment. If you look closely at the randomization scheme above, you will notice that each block of six subjects has three people in each treatment group. This is called randomization in blocks. It is important that the subjects, the investigator and the CRA do not know this assignment pattern. If they did, it could effectively unblind them to the treatments, which might introduce bias and negate the benefits gained from randomizing and blinding.

Randomization and blinding are usually used together and constitute the best defense against bias in clinical trials.

Common Study Designs

There are many different statistical study designs used, but most of the clinical trials that CRAs work on employ only two designs, or variations of them, that are briefly discussed below. If you are interested in reading more about study design, the *Guide to Clinical Trials* by Bert Spilker has a good basic discussion on this topic.

Parallel Design

This is the most common and straightforward statistical design used in clinical trials. In parallel design, each subject is assigned to a treatment group, with all subjects following the same schedule and activities. The groups are followed in parallel. There may be two or more treatment groups. (See Table 3.) The analysis will compare the groups to each other.

Table 3: Parallel study

Group 1	Drug A	
Group 2	Drug B	
	Start	Finish

Crossover Design

A crossover design is somewhat more complicated in that each group will receive both treatments. It starts off like a parallel design study, but halfway through the groups switch to the other treatment. Frequently, there is a wash-out period between the two treatments. A crossover study in its simplest form is shown in Table 4.

In this design, each group can be compared to itself as well as to the other group. There is less variability in a crossover design as compared to a parallel design. However, many drugs have a carryover or residual effect after they are stopped, which is difficult to measure. This design is frequently seen in bio-availability trials, which allow a period between the treatments of usually 10 or more half-lives of the drug to combat the carryover effect. There are many variations of crossover designs, but the general premise remains the same.

Table 4: Crossover study

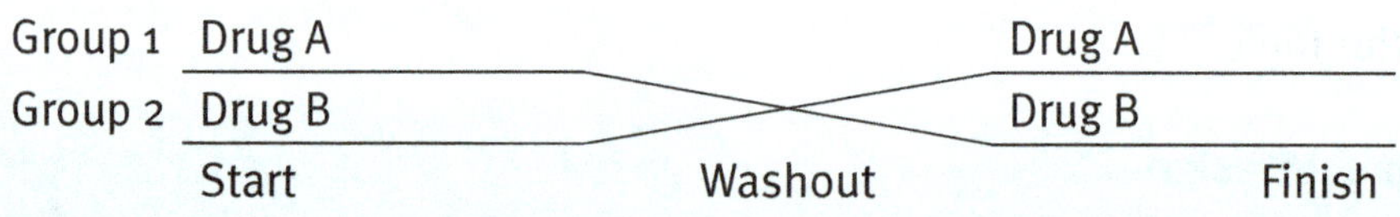

Adaptive Design

Adaptive protocol design is being adopted more frequently by sponsors conducting clinical trials. A November 2019 FDA guidance on adaptive design studies, titled Adaptive Designs for Clinical Trials of Drugs and Biologics, defines adaptive design as follows:

> For the purposes of this guidance, an adaptive design is defined as a clinical trial design that allows for prospectively planned modifications to one or more aspects of the design based on accumulating data from subjects in the trial

Some COVID therapy studies used adaptive trial designs successfully during the pandemic.

Decentralized Clinical Trials

The FDA defines decentralized clinical trials as those in which some or all of the trial-related activities occur at locations other than traditional clinical trial sites. The Clinical Trials Transformation Initiative—an organization co-founded by Duke University and the FDA in 2007—defines DCTs as "those executed through telemedicine and mobile/local healthcare providers, using procedures that vary from the traditional clinical trial model." For example, the investigational medical product may be shipped directly to the trial participant.

The FDA guidance document Conduct of Clinical Trials of Medical Products During the COVID-19 Public Health Emergency released Aug. 30, 2021, includes a Q&A appendix that describes alternate visit methodology during COVID in question five:

> Can a sponsor initiate virtual clinical trial visits for monitoring patients without contacting FDA if there is an assessment by the sponsor and investigator that these visits are necessary for the safety of the trial participant and it will not impact data integrity?
>
> Answer: FDA regulations allow for changes to be made to the investigational plan or protocol without prior FDA review or approval, if the change is intended to eliminate an apparent immediate hazard or to protect the life and well-being of trial participants (11 See 21 CFR 56.108(a)(4), 312.30(b)(2)(ii), and 812.35(a)(2).) Therefore, changes in protocol conduct necessary to immediately assure patient safety, such as conducting telephone or video contact visits for safety monitoring rather than on-site visits, can be immediately implemented with subsequent review by the IRB and notification to FDA. Since this reflects a protocol deviation (until the amendment is approved), documentation of the required deviations, as described above, would generally be acceptable (i.e., a document that lists each deviation, study reference ID, patient ID, and date). For example, documenting that all protocol-specified visits will be done by telephone contact rather than on-site visits, and that procedures requiring in person visits will either not be conducted, or performed by other means (specified, as appropriate). Since the change to telephone or video contact visits would likely result in some protocol-required procedures not being conducted (e.g., vital signs, blood samples for safety laboratory studies), the sponsor must evaluate the potential impact on patient safety, and consider how to mitigate risks to patients, including the need to discontinue the investigational product.
>
> For [investigational device exemption (IDE)] studies, sponsors are required to report deviations implemented to address the imminent safety risk to FDA within five working days after learning of the deviations. We recognize that challenges related to the COVID-19 pandemic may make it difficult to meet this timeframe.
>
> Sponsors may consolidate implemented deviations when submitting 5-day reports and should update FDA as soon as possible.

DCT trials make use of home health/mobile providers to conduct study visits in a patient's home, completing such procedures as physical exams, lab draws, vitals signs, ECGs, etc. These home health providers are trained on the protocol and study procedures and have tools/supplies to facilitate assessments. As an option, they can be part of the sponsor provision of the study vendors/package to sites. Alternatively, some investigational sites have research nurses or study coordinators who can complete study visits. The study patient consents to home study visits and these providers document study visits completed, patient status and such activities and inform the investigator of the status. Telemedicine is also used for the investigator and/or study coordinator to speak to/see the study patients and complete visit portions via that medium. DCTs also use technologies such as e-consent, e-diaries, electronic patient-reported outcomes, wearables to collect data, etc. There are also measures to have study drug shipped to a patient's home, etc.

DCTs can be fully remote or they can be a combination of remote and onsite. It depends on the study design, study visit requirements, site capability and patient preference. Consistency, uniformity, communication and training are of paramount importance in DCTs that involve the use of mobile/home health providers performing study visits to ensure quality of data and patient safety. There are obvious benefits to the patient: convenience, less travel and burden. DCTs have been implemented in industry for several years. DCTs are increasing and becoming more accepted, as speculation eases, like with the introduction of EDC and risk-based monitoring, now accepted industry standards but first heralded as nontraditional and generally unacceptable.

The number of trials with decentralized components increased dramatically during the pandemic, climbing from 1,141 in 2016 to 2,642 trials by 2021 and including 13.9 million patients, according to data compiled by WCG. Therapeutic areas using DCT components most frequently included central nervous system disorders, and mental and behavioral disorders.

Author's Story

Home visits

I worked on COVID studies during the pandemic and some studies had patient home visits and patients providing home samples (swabs, etc.). It is interesting now to see how many new trials are incorporating home visits and measures post pandemic.

–Elizabeth

Other Statistical Issues

Intent-to-Treat

In general, there are two groups of subjects analyzed in a clinical trial. The primary analysis is performed with the intent-to-treat (ITT) study population, which includes all subjects who met the inclusion/exclusion criteria, provided written informed consent, and were enrolled and received treatment, even if the treatment was incomplete. Subjects who drop out during the trial (e.g., lost to follow-up) are still included in the ITT analysis. Note that if there are many drop-outs, it can bias the trial, so CRAs should work with their sites to help minimize the number of subjects who do not complete the entire trial.

Additional analyses of study endpoints also will be performed on the per protocol (PP) study population. The PP study population consists of all study subjects who met the ITT requirements and who completed the entire study.

Missing Data

Missing data is a problem when it comes to the analysis of a clinical trial, especially if there is a lot of it. It can be handled in various ways, but none of them make statisticians very happy. One common way is called "last value forward" (LVCF). In this case, the last value preceding the missing value is used as the value of the missing data. Another method is to average all the data points that are present, then use that average data value for each missing data point. An example is shown in Table 5.

Table 5: Missing data example

Original data	1.6	1.3	1.3	—	1.8	1.9	1.8	—	—
LVCF	1.6	1.3	1.3	1.3	1.8	1.9	1.8	1.8	1.8
Average data value	1.6	1.3	1.3	1.6	1.8	1.9	1.8	1.6	1.8

As you can see, the imputed values differ with the two methods, and there is no guarantee that either method is close to what the actual values might have been. A CRA who works with his or her sites to eliminate missing data will make the statistician very happy and will increase the chance of a successful study.

Primary Outcome Measures

It is best to have primary outcome measures that are simple and easily measured. If your primary outcome measure has multiple components, it muddies up both the analysis and the interpretation of the results. You can look at multiple things and analyze them, but try to keep them separate.

For example, a primary outcome measure:

- A 50 percent reduction in the depression rating scale total score.

This is a "yes" or "no" answer, where "yes" is success and "no is failure." Secondary outcome measures might be:

- Change in the total score on the somatic section of the depression scale.
- Change in the total score on the anxiety scale.
- Change in the total score on the quality-of-life instrument.

These are easy to measure and easy to interpret.

- A 50 percent reduction in the depression rating score total and a score of no more than one on the suicide cluster and an improvement of at least 30 percent on the anxiety scale.

Keep it simple and the results from the study will be much easier to interpret.

Summary

Clinical trials are complex and have their own rules and terminology. CRAs should be familiar with at least the basics of trial design and the terminology used. When the basic design elements have been determined for a trial, it is time to write the protocol. Protocol development is discussed in the next chapter.

Key Takeaways

- Determining the sample size for a study is a statistical computation based on the expected effect size, variability and power.
- Both placebo response and placebo effect have an impact on clinical trials and must be considered when a trial is designed.
- Placebo controls and active controls are most often used in clinical trials. Historical controls are also used but much less frequently.
- Randomization and blinding are the two primary methods of reducing bias in clinical trials.
- In blinded trials, it is important that the subject and the investigator (and usually the CRA) do not know which treatment individual subjects are receiving.
- The most commonly used statistical design in clinical trials is the parallel group design. Crossover designs are also used, especially in bioavailability trials.
- CRAs should be familiar with the common designs and terminology used in clinical trials, as well as the reasons for the use of these various methodologies.
- Analysis might be done on both an intent-to-treat (ITT) study population and a per-protocol (PP) population.
- Missing data can be an issue in clinical trials.
- Outcome measures used in a clinical trial need to be carefully determined.
- Decentralized Clinical Trials are on the rise and increased during COVID.

CHAPTER 11

Preparing for a Study

Protocols, Case Report Forms, Electronic Data Capture Systems and Electronic Patient-Reported Outcomes

This chapter discusses some of the primary activities that must be considered before starting a study, including writing the protocol, developing case report forms (CRFs), the use of electronic data capture (EDC) systems/eCRFs (eCRF and EDC are used interchangeably as they are essentially the same) and the emergence of more types of ePROs. Protocols, ePRO devices and eCRFs/CRFs are critical parts of a CRA's job, and the CRA must have a good understanding of each of them, even if he or she is not involved in writing protocols or developing CRFs or ePROs. This chapter begins by discussing protocols, followed by a discussion of CRFs, EDC systems and ePROs.

The chapter is designed to give you basic information. Much of the material that follows is in the form of an annotated outline that gives you the basic considerations for these documents.

Developing a Protocol

In this section, we will look at how protocols are developed and what is included in them. The protocol is the blueprint for a study and describes how the study will be conducted. If the protocol is well written and the study design is sound, the study will be able to generate valid data that are acceptable to the scientific community, including the FDA.

CRAs will almost never write a complete protocol, but in-house CRAs may be asked to prepare sections of protocols or draft a protocol plan, sections of which will be completed by others on the drug development team, such as the medical monitor and biostatistician. Even if CRAs are not involved in writing protocols, it is important for them to have an understanding of protocol basics. The protocol is the basic tool of clinical trials and will be used in every study that a CRA monitors. Knowing the basics of a protocol makes the CRA more effective and the job easier.

A CRA should be able to read a protocol and determine whether or not it contains all the elements important to a trial, as well as the critical medical information. A CRA should be able to determine if a protocol is realistically feasible to do, at least from a logistics standpoint. There is no other study document so important for a CRA to be knowledgeable about. (It is also a pet peeve of site personnel when the CRA does not thoroughly understand the protocol.)

Designing a study and writing a protocol require knowledge of the scientific method, regulations and the medical condition being addressed. Bert Spilker has written a complete text on developing protocols for those who want a more in-depth dissertation on the subject—*Guide to Clinical Studies and Developing Protocols* (Raven Press, 1984).

Contents of a Protocol

Many sponsors have a pre-defined format for protocols dictated by their SOPs, but no two protocols are the same. Formats will vary from company to company and among different authors within the same company. The content will vary depending on the therapeutic area of investigation.

There are also differences in protocols because of the development phase of the compound. Phase I protocols are more flexible and less detailed than those for phases 2 and 3, because phase 1 studies are early in the development program and not much is known about how the investigational drug acts in humans. A phase 1 protocol is primarily an outline of the study and should include:

- A description of the number of subjects to be studied.
- A description of safety exclusions.
- The dosing plan, to include duration and dose or method being used to determine dose.
- A detailed description of the safety procedures, such as vital signs and laboratory evaluations.

Phase 2 and 3 protocols are very detailed and describe all aspects of the investigations. The FDA defines some minimal requirements for these protocols, which must contain at least:

- A description of the objectives and purpose.
- The name, address and qualifications of each investigator.
- The names of all sub-investigators working under the direction of the investigator.
- The institution where the research will be done.
- The name and address of the IRB.
- The inclusion and exclusion criteria for study subjects.
- The number of subjects to be evaluated.
- The design of the study, including the type of control group being used, if applicable.
- The methods employed to minimize bias (usually randomization and blinding).
- The method used to determine the dose(s) used, the maximum dose and the duration of administration.
- A description of the observations and measurements being used.
- A description of the measures (laboratory evaluations, procedures, etc.) being used to monitor the effects of the investigational drug and minimize risks to subjects.

These are minimum requirements; almost all protocols will contain additional elements as well. The common elements of a protocol and the order in which they usually appear are:

- Title page.
- Protocol summary/synopsis.
- Abstract (optional).
- Table of contents.
- Introduction.
- Study objectives.
- Study design.
- Randomization and blinding.
- Subject selection.

- Subject enrollment.
- Informed consent.
- Screening procedures.
- Replacement of subjects.
- Treatment.
- Concomitant medication.
- Study activities and observations.
- Adverse events.
- Data recording instructions.
- Data quality assurance.
- Analysis plan.
- Risks and benefits.
- References.
- Appendices.

A brief description of each of these elements in a typical protocol follows.

Common Elements of a Protocol

1. **Title Page.** All protocols will have a title page. Essential information for the title page includes:
   - Title: The title should be specific enough to distinguish the protocol from those for similar studies. It should be a concise description of the study providing the reader with the drug, disease, design and study phase.

     Example: A randomized, double-blind, phase 3 trial of (drug under study) in subjects with generalized anxiety disorder. A placebo-controlled, fixed-dose, parallel-group, multicenter study of 12 weeks.
   - Protocol Number: This should be a unique number that identifies the protocol. Most sponsors have a specific procedure for determining this number that identifies the drug, as well as the study.

     Example: 12AB345/0021, where 12AB345 is the drug identifier and 0021 identifies the protocol within that drug development program.

- IND Number: The IND number of the drug for studies conducted under an IND.
- Date: All protocols should be dated as part of their identifiers. This also allows various versions to be readily identified.
- Sponsor Medical Monitor: the name and contact information for the sponsor's medical monitor.
- Principal Investigator: the name and address of the investigator doing the study.
- Some protocol cover pages include the statistician, CRA, sub-investigators, study coordinator and laboratory contact information, but these are optional.

2. **Protocol Summary/synopsis.** The protocol summary should give a good overview of the study and is highly recommended. CRAs can use the summary when they are interviewing potential investigators, even when the entire protocol is not yet complete. The summary will provide enough information for potential investigators to determine if they are interested in and have the capability to do the study. The summary is usually two to ten pages long and typically includes:
    - Protocol Title: repeated from the title page.
    - Study Objective: a statement of the main objectives and purpose of the study.

      Example: The primary objective is to show that (study drug) is more effective than placebo in the short-term (12 weeks) treatment of generalized anxiety disorder. The secondary objective is to gain information on the short-term safety of (study drug).
    - Study Population: a brief description of the type of subjects to be included and the inclusion/exclusion criteria.
    - Study Design: a brief description of design, (e.g., single-dose, multiple-dose, pilot, safety, efficacy, randomized or not, single- or double-blind, open-label, parallel, crossover, etc.

      Example: The study is a randomized, double-blind, fixed-dose, placebo-controlled, phase 3, multicenter trial.
    - Study Medication, including the:

  - Generic name and trade name (if known) of the compound. Example: alprazolam (Xanax).
  - Dosage form. Example: 0.25 mg tablets.
  - Route of administration. Example: oral.
  - Dose and regimen. Example: 0.25 mg three times a day.
- Duration of Treatment: the time period during which the study medication will be administered to the subjects. If the treatment is not continuous, it should be described. Example: Subjects will be treated for 10 weeks, followed by a two-week, single-blind taper period.
- Methods and Materials: a general description of the procedures, tests, etc., required.
- Duration of Subject Participation: total duration of subject involvement in the study, including screen and any follow-up.

  Example: Subjects who complete the study will have 12 weeks of study involvement.
- Anticipated Maximum Number of Subjects: total number of subjects in all treatment groups.

  Example: There will be 440 subjects in each treatment group for a total of 880 subjects.
- Number of Centers: if known.

3. **Abstract.** An abstract is optional. An abstract should be limited to one or two paragraphs describing the objective, design, population, sample size and major study activities.
4. **Table of Contents.** A detailed table of contents should be included in all protocols.
5. **Introduction.** The introduction should identify the reason for doing the study and place it in context with previous investigations and in the overall development plan. If the introduction is lengthy, subheadings should be used. Abbreviations and acronyms should be avoided when possible. Each abbreviation or acronym should be identified in full the first time it is used. Example: Hamilton Rating Scale for Anxiety (HAM-A). The introduction usually contains:

- A brief discussion of the study medication, including the medical need and rationale for use.
- A description of the design and major endpoints, including the rationale for use.
- A description of how this protocol differs from other similar protocols for the same treatment.
- An identification of the setting in which subjects will be studied (outpatient, hospital, etc.).
- The rationale for the dose and regimen, citing supporting data.
- A description of the study control (e.g., placebo) and/or comparator drug, plus the rationale for use.
- A general description of procedures and length of the study.

6. **Study Objectives.** These should clearly state the primary and secondary objectives and identify the endpoints that will be used to satisfy them. Primary endpoints are usually the key efficacy parameters to be studied. Secondary endpoints usually consist of efficacy variables of lower clinical significance and the safety parameters of the trial. State whether the study is intended to show a difference or similarity between treatments (this also could be included under study design).
7. **Study Design.** This section should include a description of the study design, including:
    - Type of study (methodology, pilot, tolerance, efficacy, pharmacokinetics).
    - Controlled or uncontrolled.
    - Single or multiple dose (fixed or variable).
    - Single site or multicenter.
    - Open-label or blinded.
    - Randomization scheme.
    - Design (parallel, crossover, matched pair, block, sequential).
8. **Randomization and Blinding.** This section should describe the randomization and blinding procedure, including any stratification. It should also contain instructions for breaking the blind, if it becomes necessary.

9. **Subject Selection.** This section will include a description of the study population, indicating the number of subjects to be enrolled. If appropriate, it will differentiate between the maximum number of subjects to be enrolled and the minimum number of subjects required to meet protocol objectives. The subject selection criteria (inclusion and exclusion criteria) should include:

   - A description of each requirement for subject eligibility. If there are any exceptions to a criterion, they should be stated.
   - Specific disease-related criteria.
   - Willingness to sign an informed consent form as an inclusion criterion.
   - Allowed and disallowed concomitant medications.
   - Specific contraceptive requirements (as applicable).
   - Criteria that will exclude subjects.
     - Subjects who are taking another investigational medication or who have recently taken an investigational medication within a specified time period (e.g., 30 days) are almost always excluded.

   This section should also include an explanation of when the entry criteria must be met (e.g., before or following a screening period, after a washout period, etc.).

   In some trials, subjects who meet some basic study criteria are enrolled in a screening period. During this time, various tests are done (e.g., physical exam, laboratory tests) to determine if the subjects meet the criteria for entry into the entire trial. A washout period is a time when subjects are taken off their current (non-study) medications. When the carryover effect from these medications has had time to dissipate, subjects are entered into the main part of the trial.

10. **Subject Enrollment.** This section should identify the point at which a subject is considered enrolled. For randomized studies, this is usually at the time of randomization. Other possibilities might be after the informed consent form is signed or after successful completion of a screening period.

11. **Informed Consent.** The section about informed consent is sometimes located in the body of the protocol and sometimes in an appendix. It is always a good idea to provide the investigator with a draft consent form, instead of expecting each investigator to write one separately. Consent forms

were discussed in detail in Chapter 9. The protocol section on informed consent should include:

- A complete description of informed consent requirements, emphasizing the requirement for obtaining consent prior to a subject's involvement in any study-related activity.
- The investigator's responsibility to obtain IRB approval of the consent.
- Specific instructions if vulnerable populations, such as minors, will be included in the study.

12. **Screening Procedures.** This section should contain the following:
    - A description of all activities and tests related to the screening of subjects for study enrollment.
    - Specific timing relative to tests, meals or the start of treatment.
    - If results of any screening tests will be used as baseline for group comparisons, this should be stated.
    - A description of discontinuation of any concomitant medications, if required.
13. **Replacement of Subjects.** This section should specify whether subjects who drop out will be replaced and any conditions associated with replacement. If replacement is allowed, the protocol should specify how replacement subjects would be assigned to treatment groups.
14. **Treatment.** This section should provide the following information about the investigational medication and any comparator medication, including a placebo.
    - Generic, chemical and trade name (if known).
    - Formulation of the placebo.
    - Dosage forms and formulation, in general terms. If any medication contains excipients to which some subjects may be sensitive, such as lactose, this should be indicated.
    - Packaging (e.g., bottles, blister packs).
    - Special storage procedures and stability considerations. If the medication requires reconstitution, the stability in the reconstituted form should be specified.

- Route of administration. Include any special instructions for reconstituting medication or preparing individual doses. If it is administered intravenously (IV), specify the infusion rate.
- The dosage regimen and time schedule for each dose. Clarify the duration of administration, including any medication-free periods or washout periods. As appropriate, specify the timing of dosing in relation to meals.
- Rationale for the dose and regimen.
- Procedures for dosage adjustments, if applicable.
- Compliance parameters (e.g., so many days allowable, etc.)

15. **Concomitant Medication Prohibited, Allowed.** This section should include the policy on the use of concomitant medications, including over-the-counter (OTC) medications, herbals and vitamin supplements. Indicate that all concomitant medication must be recorded. If concomitant medications are allowed, there should be information about how they may be used and why the use will not confound the treatment effect. Interaction data should be cited, as appropriate. A listing of prohibited medications and wash-out duration and time frame before screening should also be included. If the analysis will be stratified based on concomitant medication, this should be stated, with reference to the analysis plan. If tobacco use, alcohol, caffeine or illicit drugs are prohibited or restricted, this should be mentioned in this section.
16. **Study Activities and Observations.** This section will give all the activities that are to be conducted at each study visit. It should also include an overall activity schedule that shows at a glance each event, procedure, observation and evaluation that will be conducted at each visit. An example of a protocol activity schedule is shown in Table 1. Other considerations to keep in mind for this section are:
    - Each time period should be clearly defined.
    - Avoid the use of "Day 0," as it is confusing to most people.
    - If "Time 0" is used, it must be carefully defined. This is usually the time of the initial dose of medication within a given evaluation period.

- List and describe all study activities, observations and evaluations to be made during each period (clinical, radiographic, diagnostic, laboratory/blood testing, rating scales, etc.).
- If any non-study medications are to be discontinued during a period (usually a screening period), describe the procedure.
- Specify the acceptable leeway or "treatment window" for each visit. This is the amount of time that is allowed before or after the scheduled visit date, such as the date plus and minus two days. Specify how the investigator should handle visits that occur outside the acceptable window.
- If there is a tapered discontinuation of the investigational medication, describe the exact procedures, including the specific dose adjustments and time schedule to be followed. Consider a tabular display of the taper schedule.

Clinical assessments also need to be described in this section. Things to keep in mind when discussing clinical assessments:

- Describe and provide specific criteria (as appropriate) for the various observations and assessments at each study period. To avoid confusion, be sure to use the same terminology and categories that will be used in the CRFs (See "Case Report Forms" later in this chapter). Relate the various clinical assessments to the primary study observations they support.
- If a detailed description of a particular procedure or assessment tool is needed, consider describing it in general terms in this section, but in more detail in the appendix.
- Provide the rationale for the selection of specific endpoints or assessment tools unless discussed elsewhere.
- Discuss the accuracy, precision and relevance of any nonstandard assessment tool or procedure, citing references when appropriate.
- Specify any special conditions under which assessments are to be made or specific equipment should be used. Quantify descriptions when feasible and appropriate (e.g., indicate that 15 minutes of rest should precede a "resting" blood pressure reading).

- As appropriate, identify who should make clinical assessments and indicate whether the same evaluator should be used for a given subject throughout the study or for all subjects. List any assessment forms that are to be completed by the subject.
- Specify the rules or criteria for changing the management of the subject if there is either marked improvement or worsening of the subject's condition.

17. **Adverse Events.** There should be a very explicit section covering adverse events and adverse event reporting. (Adverse events are discussed in detail in Chapter 15.)
18. **Data Recording Instructions.** This section should:
    - Indicate how data will be collected. If detailed instructions have been prepared, specify their location (e.g., study manual, appendix, etc.).
    - Discuss the use and management of source documents.
    - Discuss the procedure for correcting errors.
19. **Data Quality Assurance.** This section should:
    - Describe procedures for assessing subject compliance.
    - Describe any special training or other measures for site personnel to ensure valid data.
    - Discuss source document review.
    - Provide Good Clinical Practice (GCP) references.
20. **Analysis Plan.** Generally, the analysis plan will be developed and provided by the biostatistician. Items that may be included are:
    - Discussion of the general study design issues.
    - A statement of the planned sample size, reason for choosing it and power calculations.
    - Classification of study variables (e.g., primary versus secondary).
    - Identification of statistical model(s) to be used.
    - Description of specific analyses, including any subgroup analyses.
    - Information about the timing and purpose of any planned interim analyses.

- Handling of missing or non-evaluable data.

21. **Risks and Benefits.** This section should briefly summarize the risks and potential benefits associated with the use of the test compound or procedure. If there is any exposure to radiation, it should be discussed here. Note that this section should be consistent with the consent form.
22. **References.** Put all references for the protocol in this section.
23. **Appendices.** Appendices may be used to detail information that might be confusing if placed in the body of the protocol.
    - Include an appendix describing investigator responsibilities, including the requirements for compliance with GCPs and sponsor SOPs. (Investigator responsibilities are discussed in the next chapter.)

Table 2: Rising protocol complexity

	Total endpoints at DBL*	Total procedures*	Percent non-core procedures†
Phase 2			
2011–2015	20.7 (0.6)	219.4 (0.6)	17.9%
2011–2015	19.5 (0.7)	259.2 (1.2)	26.1%
Phase 3			
2011–2015	19.8 (0.7)	187.6 (0.7)	24.7%
2011–2015	25.8 (0.8)	266.3 (0.9)	23.1%

Notes: DBL = Database lock; CoV = Coefficient of Variation
* Mean (CoV)
† Non-core procedures are those that support ancillary secondary, tertiary, and exploratory endpoints as well as safety and efficacy procedures not associated with primary or key secondary endpoints
Source: Tufts Center for the Study of Drug Development

Protocol Complexity

Over the past several years, protocols have become more complex and more demanding in their requirements. According to a 2023 study by the Tufts' Center for the Study of Drug Development, "[d]espite growing awareness among sponsors and CROs of the importance of simplifying and streamlining protocol design, nearly every design variable has been increasing in complexity over time, particularly in costlier later-stage phase 3 clinical trials."

More complex protocols also require more comprehensive CRFs/eCRFs, at a greater expense to the sponsor, and they put an additional burden on study sites.

Not only does it take more time to develop a more complex protocol, but the time from protocol readiness until the first subject is enrolled increases, as does the time to when the final subject visit takes place. Anything that can be done to simplify a protocol while still making it adequate to meet the study goals will pay dividends to the sponsor, the site and the study subjects.

Protocol Amendments

Protocol amendments, meaning formal changes to a protocol, are very prevalent in the industry and require a huge amount of time and effort. Think about the steps that have to occur if you amend a protocol. The change has to be written, including a section showing both the old and new versions, it must be reviewed by multiple people, sent to sites for review, sent to the IRBs for review and approval, sent back to the sponsor and then implemented. If the protocol amendment includes safety updates/information, changed, added or altered study procedures, or significant changes, this will include an amended informed consent form that requires subjects to be reconsented and protocol retraining and documentation. The ability to recruit subjects may be affected, sometimes positively, sometimes negatively. The analysis plan may have to be altered. All in all, it can be a huge amount of work and will involve numerous people in the process.

In 2023, CSDD conducted a study on protocol amendments that found the number of protocols with at least one amendment had increased 20 percentage points between 2015 and 2022. The same study illustrated the impact of protocol amendments on trial timelines, saying, "The gaps between actual and plan for all clinical trial cycle times are wider for protocols with amendments than for those without."

Constant protocol amendments are also difficult for sites to manage. They are often confusing, especially when it comes to determining what the changes are and when they are to be implemented, which can make compliance to study procedures difficult at the site level. Amendments also cause sites a great

Table 3: Performance comparison with and without protocol amendments

	Mean gap between actual and planned outcome*	
	Protocols without amendments	Protocols with at least one amendment
Study start-up duration (protocol approved to FPFV)	2.8%	18.0%
Enrollment duration (FPFV–LPLV)	2.4%	14%
Number of patients screened	0.7%	8.6%
Number of patients enrolled	-6.1%	-7.8%
Drop-out rate	13.6%	27.1%
Close-out duration (LBLV–data-base lock)	27.6%	59.0%
Overall clinical trial duration (pro-dotol approved–adatabase lock)	3.8%	13.9%

Notes: FPFV = first patient, first visit; LPLV = last patient, last visit
* Calculated as 'actual' value divided by the 'planned' value
Source: Tufts Center for the Study of Drug Development

deal of extra time, especially with sponsor efforts to disseminate the study amendment to the investigational site, training the Principal Investigator, Sub-Investigator and investigational site staff on the protocol amendment and documentation of training, etc. It can also cause sites a great deal of extra time if subjects need to be re-consented, and they may make the sponsor look inept.

In conclusion, it is important to take the time to carefully review and check protocols before they are formally issued. This is usually a joint task, so if everyone involved takes the time to read the protocol carefully, think about it and make any necessary changes, it should be free from errors and flaws. This is time well spent.

Summary

A good protocol forms the backbone of the research process and is essential for conducting a high-quality study. CRAs must understand what makes a good protocol and the importance of protocols in research. For each study the CRA is monitoring, he or she must have a clear understanding of the protocol and what must be done to ensure adherence to it during the study. Amendments should be avoided whenever possible. Once the protocol is written, CRFs can be developed.

Case Report Forms

Technology has dramatically influenced clinical trial conduct, with new platforms and electronic systems managing a majority of data collection and reporting methods. Although eCRF systems have been around for more than 20 years, some clinical trials still rely on paper CRFs.

CRFs are used during a clinical trial to record the protocol-required data for each study subject. CRFs standardize the collection of study data and help assure that the medical, statistical, regulatory and data management needs of the study are met. EDC/eCRF systems are utilized in a large number of clinical trials/device trials and reflect the same approach for data collection as their paper-based counterparts.

The mere mention of CRFs/eCRFs can evoke images of seemingly endless corrections, piles of paper, query notifications from the eCRF system and query emails from data management with countless excel spreadsheets detailing the volume of queries to be resolved and outlining outstanding data entry. However, dealing with eCRFs/CRFs is a large part of a CRA's workload, and they play a major part in the performance of a clinical trial. (The CRA's involvement in monitoring CRFs is discussed in Chapter 10.)

Many sponsors have designated people or departments responsible for developing the CRFs/eCRFs or this work may be contracted out to a company that specializes in their development. Consequently, CRA involvement and input in developing eCRFs/CRFs varies considerably from company to company. However, the impact of eCRF/CRF design on data quality is so significant that CRAs should have an understanding of the issues involved in CRF design and development. Awareness of the problems with poorly designed CRFs will also help the CRA when reviewing the forms/systems at investigative sites.

CRF Design and Development

Unfortunately, sponsors often cause themselves significant problems because the design and development of CRFs are not given adequate attention. So much time and energy goes into protocol development that CRFs are sometimes an afterthought. However, taking the time to design good forms pays major dividends during the course of the study.

Past experience is extremely valuable, and time should be taken to utilize previous company CRF experiences. Try to use ideas that worked well for other studies. Get input from some of your more knowledgeable sites. Study coordinators know from experience what works well and what doesn't and are usually willing to share their thoughts about good and bad CRFs.

Good case reports come from consistent improvement over time. Since CRAs are in an excellent position to monitor the quality of CRFs during monitoring visits, they should make notes of which forms or parts of forms seem to produce the most errors and those that are relatively error-free; this information should be shared with those involved in designing forms.

Some of the issues involved in producing high-quality CRFs are discussed below.

Standardization of CRFs

Everyone in this business is busy. One way to make better use of time is the judicious use of standardization. An approach to form design that has been used successfully by many companies is "modularization," which employs the benefits of standardization while also capturing and utilizing corporate experience.

The modular process is simple. There are data that are always collected on study subjects regardless of the drug or disease being studied, such as header information, demographics, laboratory work and physical exams. There are also other procedures (ECGs, stress tests, etc.) for which the information gathered is standard across different disease areas. When the group of fields is created for a study to collect the information for one of these items, it should be saved as a form module that can be used for other studies.

Over time, the catalog of form modules will become comprehensive. When new studies are planned, those involved in designing the CRFs can check the catalog to see which form modules will be appropriate for the study in question. Not only does this save design time, but the modules can also be pre-coded by data management, which saves additional time.

Terminology Used in CRFs

Always use standard terminology that is familiar to clinicians. Industry jargon will not be understood in a clinical setting.

Selection of the Media for CRFs

A decision must be made about whether a paper or electronic system will be used. The entire process for designing and implementing an eCRF/EDC system will not be covered in this chapter, which will focus on high level information about EDC systems.

EDC is an electronic system for collecting, managing, auditing and reporting study subject clinical trial data. Most EDC systems are cloud-based, which ensures secure access/use from anywhere. Web-based EDC systems allow site users to enter subject data from the source documents/medical record into the EDC system's CRF pages (electronic forms with similar fields as paper CRFs). Once a form is completed, it is checked off and verified as completed by the user, which essentially notifies the data manager or CRA at the sponsor or CRO that the data is ready for review. The type of EDC system used will help define the CRF. Many of the concepts and principals discussed for paper CRFs are also applicable to electronic forms. This is important, as the majority of studies are using web-enabled systems for CRF capture and collection.

Determination of the Data that Need to be Collected

One of the first things to be done is the determination of what information should be collected on the CRFs and how it will be coded, including acceptable ranges and any exceptions. The best way to do this is to go through the protocol and list all the data that are required, keeping in mind that the forms must collect these data in a way that allows for appropriate analyses. When this has been determined, the forms design process may start. For example, it is never a good idea to ask for the same data in more than one place in a CRF because, when this happens, the data do not always agree. Sometimes the

CRFs ask for both date of birth and age, for example, and they frequently do not match when calculated; it is better to ask only one question.

Determination of CRF Layout

If a module catalog is available, the next step is to determine which modules are appropriate for the study. If not, or if the modules do not cover all of the necessary information, then the necessary fields to collect the remaining data must be laid out. Some things to consider during this process are:

Header and footer information.

There should be standard header information on all forms. The sponsor's name or ID, the protocol number, the page title and a place to enter subject identification information should be pre-printed on all forms. All forms also should be annotated as CONFIDENTIAL. Each form should have a place for a signature and date; this usually appears at the bottom of the page in a footer.

Number of fields per page.

It's tempting to crowd as much information on a page as possible to save costs. However, this approach usually turns out to be "penny wise and pound foolish," as crowding increases the chance for error. There is no easy way to quantify form density; it is a judgment call. The best way is to develop a feel for the optimal amount of information on a page and count the number of fields. Then try to stay within 10 percent of that number on all forms.

Font size.

Use a font size and style that is easy to read.

Spatial relationships.

The fields on a page, particularly the check boxes, should be lined up as much as possible. It is easier to enter data and to notice missing data when the alignment is straight.

Location of fields on a page.

Something that is almost never considered during form design is where on the page to put specific fields. It is beneficial to put primary endpoints and other critical data on the top third of the forms.

Another consideration related to the position of fields on the form is the use of a logical layout. The material on the form should be organized in a manner that makes sense relative to medical practice. Group fields together for activities that are usually done together or in sequence in a clinic setting. For example, a module for collecting data on eye exams should not be put in the middle of a page that is collecting data from a physical exam and vital signs. In addition, vital signs—pulse, heart rate and respiration rate—should be grouped together rather than in different locations. Remember that the "customers" for your CRFs are the site personnel who must fill them out. Make your forms as user-friendly as possible to help reduce errors.

Narrative fields.

As much of the data as possible should be collected using numeric fields or check boxes. Include a check box for "other" as appropriate, because exceptions do occur.

Comments on CRFs are a problem because it is difficult to computerize and analyze comments. Everything on a CRF must be coded for computer entry and analysis; consequently, comments need to be interpreted and converted to code. The true nature of the comment is often lost or distorted during the translation. On the other hand, there may not be a better way to document an occurrence than by a comment. There should be places for comments on CRFs, but only when really necessary and valuable.

It is incumbent on the CRA to instruct site personnel on the use of comments on CRFs. Many CRF designers intentionally reduce margin space on CRFs to discourage comments. It is a difficult issue, but one that can be dealt with effectively if appropriate attention is given to it.

Cross-visit forms.

The most difficult forms to design are those that collect data across visits, such as adverse event and concomitant medication report forms; consequently, a lot of care should be given to the design of these forms. Based on our experience, almost 75 percent of the errors occurred on about 15 percent of the CRFs, including the adverse events and concomitant medications cross-visit forms.

Miscellaneous Issues

CRF design and production are complex and time-consuming tasks. Based on your company's capabilities and the specialized equipment required for the production of them, it is often cost-effective to contract this function to outside vendors.

During a course taken many years ago called Managing Accelerated Performance, the instructor said something applicable to CRF design. We were discussing things that could be done to significantly improve performance and/or productivity (the "silver bullet"). He told us not to think that way because the silver bullet is seldom there. Instead, usually small improvements done consistently over time will have major impact. So, as a CRA, when you are monitoring your studies, notice what kinds of errors are occurring and where. Think about what could be done in the design of the form to help prevent them. Take notes. Help your company capitalize on good design features and eliminate bad ones. These are the small steps that lead to continuous improvement.

Electronic Data Capture

It was reported that as of December, 2018, that 75 percent of clinical trials used electronic data capture (EDC) systems. Paper CRFs and questionnaires are still used in a variety of studies, so we wanted to provide details on both electronic and paper CRF systems. EDC systems facilitate efficient data entry and review. Source data is transcribed to the patient's eCRF with essentially the same fields of entry and pages as with paper CRFs (medications, medical history, AEs, visits, etc). However, the data is entered faster in the EDC by site staff. Both data managers and CRAs can review the data instantly after entry by site personnel, and they can issue queries to address data errors or inconsistencies early on to prevent further error. Automated validity checks can be run while the data are being entered, so that the coordinator is "not allowed" to make some kinds of errors, such as out-of-range entries or missing data. Additional automated validity checks can be run by the sponsor immediately upon receipt of the data, so queries can be sent to the site in a timely manner.

The creation and management of queries is also more efficient using EDC systems. The CRA or data manager reviews the data and then is able to flag questionable or incorrect data by creating a query field, prompted by the system. The query field allows the creator to populate text that describes the question about the data entered. The field is flagged after query creation, indicating a query has been generated that needs to be addressed by site personnel.

CRAs are able to review data and issue queries in between monitoring visits. Site personnel can address queries quickly and not have to wait for monitoring visits to resolve them. With the EDC data entry and query model, the data manager, remote monitor and the CRA share responsibility for timely data review and correction. With paper CRFs, it takes extra time for query resolution.

Using EDC, error patterns can be looked at more easily across all sites, which can help define protocol problems, CRF problems or common misunderstandings that pinpoint the need for further training or revisions in study procedures. Catching problems early can greatly enhance study quality.

With EDC, the CRA can review the actual data, including queries, in-house or remotely before making a monitoring visit, so that he or she will be more knowledgeable about any study problems upon arrival at the site. The CRA can check the EDC for diary entries that may look like adverse events, look at the EDC for supporting information about site compliance with screening and enrolling patients, and associated procedures and to ascertain what sites are and are not meeting data entry deadlines (e.g., if the CRA was informed a site enrolled three new patients but no data has been entered in the EDC to verify this). When initial data review is done in-house, the CRA does not have to do it at the site, which allows more time for verifying the data (source document review), training and performing other study management activities. With the emerging role of the remote monitor, remote review of a site's EDC occurs more frequently. This increases data quality, timely data entry with reminders to sites and can help meet any study data deadlines with additional data review, communication and query resolution with the sites by the remote monitor.

If study data are cleaned as the study progresses, EDC can minimize the time between the last data being transmitted and achieving a clean database. An earlier database lock allows the final report to be written sooner.

Electronic Patient-Recorded Outcomes, Questionnaires, Diaries and Assessments

The use of ePROs, electronic diaries and electronic systems for study subject data collection and reporting is prevalent in today's clinical trials environment, although paper PROs and questionnaires are still used in some trials. The landscape continues to evolve with more innovative and convenient means for patients to report data.

The different reporting measures include:

- Electronic patient diaries to report symptoms or pain or track study drug compliance.
- Interactive Voice Response (IVR)/telephone systems to report symptoms.
- Electronic patient questionnaires, clinician-administered rating scales or cognitive testing. Delivery systems include tablets, computers or mobile devices for patients to record study drug receipt and compliance and to answer questions and report symptoms. There is even the option for the integration of the ePRO system with the study subject's smart phone.
- Wearable devices may be used by study patients to report/record data—pedometers, smart watches and patient wearables are used to record activity, heart rate, vitals, oxygen, etc.

Below are examples of digital or electronic means of recording and reporting patient data from the subject and clinician perspective.

Study Subjects:

- Patients call in to an IVR system that uses keypad or voice prompts for patients to answer questions about symptoms or medication compliance.
- Mobile device or tablets for subjects to enter symptom information, medication compliance information, diary symptom or adverse event information, or to answer quality-of-life or disease-related questions.
- Mobile devices to track and record study drug shipments or device shipments that go directly to a study patient's residence.
- Wearable devices that record physiologic data (walking, blood pressure, heart rate, sleep patterns, oxygen).

Study Clinicians:

- Clinicians are able to administer study cognitive or rating scales to study patients via web conferencing, computer systems or computer tablets.

The advantages of electronic recording and reporting of data are numerous:

- Sponsor-provided equipment ensures consistent collection, evaluation and validation of data.
- System-generated queries for incomplete or untimely data entry are available.
- Electronically-generated patient reminders to call in for data reporting or data entry at specific time points.
- Investigator and site staff afforded real-time access to data reports and entry by patients.
- Devices and ePROs help facilitate the conduct of DCTs

There are disadvantages:

- Site staff require training on electronic devices and systems, which requires time and additional cost.
- Site staff, in turn, have to train study subjects on the use of electronic devices and systems, which also requires time and additional cost.
- Sites have to store equipment provided by sponsors for this purpose, and sites that conduct multiple sponsor studies with a variety of electronic equipment need additional space to store it.
- Some study subjects or clinicians are not tech savvy and are resistant to the use of electronic devices in lieu of paper.
- Study subjects lose or do not return tablets or study devices.
- Issues with device entry, uploading or reporting data, or with internet access can impede study data collection.

In an *Applied Clinical Trials* October 2015 blog entry, titled "Mobile, the Future of Patient-Reported Outcomes," author Chris Watson discusses some benefits of more efficient data collection and the facilitation of confidentiality and patient engagement via ePROs:

> Incorporating mobile electronic clinical outcome assessments (eCOA) into clinical studies has a myriad of benefits. Native apps facilitate the collection of objective data from medical devices (e.g., spirometers and glucometers) and wearable technology such as activity trackers alongside patient diaries.

> Data from these devices can be transmitted directly into an app via Bluetooth, removing the requirement for transcribing results manually. Furthermore, date and time stamps for each data point can be captured from a patient source through to an EDC database, and fraud can be eliminated by introducing two-factor authentication. Mobile eCOA has another practical advantage, which is to provide more efficient patient engagement. A patient who has missed diary completions can be reminded of the importance of taking part in the study, and should it not improve future ePRO compliance rates, sites can follow up immediately. Site staff can discuss any difficulties or misunderstandings with patients and provide additional timely education and support to enable continuation in the study before they are lost.

The author noted that, "The rapid evolution of this technology combined with patient-centric data generation provides cost effective options for drug development. On the other hand, reliability and validation of devices and data, privacy concerns and regulatory acceptance are slowing the integration of these valuable tools as novel endpoints into clinical trials. Despite that, wearable devices and smart technology are transforming the drug development process."

Increasingly, decentralized clinical trials are using ePROs that enable patients at home to integrate the software onto their personal smart phone to report symptoms and data.

Summary

Writing good protocols and developing appropriate CRFs are the backbone of study preparation. Being familiar with all means of electronic data recording and reporting is essential for CRAs. Completion of these activities will help to ensure the success of the trial. Since CRAs work with these elements at every investigative site they monitor, they should have a good understanding of the issues and processes involved.

Key Takeaways

Protocol

- The protocol is the blueprint for a study. It contains all the information necessary to conduct the study correctly.
- CRAs must have a thorough understanding of the protocol for each study they monitor.
- The writing of a protocol is usually a team effort, involving the medical monitor, the statistician and others.
- Protocols for phase 1 studies are relatively flexible, while those for phases 2 and 3 are more rigid and detailed.
- Certain information is required by regulation to be in protocols.
- As protocol complexity increases, there is a cost to the sponsor (and to the sites) in terms of both time and money.
- Amendments to protocols are very costly in terms of both time and money.
- Care should be taken to avoid amendments whenever possible.

Case Report Forms

- CRFs have a significant impact on data quality.
- Standardize and use modules as much as possible.
- Shading, aligning and limiting the number of fields per page can reduce errors.
- Remember that the investigative site is the customer for your CRFs. Design them with the site in mind. Make them medically and clinically sensible.
- Continually improve your forms by noting good and bad design features.

Electronic Data Capture

- EDC can significantly reduce errors, cut the time for sponsor receipt and management of the data, and greatly lessen the time between the last subject's final study visit and the "lock" of the clean database.

- CRAs, data managers and study coordinators at the site all share responsibility for data quality when EDC or electronic devices for PROs are used.

Electronic Patient-Reported Outcomes

- The use of ePROs is being integrated more and more into clinical trials, though there still may be some regulatory, data privacy and device reliability challenges to overcome.

CHAPTER 12

Clinical Investigators

The conduct of studies at investigative sites is the responsibility of the investigator. In the first part of this chapter, investigators and their responsibilities are covered. In the second part, the evaluation and selection of investigators and investigative sites is discussed. How a CRA can help investigators meet their responsibilities during clinical trials will be discussed in subsequent chapters.

Investigators and Their Responsibilities

What is an "Investigator"?

According to the regulations (21 CFR 312.3), investigator means "an individual who actually conducts a clinical investigation (i.e., under whose immediate direction the investigational drug is administered or dispensed to a subject). In the event an investigation is conducted by a team of individuals, the investigator is the responsible leader of the team." Sometimes the investigator is called the principal, or primary, investigator (PI). Other members of the team may be referred to as Sub-Investigators, especially in the case of other physicians who are involved with the study. On occasion, there will be co-investigators for a trial. In this case, both individuals are equally responsible for the trial.

Usually, but not always, the investigator is a physician. Sometimes, a person with a Pharm.D. or a Ph.D. degree may serve as an investigator; in that case, there should be (at least for FDA-controlled studies) a physician as a Sub-Investigator.

With primary care and specialty physician practices (at public and private healthcare organizations) incorporating the services of mid-level practitioners such as Physician's Assistants (PA) or Nurse Practitioners (NP) into the patient treatment dynamic, it has become more common and acceptable for PAs and NPs to also serve as Sub-Investigators on clinical trials. There are several scenarios: A PI may have several Sub-Investigators under his or her oversight. a combination of physicians, NPs and PAs. Alternatively, the physician PI may only have one Sub-Investigator, either a NP or PA, without another physician Sub-Investigator. The setup is dependent upon investigational site model, institutional requirements, clinician scope of practice and sponsor approval.

Some sponsors approve the use of an NP or PA as a Sub-Investigator, provided there is also another physician Sub-Investigator supporting the PI's effort. Other sponsors approve a sole NP or PA as a Sub-Investigator under the PI, without the need for another physician as Sub-Investigator. Some PIs will utilize the NP or PA Sub-Investigator for responsibilities such as cognitive assessments or physical exams, provided they have appropriate training and experience. Other PIs will use the NP or PA Sub-Investigator for a broader scope of responsibilities: laboratory or ECG results review, confirmation and documentation of study eligibility criteria, adverse event causality, etc. Again, it depends on institution and sponsor requirements.

No matter the dynamic, the CRA must confirm that the PI is providing adequate oversight of responsibilities delegated to Sub-Investigators.

Regular communication must occur between the PI and Sub-Investigators to ensure the PI remains apprised and aware of subject status and treatment by Sub-Investigators. Some investigational sites will have weekly or bi-weekly meetings between the PI, Sub-Investigators and study coordinators to discuss subjects' status and other important study topics. This is a formal meeting at regular intervals, often with documented meeting minutes taken. Other sites have informal communication practices between the PI, Sub-Investigators and study coordinators, such as in a smaller clinical trials practice where the PI, Sub-Investigators and study coordinators work the same days or see each other consistently. Both examples of communication practices are acceptable, provided they are consistent. When there is a communication breakdown between the PI, Sub-Investigators and the study coordinator, the impact on study conduct can be detrimental.

Some investigators review all assessments and procedures/notes completed by the NP/PA Sub-Investigator to show oversight and document this review. This is not done by all investigators.

The CRA and PI/site must ensure that the PI has appropriately delegated responsibilities to the Sub-Investigators; that the Sub-Investigators are appropriately trained, licensed and experienced for the tasks to which they have been assigned (maintain CVs, licenses and training documentation in the regulatory binder); and all delegated Sub-Investigators responsibilities are documented on the delegation of authority log/site signature sheet the site maintains.

The Statement of Investigator (FDA Form 1572)

The Statement of Investigator (FDA Form 1572) must be completed and signed by the investigator before he or she may begin a study. The investigator then sends the form to the sponsor, and the sponsor submits it to the FDA.

The 1572 form contains:

- Name and address of the investigator.
- Title (and number, if any) of the protocol, including the IND number.
- Name and address of the facility where the research will be conducted.
- Name and address of any clinical laboratories that will be used.
- Name and address of the IRB used to approve the study.
- Names of any Sub-Investigators who will be associated with the study.
- Investigator commitment section (discussed below).

There is also a section of the 1572 that lists responsibilities of investigators. These include a commitment by the investigator that he or she will:

- Conduct the study according to the protocol.
- Comply with the regulations.
- Personally conduct or supervise the trial.
- Ensure the IRB complies with regulations.
- Obtain informed consent from subjects.
- Report adverse events properly.
- Read and understand the material in the Investigator Brochure before starting the trial.
- Assure that other people assisting in the trial are aware of their obligations.
- Maintain adequate and accurate records.

When the investigator signs the 1572 form, a legally binding commitment has been made to conduct a study according to the regulations and constraints of the 1572. CRAs should be very familiar with the 1572 form and should be prepared to discuss the commitments in depth (section 9, investigator commitments) with potential investigators, as applicable, during monitoring visits. CRAs will also need to assure that these forms are properly completed and signed and dated by the investigator before a study commences.

For device studies, the 1572 is not used. Instead, a sponsor must obtain a signed agreement from each investigator that includes the following, as per 21 CFR 812.43:

- The investigator's curriculum vitae (CV).
- A statement of the investigator's relevant experience.
- If the investigator was involved in an investigation or other research that was terminated, an explanation of the circumstances that led to termination.
- A statement of the investigator's commitment to:
  - Conduct the investigation in accordance with the agreement, the investigational plan, the applicable regulations and the conditions of approval imposed by the IRB.
  - Supervise all testing of the device in humans.
  - Ensure that the requirements for obtaining informed consent were met.
- Financial disclosure information.

Investigator Responsibilities

The investigator has the ultimate responsibility for the safety of participants in a clinical trial. Research participants are under the immediate care of the investigator and subject to the judgment and professional abilities of the investigator. For this reason, investigators must be qualified through training and experience before beginning to study a drug or device.

The general responsibilities of an investigator during a trial include ensuring that the trial is conducted according to the signed investigator statement (FDA Form 1572), following the protocol and regulations, and protecting the rights, safety and welfare of subjects in the trial. In the next sections, we will discuss some of the other specific responsibilities of an investigator during a trial.

Control of the Investigational Drug

One of the important responsibilities of an investigator is maintaining control of the investigational drug at all times. The drug may not be used by anyone other than trial subjects, who are under the supervision of the investigator or Sub-Investigators. Remember that the investigator has responsibility for any Sub-Investigators assisting in the trial.

If the investigational drug is a controlled substance, then the drug must be stored in a double-locked area with limited access. This is a good idea for the storage of all investigational drugs, when possible, as it eliminates potential problems. When not controlled properly, there is a risk of study drugs being used for patients who are not in the trial or being used by other physicians for non-trial purposes. Losing track of the study drug supply can be a major problem and have a negative effect on the trial.

The CRA will want to ensure that the study drug is properly stored at an investigational site and that provisions have been made to properly administer and account for the drug.

Investigator Recordkeeping and Retention

An investigator must maintain case histories of all subjects and data collected during a trial. These case histories include the case report forms and all supporting documents such as patient charts and progress notes, signed and dated consent forms, laboratory reports, EKGs and any other relevant patient-related documents. The histories must show that the consent form for each subject was signed and dated prior to participation in the study.

The investigator must also maintain complete records of the dispensing and disposition of the study drug, including dates, quantities, use by study subjects and amounts returned.

All study documents must also be maintained and retained, including copies of the signed 1572, the protocol and consent forms, the IRB approval letters, CVs for the investigator and Sub-Investigators, laboratory normal ranges and correspondence with the IRB and the sponsor. A complete listing of this documentation is found in Appendix C.

All of these records must be maintained for a period of two years after the approval of the drug for marketing or two years after the investigation is closed and the FDA is notified that the company is not pursuing further investigation of the drug. In reality, most sponsors expect the investigator to maintain the records for a much longer period, if not indefinitely. Most contracts between the sponsor and investigators require the investigator to retain all study documents until the sponsor has informed the investigator in writing that they may be destroyed. Although this is discussed in more detail in another chapter, the CRA should make it very clear to the investigator that the records must be kept until written notification is received from the sponsor that they may be disposed of.

Investigator Reports

There are reports that the investigator must provide to the sponsor throughout the duration of the trial. They include regular progress reports, which usually consist of the completed eCRFs/CRFs, plus periodic updates on enrollment and study status. Safety reports must also be furnished to the sponsor, including reports on any adverse events that may reasonably be regarded as having been caused by the study medication. Serious adverse events, those that are immediately life threatening, or deaths must be reported to sponsors immediately. A final report must be provided to the sponsor shortly after completion of the study. These reports are necessary to allow the sponsor to meet the regulatory requirements for reporting study progress to the FDA.

IRB Review

The investigator is responsible for assuring that the IRB he or she is using for the study meets the requirements for IRBs found in 21 CFR 56. The investigator must submit and wait for approval of a protocol and informed consent form before beginning a study, as well as promptly reporting to the IRB any changes in the protocol or any unanticipated problems involving risk to study subjects or others. The responsibilities of the investigator with respect to the IRB were delineated in detail in Chapter 8.

Disqualification of Investigators

Investigators who do not comply with the regulations governing clinical research or who falsify data in the investigation or reports to the sponsor and/

or the FDA, may be disqualified from receiving investigational drugs and doing studies in the future. The FDA maintains a list of restricted and disqualified investigators, known in the business as the "black list." This list is available on the FDA website (fda.gov). Once an investigator is put on the list, the name stays there forever, even if all conditions for reinstatement are met and the investigator is allowed to do research again. Most sponsor companies will not use an investigator who is on this list, even if the person has been reinstated to do research. More information on this topic is included in Chapter 19. CRAs should always check the "black list" before contacting a potential investigator. There is also a listing on the FDA website of all investigators who have been audited by the FDA with one of three classifications:

- **No Action Indicated (NAI)**—no significant objectionable conditions or practices found.
- **Voluntary Action Indicated (VAI)**—insignificant objectionable conditions or practices found that do not require enforcement but that the FDA expects the investigator to remedy voluntarily.
- **Official Action Indicated (OAI)**—objectionable conditions or practices found are significant enough to warrant FDA enforcement action.

In summary, investigators have enormous responsibility when they agree to participate in clinical research. A good investigator will enable the research to proceed smoothly, while a study conducted by a poor investigator most likely will be fraught with problems. Consequently, the selection of investigators is a crucial element of the research process.

Evaluating and Selecting Investigators

One of the most important tasks that CRAs undertake is the evaluation and selection of investigators. The success of a study depends in large part on the investigator—his or her experience, expertise, commitment, staff, resources and facilities. In this section we will discuss the qualities of a good investigator/investigative site and how a CRA can locate and evaluate sites for successful studies.

Author's Story

Pre-study evaluation visits are important because they allow sites to showcase their capabilities: staff experience, recruitment prowess, facilities/equipment. The CRA and the site theoretically each need something from the other: the site wants to be selected for the study and the CRA conducting the evaluation visit wants to select a strong, compliant site for the study. This reciprocal need usually dictates behavior on behalf of vested parties. Most sites are courteous and accommodating during site evaluation visits and the CRA conducting the visit maintains a professional and friendly demeanor throughout the process. Relationship development is a large part of this process. The resulting camaraderie between the investigator and CRA, initiated during the site selection process, will benefit the site management relationship during study conduct just as unprofessional behavior during an evaluation visit will contribute to a negative perception of the site by the CRA or of the CRA by the investigator.

One week, I was tasked to conduct two pre-study evaluation visits and there was a big disparity between the clinical and personal dynamic at each institution. At the first potential site, the study coordinator was extremely businesslike and informed me that the investigator did not care for small talk. We spent the entire pre-study visit without ancillary chit-chat. I made the mistake of asking the investigator if he was from the area and was informed in no uncertain terms that the "evaluation visit was not the place for personal chatter." That disappointed me, for though the site had the physical capabilities and staff experience for study conduct, the lack of positive communication would create a challenging dynamic for the CRA taking over the site and trying to build a partnership with the investigator.

The next day, I visited the second site and the differences were startling. They had the facility and experience required for study conduct and provided comprehensive answers to my questions. The level of courtesy and positive communication demonstrated by the investigator and staff at the start of the process set the precedent for a visit in which dialog flowed, information was exchanged and feedback was obtained without effort. Their demeanor confirmed their enthusiasm not just to work successfully with me through the evaluation visit but also gave insights into their willingness to work well with the monitor for their study.

A slight shift from a clinical to a personable attitude can have a huge impact on the site evaluation process.

—Elizabeth

Types of Investigative Sites

There are many types of investigative sites conducting studies. It is useful for a CRA to have an understanding of these different organizations when looking for and assessing potential sites for study placement. Some of the more common investigator site organizational types are listed below.

Part-Time Sites (single physician or multi-physician medical practice)

Investigators at part-time sites participate in research studies, but also maintain their regular practices. Sometimes these investigators do only one or two studies at a time, while others may participate in research to a greater degree, depending on their interest and their resources for conducting studies. Most sponsors like this kind of site because there is greater potential for study subjects and because the physician, if chosen, will become familiar with the drug. By the time it is marketed, he or she will be more likely to prescribe it to patients.

As a CRA, this type of site has both advantages and disadvantages. Because the site may not be as experienced, the CRA can train the site to do things in the way the sponsor would like them to be done, without having to "un-train" or change the way the site is used to doing things. On the other hand, since these sites may have less experience, they may need more training and "hand-holding" throughout the study. Some of the larger physician practices with research departments have a combination of experienced and new study coordinators, so CRAs are able to work with a variety of site staff. At these sites, study coordinators usually wear many hats (budgets, patient visits, regulatory, lab drawing and processing, etc.).

Dedicated Research Sites

These sites are dedicated specifically to conducting studies; no other medical practice is carried out. They generally are very experienced and need less help from the CRA in learning how to do studies, although they may still need instruction in how to do each particular study, with its unique characteristics. These sites are usually very productive. They also tend to be very aware of which studies they can do successfully and are less apt to accept studies for which they do not think they can enroll sufficient subjects within the given time period. These sites mitigate risk of potential staff turnover by developing guidelines/SOPs that govern research conduct at their facility. This ensures consistency in study conduct and new staff assuming study responsibilities. SOPs cover such tasks as training, consent form creation and administration, study drug storage and administration, source creation and storage, and adverse event reporting. Concerns are sometimes expressed about these sites being "study mills" and having "professional study subjects;" but, as long as they are not in violation of the protocol, this does not seem to be a problem.

These sites either are stand-alone clinics with investigators and study coordinators as direct employees or use the physician investigator's medical practice for research activities, providing research personnel to support the investigator with whom they have contracted for study conduct. These sites usually have dedicated study coordinators, data managers and lab personnel to conduct study activities.

For the CRA, these sites are usually easy to manage. Since they rely on studies for their business, they are usually accommodating as well as compliant.

There are large, dedicated research site networks, with sites across the United States, Canada and sometimes even Europe. In recent years, some large site networks have grown, merged and have been purchased by CROs.

Academic Sites

Academic sites are those located in universities and teaching hospitals. They tend to do original research on their own and government-sponsored clinical trials, as well as industry-sponsored clinical trials. Often these organizations are headed by "thought leaders," the top specialists in their fields. Clinical trials may or may not be the academic site's primary interest, although in recent years sponsors have been using academic sites more frequently. Occasionally, industry trials provide added funding to allow these sites to carry on other research. It is desirable for a sponsor to use some academic sites in its development programs. This allows thought leaders to become familiar with the new compounds and, hopefully, to become spokespersons in favor of the compound once it is marketed.

Unfortunately, these sites can present some difficulties for a CRA. It can be difficult for the CRA to meet with the busy investigator; these investigators have been labeled "phantom investigators" because they never seem to be around during the trial. It can also be difficult if industry-sponsored research is not the primary interest of the site, in which case enrollment may wane and study activities may not receive proper attention. Also, because publishing is a key issue at academic sites, sponsor policies regarding publication of the trial results should be clearly delineated prior to the initiation of the study. That being said, there are many excellent academic sites with dedicated researchers who add an extra dimension to clinical development programs. The research staff at these institutions are usually part of the same therapeutic area as the investigator with whom they work.

Other Hospitals/Health Institutions

There are hospitals/healthcare institutions (not academic) that have centralized research departments with study coordinators experienced in a variety of therapeutic indications, so one central research group helps the different physicians conduct trials.

Site Management Organizations

SMOs bring together a group of sites and organize them centrally to conduct studies. They standardize procedures across sites and often provide standardized materials (SOPs, study file procedures, etc.) to each site in the organization. Many SMOs also provide training for their sites and assist the sites in compiling and submitting the required regulatory documents. They usually provide centralized services for marketing the sites (attracting studies) and for subject recruitment. There are several types of SMOs, from those that own the sites in the group to those with other partnership agreements.

The main difference for a CRA when using an SMO is that control over study processes may not reside at the site, but may be handled centrally. If the CRA is working with only one site in the SMO, this can cause a bit of difficulty, as it requires dealing with several different individuals at more than one location for that one site; regulatory, contract and budget staff are located at the SMO, and the site clinical and research process is handled by the study coordinators at the investigational site. It may be advantageous if working with multiple sites in the SMO because of the consistency of study practices.

A variation of an SMO is the Coordinator Organization. This is usually a group of experienced study coordinators who have formed a business. They recruit investigators to conduct trials and then place an experienced coordinator in the investigator's office to manage and help with the trial. These coordinators usually act as the interface with the sponsor/CRO and manage the operational aspects of the trial; the physician is utilized for his or her medical expertise and patient base. The only difference for the CRA is that the coordinator is the main contact for all business aspects of the trial, including grant payments. (Note that the investigator is usually paid a fee by the coordinator organization.)

Regardless of how the physician's research practice is organized, the CRA must still monitor and manage the trial for the safety of the subjects and the integrity of the data.

More and more physicians are interested in entering clinical research and conducting drug studies. However, there is more to the process than finding the appropriate space and experienced study coordinators. Investigators must first decide what they would like to do: start a research site, integrate a research department into their private practice or affiliate with a dedicated research site as a principal investigator.

There are some critical elements required to establish a physician as a principal investigator, and/or to start a research site or research department, as noted below. These are non-inclusive, generalized guidances:

- Principal Investigator and Sub-Investigator credentials, specialty, training and experience.
- Appropriate funding.
- Key staff for contract, budget and regulatory activities; business development/recruitment staff for attracting studies and recruiting patients; administrative staff, clinical staff for study coordination and clinical activities/testing (vitals, phlebotomy, specimen processing and shipment, spirometry, etc.); appropriate location for patient examination and lab/imaging/specialized testing; and space for staff, etc.
- Documented research process and infrastructure such as ICFs. SOPs, drug accountability and pharmacy SOPs, training checklists, job descriptions, departmental meetings and plans.

There are many more applicable details to this process, but this is just a generalized summary.

Locating Potential Investigators

There are a number of ways to locate potential investigators. Large sponsors and CROs keep computerized databases of investigators with whom they have worked. This is the best place to start identifying potential investigators for your trial. These databases may include such metrics as enrollment rates and numbers, timelines of data submission and error rates on CRFs.

If your company does not have an investigator database, ask for suggestions from other therapeutic groups. (See Chapter 18 for examples of site metrics.) Sometimes the best way, in the absence of a central investigator database, is to ask people in your company for suggestions. People working in one medical group may not be aware of good potential investigators, and asking another group may provide good candidates.

Another excellent way to find good investigators is to ask investigators you know and/or with whom you are currently working. "Dr. Smith, you've been doing a terrific job on this rheumatology study. I have some cardiovascular studies coming along soon. Do you know any physicians who might do as good a job on those studies as you are doing on this one?" If your investigator has some suggestions for you, he or she may be willing to call the other physician as an introduction for you. Some CRAs have had great success using this technique.

There are websites that list investigators and their areas of specialty. These sites will give you names and contact information by region and specialty and make it fairly easy to start a list of people to contact. There are references to some of these websites in Appendix A.

Another successful method is to network with colleagues from other companies. Ask colleagues if they have worked with anyone in the therapeutic area in which you are interested who did competent work for them in the past. This is often a very useful method, but be sure to reciprocate when you can. Other potential methods for locating investigators are:

- Look in medical journals for articles dealing with the therapeutic area in which you are interested and contact authors of relevant articles.

- Look at regulatory submissions from other companies working in the same therapeutic area and contact the investigators they used.
- Contact professional organizations that may have listings of physicians.
- Use Google or internet searches.
- Contact patient advocacy groups that may keep lists of investigators.
- Look at clinicaltrials.gov for studies and contact information.

Once you have collected a list of potential investigators for your program, you will want to contact them.

Initial Contact

If you or anyone in your company has had no previous experience with a potential investigator, a telephone call is probably the best initial contact. Try to call the physician directly, rather than leaving messages with staff. When you call, if you say only that you are from a pharmaceutical company, the person answering the phone may think you are a salesperson, and you are apt to have a difficult time reaching the physician. You might say you are from the "research division of the XXX company" and that you are interested in talking with Dr. Smith "about becoming involved in research studies." If you still encounter some difficulty, you may want to tell the person that you are not in sales. If you have too much trouble trying to get through, call the next person on your list and forget this one—if he or she is that hard to reach, you'll probably always have trouble with direct contact.

Once you reach the physician, introduce yourself and say why you are calling. If the physician appears to be interested, give a brief overview of the program and the study to be done. Find out if the physician has research experience and, if so, the types of projects he or she has worked on in the past or is working on currently. Ask questions about the patient population, the staff and the facilities.

If interest is high on the part of the potential investigator and if you feel there is good potential for placing a study at the site, arrange a time to visit the site in person. This will enable you to better evaluate the investigator's capability to complete your project. Depending on your company policies, you may be able to send the potential investigator some materials about your drug and/or program, such as a protocol or a protocol summary, before you visit. If your company requires a signed confidentiality agreement before sharing these materials, arrange to fax/email it to the site and have it completed and returned before sending any other materials. One clue to the interest of the investigator is the speed with which the signed confidentiality agreement is returned to you.

A number of sponsor companies delegate trial responsibilities to CROs, which include study startup responsibilities such as feasibility and investigator identification/evaluation. Feasibility encompasses initial investigator vetting and contact for the purposes of obtaining investigator/site experience and site capability information. Feasibility has become such an integral part of the study startup process that there are entire departments dedicated to investigator identification and feasibility services. Initial investigator identification, correspondence and provision of information has become a streamlined, sophisticated process that is completed via online standardized investigator questionnaires with which to capture site capability information. Feasibility departments have investigator information stored in dedicated databases, and reports can be accessed to assist with identification and initial evaluation of investigative sites. This dedicated dynamic has shortened the investigator identification and evaluation timelines by streamlining process and harmonizing data collection.

After investigator information has been received and confirmed, the investigator is deemed ready for the official evaluation visit. Best practices dictate that the CRA sends an email or letter to the investigator to confirm the date and time of their visit to the site.

Site Evaluation Visits

When the CRA completes an evaluation visit to a potential investigative site, the CRA will be evaluating the investigator's experience, expertise and interest in the trial, as well as the staff, facility and potential patient population available. The sponsor company may have a specific checklist that will guide the CRA in making an assessment. The advantage of using a checklist is that the CRA won't inadvertently forget to assess some important items. A sample site evaluation checklist is found in Appendix C.

The CRA should have a good understanding of the study requirements, the schedule of assessments, preliminary protocol design, patient eligibility and logistical requirements to be able to have a sound discussion on study requirements and investigator recruitment capabilities with the investigator and staff. At the very least the CRA should discuss the following protocol components during site evaluation: trial design, inclusion/exclusion criteria, safety reporting, patient population, study endpoints, critical testing/procedures, investigator availability, specialized testing/vendors/schedule of assessments, study drug, investigator access to the study population and investigator commitments. It is optimal if the PI and study coordinator are present for this discussion.

Investigators and their staff are understandably busy with unforeseen schedule changes, and a CRA needs to be flexible and ready to discuss the study with the PI with little notice. This may be in an exam room or the study coordinator's office. However, it is imperative to remember confidentiality and never discuss the study design in front of another CRA or staff not covered by a confidentiality agreement. Ask if the meeting can be moved to another location with privacy, such as the investigator's office or an empty area.

Investigator Experience, Expertise and Interest

The investigator's CV will help you make a general assessment of the investigator's experience and expertise. Reviewing the feasibility information (listing details of the investigator and site study experience, access to the population for enrollment and information on site equipment for study conduct) prior to the evaluation visit will give you specific details to review or questions to confirm with the investigator during the site evaluation visit. Conversing with the investigator in person will allow you to determine his or her research activity, especially in the therapeutic area of interest. This is a good time to determine if the investigator has conducted trials similar to the one being proposed or has worked with similar compounds. This is also a good time to determine if the investigator's research experience matches his CV and if the study experience on the CV is as a PI or Sub-Investigator. Sometimes investigational sites will present a potential PI without research experience, which is not clear from the CV. Investigator experience is critical to clarify during the evaluation visit.

A physician new to research should not be immediately disqualified for consideration as a PI. There are many variables to consider with new investigators/sites, such as research/investigator training completed and preparation for the site evaluation visit, study design and therapeutic area.

If the study is a simpler, phase 3 design for a chronic disease such as Type 2 diabetes or hypertension, using a new investigator with expertise in the therapeutic indication and access to a large population may be appropriate in lieu of research experience. When taken into consideration during site evaluation, confirm any training the investigator has completed to learn his role (GCP training, web-based investigator training modules). Confirm if the investigator has access to another experienced investigator to provide guidance during the first subject's screening and randomization visits. Ensure the new investigator has an experienced study coordinator. There are several variables that may make an inexperienced investigator a viable candidate for study consideration. The CRA should never apply a broad stroke categorization of new investigators. Rather, each site, experienced or not, is considered on a case-by-case basis.

While listening to the prospective investigator answer your questions, be aware of any nonverbal clues being conveyed. Is the investigator actively listening to you? Asking pertinent questions? Being attentive to the conversation and materials? If an investigator professes great interest in conducting a study but is also replying to his email during the meeting, obviously his interest level isn't very high. One of the most critical factors for the success of a study is the interest of the investigator. If the investigator isn't truly interested, the study won't be foremost in his or her mind and will probably suffer because of it.

The CRA should also try to determine the investigator's commitment to actually participating in the trial, as opposed to delegating all the responsibility to others and being an investigator in name only. These absent investigators are referred to as "phantom" investigators—they assign the study activities to Sub-Investigators and study coordinators and have very little, if any, personal involvement in the trial. This is unacceptable. When an investigator signs a 1572 form, the investigator commits to personally conduct or supervise the trial or, for devices, to supervise all testing of the device in humans. This is a legal responsibility and cannot be taken lightly. Some specific questions to cover with investigator/site staff during the evaluation visit, to better determine investigator involvement and oversight, are listed below:

- How many studies is the PI currently conducting?
- What percentage of study subjects will the PI treat compared to the Sub-Investigators?
- What days of the week/hours is the PI on site and treating study subjects?

Answers to these questions will serve as a strong indicator of investigator commitment and oversight, and will contribute to the decision of investigator selection.

There are situations that mandate that study subject care be divided between the PI and his Sub-Investigators. One common situation where this occurs is when the investigator is part of a large practice with all physicians affiliated with the practice serving as Sub-Investigators. The PI and Sub-Investigators would be enrolling potential study subjects from his or her respective practice and would be the treating physician to the subjects they enrolled to ensure continuity of care and subject engagement. This is a scenario where the PI would not see the majority of the subjects, but where subject treatment would be divided between the PI and Sub-Investigators. As long as the PI ensures oversight by discussing study subjects with the Sub-Investigators, remains involved and aware of any SAEs and critical safety issues, and assures his or her commitments in accordance with section 9 of the 1572, then this is acceptable.

The CRA will also want to assess the investigator's reactions to the protocol. Is there anything in the protocol that the physician objects to doing? Is the investigator willing to follow the protocol as it is written? Is the physician comfortable with the study design and the use of a placebo, if applicable? Does the protocol match his or her clinical practice, except for study-specific parameters? Making assumptions that everything is acceptable without checking is a risky path to follow—it's better to find out about potential problems and conflicts before the study is offered to him or her.

This is also a good time to review the following differences between clinical practice and clinical research with the investigator. This is particularly important if he or she is new or relatively inexperienced. Failure to understand these differences can lead to protocol violations, which could have a serious impact on the quality of the study or lead to its termination. Some of these differences are:

- During a clinical trial, the definitions used for adverse events are regulatory definitions and are not necessarily based on usual clinical observation (See Chapter 15 on adverse event reporting).
- Concomitant medications that would normally be prescribed for the subject may not be allowed by the protocol or, if allowed, the dose and regimen may differ from standard practice.

- The protocol treatment period for the disease being studied may differ from normal medical practice. It could be longer or shorter and is apt to involve more frequent visits.
- If the study is placebo-controlled, the investigator must be comfortable using placebo in subjects with the condition being studied.

Sub-Investigators

A section on the 1572 form requires the listing of all Sub-Investigators who will be involved in the study, and there have always been questions about who should be listed. In May 2010, the FDA issued a final guidance document titled, "Information Sheet Guidance for Sponsors, Clinical Investigators, and IRBs: Frequently Asked Questions—Statement of Investigator (Form FDA 1572)." This question is discussed in this document.

The guidance states that:

> The purpose of Section #6 is to capture information about individuals who, as part of an investigative team, will assist the investigator and make a direct and significant contribution to the data. The decision to list an individual in Section #6 depends on his/her level of responsibility (i.e., whether he or she is performing significant clinical investigation-related duties). In general, if an individual is directly involved in the performance of procedures required by the protocol and the collection of data, that person should be listed on the 1572. For example, if the protocol notes that each subject needs to visit a specified internist who will perform a full physical to qualify subjects for the clinical investigation, that internist should be listed in Section #6.

It goes on to say:

> Hospital staff, including nurses, residents or fellows, and office staff who provide ancillary or intermittent care but who do not make a direct and significant contribution to the clinical data do not need to be listed individually. It is not necessary to include in this section a person with only an occasional role in the conduct of the research (e.g., an on-call physician who temporarily dealt with a possible adverse effect or a temporary substitute for any research staff.)

Different sponsors and sites have had differing opinions on whether the study coordinator should be included as a sub-investigator on the 1572. The guidance document addresses this issue directly. It states:

> Generally, a research coordinator has a greater role in performing critical study functions and making direct and significant contributions to the data. For example, a research coordinator often recruits subjects, collects and evaluates study data and maintains study records. Therefore, the research coordinator should usually be listed in Section #6 of the 1572.

Staff and Facility

It is not enough for an investigator to want to do a study; sufficient staff and an appropriate facility are also necessary for success.

It is not a good idea to place a study at an investigative site that does not have a research coordinator (also called a study coordinator). The research coordinator is essential for the administration of the study; he or she coordinates patient enrollment and visits, manages the study documentation, completes the CRFs and is the primary contact for the CRA throughout the study. The CRA will want to meet and spend some time interviewing the research coordinator during the evaluation visit. If the trial calls for other specialized site personnel (a dietician or pharmacist, for example), then the CRA should ask about these people during the evaluation visit. Is the staff experienced in conducting clinical trials? Some questions to ask investigational site staff during the evaluation visit, to determine clinical research experience include:

- How many years of experience in clinical research?
- How many years of experience in the therapeutic indication under study?
- Specific questions regarding staff educational background or medical training.
- How long have investigational site staff worked at the site?

These questions will help confirm that investigational staff proposed for the study have the appropriate experience and training to conduct the study successfully.

And don't forget to ask about turnover among the staff.

Not only must there be appropriate people available for a study, but they must have sufficient time to do the necessary work. On occasion, an investigator may assure the CRA that there are plenty of people to do the work, but when the CRA talks with the research coordinator, it is apparent that there is already too much work and that adding an additional study would severely compromise the abilities of the coordinator. Are the people in the office pleasant and friendly? If you were a study subject, how would you feel about interacting with them? Determining workload, asking specific questions about the number of studies assigned to a study coordinator, working hours, support staff and roles can help determine if the addition of this study is feasible with the current workload.

CRAs need to obtain information about site recordkeeping practices (electronic or paper medical records/study documents) and the policy of CRA access to study records during monitoring visits. If a site is using an electronic medical records (EMR) system or electronic source system for study patient data and procedures, the institution's IT or medical records department may need extra time to obtain access for the CRA to a study patient's EMR or electronic source required for the monitoring visit. This may add several days or weeks to the timeframe needed for scheduling monitoring visits. This information should be clarified during evaluation visits to plan for the subsequent monitoring visit cycle.

It is important to confirm if the site has appropriate SOPs or guidelines for study conduct, such as a documented process for informed consent, GCP training, staff training, investigational product, records retention and safety reporting. This will help determine the level of research infrastructure and established process for consistent research methodology at the site.

The CRA needs to confirm who will complete study tasks and responsibilities (PI versus Sub-Investigator versus study coordinator) to ensure that the appropriately trained, delegated individuals are completing tasks commensurate to their scope of licensure and/or responsibility (e.g., if the study coordinator is drawing study blood tests, does he or she have the appropriate phlebotomy training and certification?) If the study coordinator is giving injections, does his or her license or credentials encompass this responsibility? If the study coordinator is processing and shipping study blood specimens, does he or she have updated IATA training and certification? It is important to confirm these details as they can impact study conduct with delays, certification/completion of training required to conduct these tasks or reassignment of duties to appropriate staff.

CRAs need to confirm an investigator's site, facilities and equipment during the evaluation visit to ensure they are equipped to complete all required study procedures. Examples of things to confirm during a facility tour are:

- Space to store the study drug and other supplies.
- Secure area for the study drug with adequate temperature monitoring systems and limited access to appropriate staff. (Discussions with the pharmacist or study coordinator responsible for the study drug are crucial to ensure appropriate study drug storage, documentation, dispensation and compliance practices at the site).
- Treatment areas (examination rooms, vital signs equipment, EKGs, scale, specialty equipment).
- Laboratory area for ranges, certifications, freezer, centrifuge.
- Imaging and Safety Testing (ophthalmology and pulmonary testing, for example) as required by the protocol
- Records storage area.
- Adequate monitoring area (desk or table space, chair, power outlet, fax and copy machine access, internet access).
- Adequate study coordinator working area.
- Clean and well-maintained facility.

The CRA should use a checklist, modified to study requirements, to ensure all equipment and required areas are assessed during the tour, including ancillary facilities that may be used for study evaluations, such as imaging or safety testing (dermatology, ophthalmology, etc.).

The CRA needs to determine if there are any clinic or hospital policies that would limit the CRA's ability to review source documents, such as patient charts or EMRs.

Patient/Subject Population

One of the primary problems facing the smooth execution of clinical trials is enrolling appropriate patients within the allotted enrollment time. Consequently, when interviewing possible investigators, the CRA should thoroughly

The "halving" technique

The investigator says, "I have 500 patients with the disease of interest in my practice." Your protocol has five major exclusion criteria. Cut the 500 in half for each one.

500 ▸ 250 ▸ 125 ▸ 63 ▸ 32 ▸ 15–16

This is probably about the number of subjects you can plan to enroll.

assess the enrollment potential of the site. The CRA will want to ascertain if the subjects will come from the investigator's current patient population or if they will be drawn from elsewhere. Will the investigator be able to draw patients from other physicians in the same hospital or clinic? Will the site need to advertise for patients? (Advertising will be discussed in Chapter 16.) Will the investigator be conducting any competing studies; and if so, how will the investigator demonstrate enough access to the study population at the site to adequately enroll all studies?

It is usually easier to assess enrollment potential for chronic disease studies than it is for acute disease studies. For chronic diseases such as arthritis or diabetes, the investigator should already have appropriate patients among his or her current patient base. It does not necessarily follow that these patients will qualify for or want to participate in the research study, but it provides a base from which to start. For acute studies, one must rely on past statistics. For example, if a pneumonia study is being discussed, the CRA will want to know how many patients with pneumonia the investigator saw over the past year. In either case, the more thorough the records are concerning the patient population, the better the enrollment estimates will be.

The CRA needs to assess who will be identifying/recruiting for patients, such as dedicated recruitment staff or study coordinators. The CRA needs to assess how the PI and his recruitment staff communicate and methods used to identify patients (review of the EMRs, medical records, review of the clinicians practice schedules, utilization of recruitment companies, internet searches, email or paper correspondence to study patients). A successful site will have a diversity of enrollment tactics specific to their site model and target demographic.

Unfortunately, estimates of subject enrollment are almost always too high. Some CRAs use the "halving" technique to arrive at a final estimate: For each major exclusion criteria in the protocol, cut the original number of patients in half. The final number will be much closer to the enrollment you can actually expect to achieve.

During the pandemic, patients for COVID studies were identified from investigator or institution relationships with COVID testing facilities, positive COVID test results from hospitals with which the investigators were affiliated, etc. This has evolved to include COVID studies that allow the use of rapid COVID testing.

Miscellaneous Factors

There are several other items a CRA will want to discuss during an evaluation visit. One is whether or not the site is conducting, or is planning to conduct within the same time period, any competing studies. A competing study is usually one in which similar subjects are to be enrolled. In order to meet the enrollment targets, it's important that your study does not have to compete for subjects with another sponsor's study. In assessing competing studies, it is not enough to assess only those studies being done at the investigator's site, but those being done in the same community. Those studies will also be in competition for subjects and can have a great impact on the ability to meet enrollment targets.

Another factor is the timing for the study. If the site has too many active studies at the same time, your study may not get the attention it needs to be conducted well.

The CRA also needs to confirm whether any regulatory agency or FDA audits of the investigator or site have occurred, and whether a 483 was issued for any audit findings. All accompanying FDA audit documents and site audit responses/corrective action need to be obtained and reviewed by the CRAs during the site evaluation process because this can influence the selection decision, especially if the audit findings were significant. The CRA can also check the FDA website and the clinical investigator inspection list, to determine if a PI has been audited by the FDA and if a 483 was issued.

The CRA should be certain that the investigator is familiar with the IRB process and should determine which IRB will be used for the study. How often does the IRB meet and how long does it usually take for the IRB to review and approve a study? The time it takes to review and approve a study or documents related to a study is called "turnaround time."

Some preliminary budget discussions can take place at an evaluation visit. The CRA can discuss with the investigator how the sponsor prefers to work with respect to the budget and payments for trials. The CRA may also want to find out how the investigator normally puts together a budget. If the site looks promising, it might be appropriate to talk about the grant range the company is willing to pay to ensure that both parties are at least in the same ballpark. Details can be left until the CRA is sure that the site is desirable to use for the study.

The CRA should be sure that a thorough evaluation of the site has been made before leaving, including notes for future reference to include in the required pre-study visit report/recommendation. It is appropriate to send a thank you letter to the site within a few days of the visit. If the investigator is selected to do the study, a telephone call can be made to finalize the site's willingness to participate, followed by a confirmation letter.

Pre-study Visit

If a study starts soon after an evaluation visit for a selected investigator, the evaluation information is current. Sometimes, however, several months can pass between the evaluation visit and the actual start date for a study. In this case, it can be valuable to do a pre-study visit to reevaluate the site's capability to do the trial. This visit does not vary much in content from the evaluation visit, except that the investigator is already committed to conduct the trial. The purpose of the visit is to assure the sponsor that the site is still appropriate for the work.

At this meeting, the CRA should take time to go over the protocol in detail with the investigator. Does the investigator have a good understanding of what needs to be done, when it needs to be done, subjects that are suitable, etc.? Has the investigator changed his or her mind about any aspects of the medicine or clinical aspects involved? Are there any problems with using a placebo control or with using the comparator medicine? Sometimes if there has been quite a long time between when the protocol was written and when the study is due to start, other new medications might have become standard treatment for a condition and physicians may not want to use an older drug as a comparator in a trial.

Pay close attention to the investigator's attitude, interest and reactions during your discussions. The investigator may be saying one thing but communicating something much different. Interpreting nonverbal clues takes experience and good human relations skills; over time, a CRA can become very adept at "reading" people.

It is much better for an investigator to back out of a program before it starts than to fail at it later. An experienced CRA will let investigators know that saying a project is not right for his or her site is not a negative; saying it can be done and then not following through means a sponsor rarely will come back.

Reassess the staff and their ability to do the study at this visit. Are the same people at the site? Has there been any major staff turnover? Ask the investigator and the staff if there are plans for anyone to be away for an extended period of time during the study—you might be surprised by what you hear.

Check again for competing studies. The site may have started other studies in the several months that have passed since the last evaluation visit It is important to ascertain if these studies will be competing with your study for patients, coordinator time or other resources.

Be sure that the facilities are still acceptable, including storage areas for the study medication and supplies. Ensure that the pharmacy and laboratory are aware of and ready to handle their study responsibilities. If a pharmacy is to be used, find out how much storage area it has for the study drug. It may be necessary to make multiple drug shipments over time instead of sending it all at once if space is limited. (Space in pharmacies is almost always at a premium.) Be sure that the storage requirements for the study drug are clearly understood and that appropriate storage conditions are available. If, for example, your drug requires refrigeration, there should be enough capacity to store an adequate supply of the drug.

The CRA should discuss with the investigator the subject population for the study. This is a good time to review the inclusion and exclusion criteria of the protocol in detail. There may have been changes in the physician's practice since the last evaluation that could adversely affect the site's ability to enroll subjects in the trial.

Hopefully you will have all the documents necessary to start the study in-house by this time; but if not, try to collect the rest of them at this visit. If the IRB has approved the study, the investigator should have a copy of the approval letter. Retrieve a copy for your company while you are at the site if you do not have it already. If the study has not yet been approved by the IRB, find out when the IRB is meeting and when approval can be expected. If there have been any changes in the study team personnel, be sure that the correct people are listed on the 1572 form. If they are not, have the site revise the 1572 and give you a copy while you are there.

Usually the grant for the study has been agreed upon prior to this visit but, if not, now is the time. You don't want any last-minute delays in a study initiation because of stalled grant negotiations. Large organizations (hospitals, university medical centers) may have a separate office that handles grants and contracts. If so, the savvy CRA will get to know this office staff, which may smooth the way for speedier negotiations.

The bottom line is whether you still feel comfortable about using this site for your study. If you are having doubts, pay attention to them. Chances are that if something doesn't feel quite right, it isn't. You will always come out ahead dealing with problems before the study starts rather than later.

If the evaluation and any pre-study visits have gone well, if you have thoroughly and accurately assessed the site's ability to complete your study and if you feel comfortable about conducting a study at the site, you have done the best you can to ensure a successful study start.

Key Takeaways

- The investigator is the individual who actually conducts and is responsible for a clinical investigation.
- The Statement of Investigator (FDA form 1572) contains pertinent investigator and site information, as well as a listing of investigator responsibilities. The signed investigator agreement is the equivalent document for device trials.
- Investigators have the ultimate responsibility for the safety of subjects in a clinical trial.
- Investigators must be qualified by training and experience to study a drug or device.
- The investigator must have a suitable facility and qualified staff for study conduct.

- Investigators may be disqualified if they do not comply with the regulations concerning clinical research, or if they falsify data or reports of the trial.
- Some of the best ways to locate potential investigators are:
  - Databases maintained within your own company.
  - Suggestions from current investigators.
  - Colleagues from other companies.
- Most CROs have feasibility departments dedicated to finding and confirming an investigator's preliminary capabilities for study participation and readiness for a site evaluation visit.
- A site evaluation visit is the best way to assess a site's capability to conduct a clinical trial.
- A pre-study visit should be done to reassess a site if there has been a long time between the evaluation visit and the start date for a study.

CHAPTER 13

Study Initiation

This chapter discusses a number of activities that must be completed before a study site can begin enrolling subjects. Topics include: study initiation documents, financial disclosure, investigator meetings, study initiation meetings, investigator study files and grants, and contracts. CRAs are very involved in these activities and need to have a thorough understanding of them.

Study Initiation Documents

Before a trial can begin, a number of documents must be collected for each site. Most of these are required by FDA regulations, although some sponsors may require their own additional documents. Both the sponsor and the investigator must have copies of each document; usually, the originals are kept at the investigator's site while copies are sent to the sponsor. It is recommended that the CRA also keep copies of most of them, in case one is misplaced or disappears and needs to be replaced during the study. The documents listed below are what a sponsor must have before the trial may start. Note that most sponsors will not ship the study drug before receiving all of the documents.

- Signed IRB-approved protocol and any amendments.
- IRB-approved informed consent, preferably containing an IRB-approved stamp.
- IRB approval letter, verifying approval of both the protocol and consent document.
- IRB approval of advertising and subject recruitment materials including subject compensation, if applicable.
- Signed, completed FDA Form 1572 (Statement of Investigator). (Note: for device studies, form 1572 is not used; instead the sponsor

obtains a signed agreement from the investigator that includes statements similar to those on form 1572.)

- Financial disclosure forms for the investigator and any other study personnel listed on form 1572.
- Appropriate CVs of everyone listed on form 1572.
- Current laboratory certification and laboratory normal ranges.
- Signed contract or letter of agreement (not required by regulation, but required by most sponsors).

Some sponsors have specific employees whose primary responsibility is to work with sites in collecting, submitting and maintaining these documents (central IRB submissions). In other companies, the CRAs gather the documents for their sites. The CRA is the person who visits the site, so he or she will probably be involved in the collection and maintenance of documents even if another internal group has primary responsibility.

The document that generally takes the longest time to receive is the IRB approval letter. This is the only document not under the direct control of the investigator. The IRB may have approved the study, but until the investigator receives written notification, it is not official. The CRA may need to encourage the investigator to keep contacting the IRB, as some are slow to issue approval letters.

Most sponsors will not ship the study drug until all the documents have been received. Note that some companies do ship nondrug supplies, lab kits, and CRFs if applicable before receiving all the documents in an effort to speed up the process, while others wait and ship everything only after documentation is complete.

Financial Disclosure

In 1998, the FDA published a final rule on financial disclosures by clinical investigators. This requirement became effective in 1999 and applies to any study of a drug, biologic or device that is used to support a marketing application (21 CFR 54). The regulation requires that sponsors certify the absence of certain financial interests of clinical investigators, disclose these financial interests or certify that the information was impossible to obtain. If a sponsor does not do this, the FDA may refuse to file the application.

In a February 2013 guidance on financial disclosure by clinical investigators, the FDA noted that the dollar amounts that trigger reporting are the combined financial interests of the investigator, spouse and dependent children, including:

- Any compensation made to the investigator by any sponsor of the covered clinical study in which the value of compensation could be affected by study outcome.
- A proprietary interest in the tested product including, but not limited to, a patent, trademark, copyright or licensing agreement.
- Any equity interest in any sponsor of the covered clinical study (i.e., any ownership interest, stock options or other financial interest whose value cannot be readily determined through reference to public prices). The requirement applies to interests held during the time the clinical investigator is carrying out the study and for one year following completion of the study.
- Any equity interest in any sponsor of the covered study if the sponsor is a publicly held company and the interest exceeds $50,000 in value. The requirement applies to interests held during the time the clinical investigator is carrying out the study and for one year following completion of the study.
- Significant payments of other sorts (SPOOS) that have a cumulative monetary value of $25,000 or more and are made by any sponsor of a covered study to the investigator or the investigator's institution during the time the clinical investigator is carrying out the study and for one year following completion of the study. This would include payments that support activities of the investigator (e.g., a grant to the investigator or to the institution to fund the investigator's ongoing research or compensation in the form of equipment), exclusive of the costs of conducting the clinical study or other clinical studies, or to provide other reimbursements, such as retainers for ongoing consultation or honoraria. See Section IV, Questions C.4, C.5, and C.6 for additional information on SPOOS.

A financial interest in a company or product does not mean that an investigator cannot be involved in a trial; it simply means that all parties must be aware of the potential for conflict of interest. The sponsor will want to evaluate the potential for bias based on an investigator's financial interest before deciding whether or not to use that investigator. The FDA will do the same when reviewing an NDA.

Financial disclosure applies to all of the people listed on form 1572 for a study, plus their spouses and dependent children. This is a good reason to not list unnecessary people on the 1572 form.

Financial disclosure information must be collected at the start of the study. Any changes that result in exceeding the threshold(s) must be reported during the course of the study and for one year following its completion. There is no required form for the collection of this information from the investigator. Consequently, sponsors develop their own forms and ways of collecting and maintaining this information.

Financial disclosure information must be reported to the FDA on FDA forms 3454 (certification of absence of financial interest) or 3455 (disclosure of financial interest). These forms are submitted as a part of the NDA.

Although not popular with investigators or sponsors, financial disclosure information is required to be collected, and usually CRAs are involved in its collection. Because of their involvement, it is recommended that CRAs read the FDA guidance on financial disclosure, referenced at the start of this section, which is available on the FDA's website.

The Investigator Meeting

For a clinical trial with six or more sites, most sponsors hold an investigator meeting. Although not required by regulation, this meeting, which includes all investigators, their coordinators and appropriate sponsor representatives, is one of the most important activities pertaining to the conduct of a good trial. This meeting is often the first time the investigators and study coordinators meet the sponsor personnel; it creates an initial impression and sets the tone for the rest of the study.

Investigator meetings may also be web-based virtual meetings, which are more cost effective and less time-consuming than traditional investigator meetings that require attendees to take time off of work (which is difficult for physician investigators with private practices and other employees with large workloads) and travel to an agreed-upon meeting site to attend. The PI typically only needs to give 3-4 hours to attend their required portion of the meeting, with a larger commitment from the study coordinator or research staff. The downside to web-based investigator meetings is that they may be less interactive and engaging for those who prefer live meetings. During COVID, all in-person meetings were cancelled due to social distancing restrictions. Resuming in-person meetings was a very positive and gratifying experience for investigational site staff forced to work remotely for more than a year due to the pandemic.

Investigator meetings may be held when there are fewer than six sites, depending on the complexity of the study. Six sites in a clinical trial is merely a rule of thumb. Some investigator meetings include 200 or 300 people, if the trial is very large. Frequently, if the meeting were to be very large (e.g., over 150 attendees), two or three smaller meetings would be held instead. Smaller meetings allow for more opportunity for questions and interaction among the participants. These smaller meetings may be held regionally to lessen travel. Division may also be based on which sites are ready to start the study and which sites still have documents outstanding. It is also common to hold an investigator meeting specific to participating countries or regions; North America, EMEA, Asia Pacific. These are also impacted by when the study conduct is approved for a country.

Investigator meetings are scheduled and conducted by the sponsor (sometimes with the help of a contract company). The purpose of these meetings is to allow participants to get to know one another, which facilitates communication throughout the study. It is also an opportunity for the sponsor and investigator/staff attendees to review study design, conduct and all study information and engage in question answer/informative discussions. The major advantages of holding these meetings are that everyone hears the same thing at the same time and people become acquainted. If done properly, the investigator meeting can also be a powerful motivational and training tool.

Due to the meeting's importance to the success of a trial and frequent involvement of CRAs in these meetings, both in the planning stages and as attendees, the investigator meeting will be discussed in further detail.

There are a number of items that require serious thought and planning when it comes to investigator meetings. These include when to hold the meeting, the location, who should attend, social activities and the agenda.

Author's Story

I will never forget my first investigator meeting. It was in the Spring of 2000 and I had only been a study coordinator for two months. My PI informed me we were going to an investigator's meeting in Orlando and I was so excited. We booked our travel, I reviewed the protocol and all study documents to prepare, and then the day before the meeting my PI informed me that she would be unable to attend due to a family emergency. She, however, still wanted me to attend, which worried me to no end. How could I attend this meeting without her when I was brand new to my role as a study coordinator and still had no idea what I was doing (or so I thought). My PI told me I would be fine (she had way too much confidence in me) and on to Orlando I went. On the plane, I met another study coordinator from San Diego, who served as my unofficial escort and mentor throughout the meeting. She was kind, supportive and funny and made the time pass wonderfully. Though I was intimidated, the meeting was very interesting and the sponsor personnel were friendly and informative. Meeting other investigators and study coordinators really validated my decision to enter the industry and helped me realize just how important this work was. I stayed in touch with the study coordinator who befriended me and 15 years later loosely based a character on her in the clinical research novella I wrote about being a study coordinator. Relationships in clinical research can develop into friendships that mentor and support us in the most challenging times.

–Elizabeth

Timing and Location of Investigator Meetings

The first decision to be made is when to have the investigator meeting. These meetings are expensive, so CRAs must make every effort to ensure that all their sites are ready to start the study before the meeting. Sites that start the study more than a month or two after the investigator meeting may need to be refreshed on much of the information before work can begin. Ideally, the study drug is shipped while the meeting is taking place and the motivated investigators and their coordinators return home to immediately enroll the first patients. Unfortunately, this rarely, if ever, happens.

A nearly impossible task involves gathering numerous sites for a multi-center trial that are ready to start at the same time. Given this scenario, the sponsor should try to hold the investigator meeting when as many sites as possible are ready to start and within a month of when the last site will be ready. The problem of determining when to hold the meeting is compounded by the fact that the meeting has to be planned so far in advance that good estimates of site readiness may not be available.

The meeting location requires a balance between business and pleasure. Everyone wants to go to a nice place for a meeting, preferably warm, with lots of things to do or see. However, from a business standpoint, the ideal place is probably at the sponsor company or at least in the same town.

If the meeting is held at the sponsor's primary location, there will be few budget restrictions on company representatives attending. Consequently, all the clerical personnel needed to make things run smoothly will be available. It will also be possible to have the professional support needed from groups such as Quality Assurance and Regulatory who attend infrequently when travel is involved. CRAs not involved with the study and other clinical or support people can attend as a learning or training experience. In addition, the investigators and coordinators can see the company and meet more employees than they would if the meeting were held elsewhere.

Another popular location for the investigator's meeting is at a large hotel near the airport of a large, centrally located city. A centrally located hub city is very convenient for attendees flying in from various areas across the country and for those who can only attend part of the meeting. These venues are sometimes less costly and provide less distractions for attendees as opposed to holding the meeting at an elegant downtown hotel or historic site.

Planning and Logistics

Once the date and location have been determined, it's time to start making arrangements. Many sponsors have meeting planners who put these meetings together, so CRAs are not usually involved in this aspect. If you have input, remember that the meeting should be informative, yet pleasant, for those attending.

An agenda and general information regarding transportation, hotel information (swimming, tennis, golf, etc.) and reimbursement procedures should be sent to all investigators at least a month prior to the meeting. If the sponsor is arranging travel, travel plans/itineraries should be sent well in advance of the meeting date. Additional information and handout materials should be available for participants when they check into the hotel.

One important consideration to keep in mind is the duration of the meeting. One day is usually sufficient unless it is a large, complicated trial. Physicians may not be able to afford to be away from the office for more than one day. If one day is sufficient, the meeting could be held on the same day or split between the afternoon of one day and the morning of the next. Each has its advantages and disadvantages. Many prefer the split-day format as it allows attendees to arrive the morning of the first day and because it is split into two shorter sessions. If the agenda is planned properly, investigators may leave after the afternoon session if they need to. The primary disadvantage is that there is little time to relax or rest prior to the start of the meeting and it may make leaving that same night difficult. Airline departures and connections for investigators must also be considered.

It is appropriate to plan a social event, such as a dinner or reception, so the site and sponsor staff can get to know each other in a less formal environment.

Another meeting option that has become more popular in recent years, is to host a welcome dinner the evening prior to the meeting. This presents a less formal "first meeting" for investigators and CRO/sponsor personnel, and the dinner is an entertaining ice breaker to an otherwise formalized, sometimes rigidly structured, meeting.

Table 1 summarizes the major activities required in planning. Note that planning starts about four months in advance of the actual meeting date. The bigger the meeting, the more time it will take to plan and execute the preliminary activities.

Table 1: Example of protocol activity schedule

Study activity	Month 4	Month 3	Month 2	Month 1
Budget	✓			
Select location	✓			
Contact hotels	✓			
Prepare reference/instruction manuals		✓		
Letter of invitiation		✓		
Rooming lists/requirements			✓	
Final agenda				✓
Follow up letter with agenda				✓
Rehersal				✓
Meal selections/reception				✓
Ship materials to hotel				✓
Final transportation reservations				✓

Preparation for Meeting Presentations

Frequently, presentations held during investigator meetings get the least attention, which can spell disaster. First, the person presenting material from the sponsor must be determined. If key personnel from the sponsor choose not to present, a replacement must be found. It is hoped that said key personnel will attend the meeting regardless.

Remember, Chapter 1 stressed that good CRAs must have good communication skills. Investigator meetings are one activity for which that is very important. CRAs frequently present topics during the meeting. If you are asked to do this, you should be prepared and follow basic presentation procedures (e.g., speak clearly, engage the audience, practice pronunciations [this is critical] and use visual materials effectively).

Another key part of preparation is rehearsal, a full run-through. Unfortunately, very few companies take the time to do this. At a minimum, everyone who will be attending the meeting should be present for the rehearsal so that everyone gets a chance to hear what the others have to say before the meeting.

One of the most embarrassing things that could happen at an investigator meeting is the possibility of the speaker being interrupted by one of his colleagues who says, "That's not right, we don't want it done that way." Not only could it be embarrassing for the presenter but the sponsor representatives, as a group, very well may immediately lose credibility. Rehearsals can help prevent embarrassing situations.

Another benefit of a rehearsal is that it allows the presenters to run through their material in front of an audience and check the timing, both for individual presentations and the entirety of the meeting. This allows for editing and overall planning.

The rehearsal should be open to people other than the attendees, because it is a good learning opportunity for less experienced employees and will help prepare them to become involved as a presenter, if they so choose. Everyone, including CRAs, should try to attend a rehearsal or an actual meeting before having to organize and/or participate in one. It is also valuable to have some experienced people from other units or divisions attend to act as advisors. Their experience and ability to look at presentations with a fresh view are very useful.

It is recommended that a moderator be used for an investigator meeting. Companies that use moderators seem to hold better meetings. The moderator should be a good speaker and a "people person." He or she usually opens the meeting, makes introductory remarks about the company, gives an overview of the meeting, makes administrative announcements, introduces company speakers and injects humor when appropriate. The moderator is a huge asset in regard to keeping the meeting running smoothly and on time; this allows the medical monitor and other presenters to concentrate on their

Table 2: Investigator meeting agenda—Basic

- Introduction of attendees
- Introductory remarks about the company in general
- Background of the project
- Discussion of the protocol
- Administrative responsibilities of investigator and sponsor (and/or CRO) personnel involved in the study
- Sponsor procedures and expectations
  - Monitoring
  - Data collection
  - Adverse event reporting
  - Other sponsor-specific issues
- Financial matters
- Miscellaneous

Table 3: Investigator meeting agenda—Expanded

- Welcome
  - Introductions
    - The company (very brief overview)
    - Individuals and their roles
    - Investigators and their staff members
- Overview of the drug development program (include significant timelines, dates)
- Discussion of the protocol (avoid a page-by-page review)
  - Objectives
  - Study overview
  - Main protocol areas
  - Design
    - Primary efficacy endpoints
    - Entry criteria
    - Drug (formulation, dosing and regimen)
    - Risk/benefit
    - Medical events
    - Methods and materials
    - Any special procedures that may be required
- Administration
  - Responsibilities and obligations of the investigator
  - Informed consent
  - The IRB
  - Forms requiring signatures
  - Study documents
    - Protocol, IRB approvals, etc., and filing requirements
  - Financial matters
- Study Materials
  - Clinical supplies
    - Packaging, ordering and receipts (have sample packages if there is anything unique or unusual)
    - Drug accountability
    - Drug-dispensing procedure, forms
    - Reorder procedure
    - Storage
    - Inventory and return
- Laboratory
  - Exhibit forms, supplies, mailers, etc.
  - Demonstrate any unusual procedures
- Special Procedures and Forms
  - Diaries (if used)
  - Demonstrate special medical procedures if appropriate (treadmill, Holter monitor, etc.)
  - Training, rater certification
  - Procedures for randomization and breaking the blind
- Case Report Forms
  - Design
  - How/when to complete
  - Source document management
  - Correction procedures
- Closing remarks and questions

presentations and on meeting the investigators and coordinators without having to worry about logistical matters.

The Agenda

There is no one agenda that fits all investigator meetings. However, they will almost always contain the items shown in Table 2. An example of an expanded agenda is shown in Table 3. These can be used as starting points for planning a meeting, with other items added and deleted as appropriate.

Attendees

Who should attend investigator meetings? Key people from both the sponsor and the sites should be there; other attendees may be determined by the budget. Table 4 shows the usual cast of mandatory and optional attendees from both the sponsor and investigative sites.

Remember that one important purpose of the meeting is for sponsor personnel and site personnel to become acquainted. Sometimes, the CRAs are the only people who know attendees in both groups before the meeting. The CRA should take responsibility for the people attending from his or her sites. The CRA should also ensure that the investigators and coordinators are introduced to the appropriate sponsor representatives they may come in contact with during the study. Taking care of them includes ensuring that they have all meeting materials and that they have an informative meeting. If site personnel have any unanswered questions at the end of the meeting, the CRA should get the information to them within a few days.

As a CRA, you should act as the host for your sites. Let the physicians and the coordinators know they are critical to the success of your study. Ask your site people questions and listen to the answers. Spend time with them. This meeting is an excellent opportunity to establish good relationships with your site personnel, which can make the study go smoothly for you as it gets underway.

The CRA attending the investigator meeting must remember that this is a professional, work-related meeting; this is not an opportunity for a mini vacation. The CRA MUST act professionally at all times. Most CRO/sponsor companies have a maximum 1-2 alcoholic beverage per day rule for personnel traveling for business meetings (after work hours or for social dinners with clients), and this is a smart rule to follow during investigator meetings to ensure

Table 4: Investigator meeting attendees

Investigator site attendees

Mandatory attendees	Optional attendees
• Investigator • Clinical research coordinator	• Co-investigator • Research manager • Pharmacists • Dietician • Others as appropriate

Sponsor attendees

Mandatory attendees	Optional attendees
• Investigator • CRA(s) • Biostatistician • Project manager • Data manager • Laboratory person (usually from a central lab) • Moderator, if one is used • Designated presenters • Meeting facilitator, if needed	• Management (Medical director, etc.) • Other monitors, CRAs • Regulatory representative • QA person • Secretary • Consultants, if appropriate

appropriate behavior. Never forget that you are the sponsor representative, and your behavior will be scrutinized.

Evaluation and Critique

It is important to evaluate how the investigator meeting went and was perceived. To help with this, it is useful to have evaluation forms for attendees to complete. They do not need to be complicated. Sample evaluation forms are shown in Tables 5a and 5b.

Table 5a: Investigator meeting evaluation form

Protocol:______________________________ Date:__________

Please complete this form before you leave to help us evaluate and improve our meetings. (Include instructions for where to leave the form.) If you forget, please mail it to us at: (insert address)

Please rate the level of satisfaction with the facility:	High				Low
Accommodations	5	4	3	2	1
Food	5	4	3	2	1
Meeting room	5	4	3	2	1
Location	5	4	3	2	1
Meeting planning:	High				Low
Pre-meeting communication	5	4	3	2	1
Organization of meeting	5	4	3	2	1
Agenda	5	4	3	2	1

- ☐ Too long
- ☐ Too short
- ☐ Too little (much) time on some items (specify)

Sessions of least value:______________________________

Sessions of most value:______________________________

Suggestions for improvement:______________________________

After each investigator meeting, the sponsor should create a critique of the meeting, including a discussion of the evaluations. This should help in determining what was done well and should be incorporated at future meetings, as well as what should be changed or eliminated. Reviewing past meetings is an excellent tool for improving future meetings; each meeting should be better than the last one.

Table 5b: Session evaluations

Session:________________________________ Presented by:__________________

Please rate the presenter of this session in the following areas:

	High				Low
Speaking quality	5	4	3	2	1
Adequately established objectives at the beginning of the session	5	4	3	2	1
Presented material in a clear understandable manner	5	4	3	2	1
Material was in a logical sequence	5	4	3	2	1
Provided useful information	5	4	3	2	1
Effective use of audiovisual aids	5	4	3	2	1
Adequately summarized material	5	4	3	2	1
Provided adequate opportunity for participation/questions	5	4	3	2	1
Responded satisfactorily to questions and comments	5	4	3	2	1

Comments:____

Study Initiation Meetings

The study initiation visit (SIV) is held at the investigative site just before the study begins. The CRA (and sometimes additional sponsor personnel) will meet with the investigator, the study coordinator and the supporting staff. The purpose of the meeting is to review the study protocol, processes and procedures to ensure that all site personnel understand what is necessary to perform the study. It is an extremely important visit as it is truly the teaching visit to confirm all aspects of study conduct, to verify study supplies/IP receipt, systems access and equipment readiness. Adequate preparation by all participants is crucial for the success of the SIV.

The study initiation should be held at the point when all regulatory paperwork is complete for the site and the study drug and other supplies have been shipped, but before any subjects have been enrolled. Many sponsors will not allow the site to begin enrollment until after this meeting is held.

Deadlines are critical for cost effective site activation and study start-up. Even the slightest delay may have far reaching financial implications and cost thousands of dollars in recovery. The integration of computer systems and web-based portals into study start-up activities has made a once-convoluted process more efficient, reducing timelines and costs associated with site activation. Examples include:

- Centralized portals or databases that facilitate real-time creation and submission of essential regulatory documents between site or sponsor/CRO staff; documents are shared/edited in real-time in the database; edit changes are documented and are communicated via system-generated emails.
- Electronic submission of protocols, ICFs and accompanying documents to IRBs via a centralized portal or IRB website save time and money by circumventing the need for staff to print hundreds of copies of documents for IRB review, and it makes the IRB submission a "rolling" submission as opposed to the historical 2-3-week submission deadline prior to the IRB meeting.
- Site systems access and supplies receipt are tracked centrally at the sponsor/CRO.
- Electronic trial master files (regulatory files) for both the sponsor and site that hold the essential documents for a study filed electronically. Site staff upload essential documents to their electronic files with ease; CRAs are granted access to a site's electronic files before and during monitoring visits to facilitate document review and retrieval. CRAs are able to take pictures of and scan regulatory documents to electronic regulatory files with designated software from their smart phone during monitoring visits, saving valuable time and money by circumventing the need for copies.

The CRA must be flexible when it comes to scheduling the SIV; to maximize attendance, it may need to be held early in the morning or in the evening. A thorough, informative SIV may take half a day or even longer for a very complicated study.

The CRA is almost always in charge of the initiation meeting, although the sponsor's medical monitor and/or an in-house associate monitor may also be present. It is important that all involved site personnel attend the meeting, to include ancillary personnel such as the sub-investigators, other coordinators, pharmacist, dietician, etc.

If the investigator and coordinator attended an investigator meeting, the initiation visit will serve as a review and amplification of the topics covered during that meeting. If there was no investigator meeting, or if it was held a month or more prior to initiating the study, then the entire protocol, processes and procedure should be discussed in detail. The investigator and study coordinator are usually the only site people who attend the investigator meeting, so other site personnel will not be as familiar with the study. The initiation meeting provides an opportunity for those at the site to become familiar with the study and to understand everyone's study role.

Preparing for the SIV

The purpose of the SIV is to train study staff on protocol and procedures. It is a teaching visit and involves extensive preparation by the CRA conducting the visit; how the site staff comprehend and apply the principles learned will influence study performance and outcome. The CRA should think about how to conduct the meeting and what should be addressed. On occasion, the sponsor's medical monitor, project manager or recruitment liaison will want to attend the meeting, particularly if it is the first time the investigator has done work for the sponsor. In this case, the CRA will need to determine what roles these individuals would like/expect to play and plan accordingly. However, the CRA should act as the "lead" of the SIV and ensure coordination of travel times, meeting times and communications between the sponsor personnel attending, the internal study team and site personnel, to ensure all are on the same page and understand their responsibilities. The CRA must prepare an agenda. Much of the same material will be covered at the initiation meeting as was covered at the investigator meeting, if one was held. The agenda and the amount of detail to be covered at the initiation visit will depend on: if there was an investigator meeting and who attended; how long it has been since the investigator meeting was held; the involvement of other personnel at the site (pharmacist, etc.); the complexity of the program; and how much time you are allowed for the meeting.

The preparation that occurs ahead of the visit is extensive and critical. The CRA is involved with confirming the site's receipt of the regulatory binder, study supplies, lab supplies, any study-specific equipment being furnished, electronic systems access, etc. This requires consistent communication, response, follow-thorough and documentation.

The items to be covered at an initiation meeting are:

- Detailed discussion of the protocol, including:
  - Overview of study drug or medical device.
  - Inclusion and exclusion criteria.
  - Study rationale and procedures.
  - Study endpoints and objectives.
  - Administration of the study drug.
  - Randomization and blinding.
  - Primary outcome measures.
  - Review of the study schedule of assessments
  - Other pertinent details.
- Drug accountability.
- Adverse event reporting.
  - CRFs, eCRF/EDC systems (review of the CRF completion guidelines, logging into the EDC system to ensure access is granted to site personnel), going over each unique form or field in detail, including how to avoid errors. (See more about this in Chapter 14, "Monitoring.")
- Monitoring visits—the study monitoring model, how often, what should be ready, what will be covered.
- Regulatory requirements.
  - Investigator responsibilities.
  - IRB interactions.
  - Informed consent.
  - HIPAA, confidentiality.
  - ICH/GCP.
- Source documents/ALCOA-CCEA.

- Completion/signature of study documents such as the training log, attendee log, delegation of authority/site signature log, and any sponsor-specific investigator agreements required to be retrieved.
- Any other study-specific or sponsor-specific items of importance.
  - Periodic reports of enrollment.
- Overview of vendors participating/completing assessments/assessment requirements (central imaging, central lab, central EKG, central spirometry, central rating scales, etc.).
- Confirmation of user access and familiarity for any specific sponsor/vendor systems used, such as safety portals, central lab website, central vendor websites (ECG, ECHO, Imaging) to ensure user access and uploading capabilities are confirmed.
- Confirmation of site equipment and facility (tour of departments, pharmacy, lab, clinic areas, etc.).

It is recommended that the CRA rehearse before the meeting to check timing, word pronunciation and to be sure the material is clear and understood. It is embarrassing to find out that you don't understand or can't pronounce something at the time of your presentation. There is nothing harder than explaining a process to someone else when you don't understand it yourself.

If the CRA is not comfortable with any of the study procedures, he or she should ask for help and/or clarification before the meeting. For example, if the CRA is not comfortable with the data management and correction process, it should be reviewed with the data management people supporting the study.

If a study instruction manual has been developed, the CRA should be familiar with what is in it and how the site is expected to use it; if the site does not have one yet, plan to take it with you to the meeting. (Note: The study instruction manual is simply a guide for sites that explains study procedures in detail. It is a quick reference and will usually include practical hints and tips that would not be found in a protocol.}

The remote monitor will also help with the meeting to:

- Ensure that regulatory binders, lab kits and required supplies have been ordered for the site.
- Ensure that the study drug is in route prior to the meeting.

- Obtain any last-minute regulatory documents to release study drug.
- Order account and system log-in credentials for sites, etc.

During the SIV

This meeting involves several people. Since the CRA is the SIV lead, he or she should always be at least 20 minutes early to the SIV to ensure any set up of equipment is completed in a timely manner or to ensure all materials have been received (slides and protocol emailed to the site). Some sites have a large video screen or wall they want the CRA to use for study presentations to investigational site staff. This requires some set up between the CRA's laptop and the screen. These AV connections may be challenging and you need to ensure there is enough time allotted for these situations. Investigational site staff do not expect the CRA to be a whiz at AV connections and will have an appropriate person help with the screen set up. If you have a morning meeting and it's out of town, plan to arrive the day before. Be sure you know where you are going and how long it will take to get there to allow for problems like morning rush hour traffic. Depending on the time of day, it is a nice gesture to provide coffee or other refreshments; this should be approved by the sponsor or company management prior to the meeting.

Begin by expressing your pleasure at attending and your enthusiasm to begin working on the study. Leave time for introductions and then start the agenda.

It is important that people know they can ask questions as the meeting progresses. The main purpose of the meeting is for everyone to have a clear understanding of what is involved in conducting the study. It is far better to answer questions now than to have things completed incorrectly later. Take your time. Solicit questions periodically. Look around and see if people look perplexed or comfortable. This is an instance when a CRA's interpersonal skills are critical.

If certain attendees are not able to stay for the entire meeting (investigator, pharmacist), be sure to cover items critical to their participation while they are there. Other items, such as reviewing CRFs or systems used can be covered with the coordinators (and others who may be involved) in a smaller group.

When the formal presentation part of the meeting is complete, there are some additional activities the CRA should do before leaving. One is to check the study drug and other study supplies to be certain they arrived in good condition and are appropriate and in the proper quantities. If computer equipment was provided, be sure it is in order, set up properly and working. Check with the pharmacy to be sure that it understands the drug dispensing, if appropriate. Check the investigator's study file to be sure that all the necessary documents are present and correct. If the file has not yet been set up, the CRA can help with this. (See next section, "Investigator Study Files."). Confirm the study coordinators have started completing the required documents, if not already done (including the training log, attendance log, delegation of authority log and any other required forms).

Once everything has been covered, the CRA should be sure to thank everyone involved before leaving. One of the important intangibles at this meeting is the opportunity it gives the CRA to establish good working relationships with all of the site personnel. Do everything possible to make the people at the site feel good about you, the study and the sponsor. This will pay huge dividends as the study progresses.

After the meeting, the CRA must complete a visit report detailing what was discussed and completed during the visit. Many companies have a specific database or program for creating and writing monitoring visit reports and site communications. ICH guidelines call for a trial initiation monitoring report that documents that trial procedures were covered with the investigator and his or her staff; this report is to be kept in both the sponsor and investigator study files. The same can be accomplished by sending the investigator a letter listing what was covered during the meeting.

If questions arose during the meeting that need further follow-up, the CRA must be sure to get the needed answers and relay them to the site. A written thank you letter is a nice gesture on the part of the CRA.

Conducting this meeting well will go a long way toward helping the site complete a successful study. It deserves the full attention of the CRA.

Investigator Study/Regulatory Files

Either before or during the initiation meeting, the CRA should discuss with the investigator and coordinator how to establish and maintain an investigator study file. This file will have a significant impact on the quality assurance for a study and, subsequently, the validity and usability of the data.

If the site is experienced, this will be a routine activity. If the site is new or relatively new, the CRA should be prepared to recommend how the files should be organized and instruct the site regarding the documents that must be maintained in the file.

By regulation (21 CFR 312.62), the investigator must keep records relating to disposition of the study drug, including dates, quantity and use by study subjects and case histories, including CRFs and all supporting documentation. Supporting documentation includes the signed and dated consent form, medical records, progress notes, hospital charts, nursing notes and any other source documents. It should also be documented that informed consent was obtained prior to the subject's participation.

This is the minimum by regulation. In reality, study files contain much more information. One recommendation is to have three major categories for study files: regulatory, administrative and clinical. As noted, investigator regulatory files are maintained several ways, such as electronically or in the regulatory binder provided by the sponsor company, with tabbed sections. Or a site may maintain the regulatory binder another way, with documents maintained electronically and a hard copy file or in hanging file folders, etc. A site can maintain essential regulatory documents in whatever manner that works for them as long as it is in compliance. A CRA should never take it upon themselves to "organize" or update a site's regulatory file. The CRA can only provide guidance or cite requirements.

In the regulatory files, the following will be kept:

- Completed FDA form 1572 (Statement of Investigator).
- Copies of the CV/medical license for the investigator and sub-investigators.
- Financial Disclosure forms for the investigator and sub-investigators listed on the 1572.
- IRB-approved consent form and any translations.
- Written IRB approval of the protocol (study), consent form, advertising and subject compensation, if applicable.
- Signed copy of the protocol and any amendments.
- Copies of the laboratory certification and normal ranges.
- Investigator brochure.

In the administrative section of the file, the following will be kept:

- Correspondence, email and telephone logs, including contacts with the sponsor, CRO (if involved), IRB and the institution (if applicable).
- Instructional material:
  - CRF completion/correction.
  - Guidelines for handling adverse events.
  - Procedures for handling and storing laboratory specimens.
  - Study drug information, including instructions for storing, dispensing and accounting.
- Drug shipment, dispensing and return records.
- Sponsor/CRO contact information.
- Log of study subjects (Master Study Subject Roster).
- Records of meetings and contact with the sponsor and/or CRO.
- Monitoring log (a record of CRA monitoring visits).
- Miscellaneous.
- Monitoring Visit letters.
- Training logs.
- Manuals.

The investigator will also have a clinical file for each study subject, which will include:

- CRFs and supporting documents for each subject.
- Signed consent forms.

Files will vary depending on the site, the sponsor and the nature of the studies.

There are two items not mentioned in the list above: the grant and any reports from sponsor QA audits. This information is not routinely made available to FDA auditors and should not be kept in study files.

File retention is discussed in Chapter 17, "Study Closeout." Investigators must be aware from the start of the study that all study documents must be retained long after the study is over. The CRA can be a valuable help to the site by assisting it with setting up and maintaining its files throughout the study. The CRA must also check the files regularly throughout the study and again at study closure. Keeping the files in order during the study will ensure that they are ready in the event of a site audit by the sponsor, the IRB or the FDA. Some companies provide clearly marked containers for study files to help minimize loss after the study is completed.

More investigational sites are opting to store their regulatory files electronically or in a separate database. Some sites provide CRAs temporary username/password access to review their electronic regulatory files during monitoring visits, while some sites will provide the CRA with a flash drive of the regulatory files and a site computer with which to view the regulatory documents on the flash drive.

Grants and Contracts

Involvement of the CRA in grant negotiation and investigator contracts varies considerably among sponsors. In general, the larger the company, the less the CRA is involved; this is because large companies tend to have a separate department that handles the financial aspects of trials. However, CRAs need to have an understanding of the grant and contract process in order to work well with study sites.

Grants

A good CRA will have an understanding of how grants are determined, both by the sponsor and by the investigator. Frequently the CRA can help move negotiations along to everyone's benefit.

Most sponsors operate on a fee-for-service basis. This means they will pay for actual work performed (i.e., subjects enrolled and subject visits). Most grants are formulated on a per-subject amount and prorated for the number of visits a subject actually completes. The amount per visit will often vary, as some visits are more labor- and time-intensive than others. Sponsors feel that they are buying a service from the investigator and do not expect to pay if the work (subjects and data) is not delivered.

There are different ways in which sponsor grant figures are determined. Some companies use commercially available grant management systems that estimate costs for protocol activities. This gives the sponsor a realistic grant range to work from when determining how much it wishes to pay for per-patient grants. Other companies determine grants based on their own actual data or data gathered from other sources. Others rely on information from the investigators they are considering for the study.

Some sponsors will determine a range or a single per-subject grant figure they will pay and will not budge from this figure. Investigators either accept it or will not be able to do the study. Other sponsors will allow more flexibility, depending on experience with an investigator or geographic location. Costs differ in different parts of the country, so it makes sense to allow some flexibility.

Some companies expect their CRAs to negotiate grants with their investigators. Ideally, there will be a range or a starting figure given for the negotiations. A CRA must understand enough about calculating reasonable grants to help a site, especially if the site is inexperienced and has not done this before.

A good way to calculate a grant figure is to look at each study activity, have the investigator attach a cost to it, add an additional amount for overhead and other required activities and total it up. An example of a grant worksheet for a hypothetical study is shown in Table 6.

For this hypothetical study, there are eight visits. One common way to determine a prorating schedule is to look at the number of visits and the amount of work to be done at each visit. If some visits demand considerably more work than others, count them as two visits; generally speaking, the baseline visit and the final visit are the most demanding.

In the example shown in Table 7, there are three visits that are more labor intensive (Visits 1, 5 and 8), which involve physical exams and stress testing. To determine the prorated dollar amount, each of these visits should count as two and the other five visits should each count as one, for a total of 11. If the cumulative amount of $5,152 is divided by 11, the cost per visit is $468.36. Based on this, the three more intensive visits should be pro-rated at $937, and the other five at $468 (with the extra dollar added to the cost of the last visit). Note in Table 7 that if a subject drops out after visit 3, the investigator would be paid $1,837. For a subject dropping out at Week 7, the payment would be $4,214, and so forth.

This is a simple way to calculate grants and prorate visit costs, but it is quite effective if the initial amounts for each procedure and activity are real-

Table 6: Budget worksheet—Protocol XXX

Study activity	Number of visits	Cost	Expanded cost
Phone pre-screen	1	50	50
Medical history	1	50	50
Physical exam	3	150	450
Labs	8	150	1,200
EKG	3	200	600
Treadmill stress test	3	250	750
Office visit—general assessments	8	75	600
Phone assessments	2	50	100
Sub-total for procedures			**$3,800**
Coordinator time	8	50	400
Pharmacy charge	8	35	280
Subtotal			**$680**
Total			**$4,480**
Overhead—15%			672
Grand total per completed subject			**$5,152**

istic. It is easy to explain and should help the CRA when negotiating a grant amount that is fair to both the sponsor and the investigator.

When a grant has been agreed upon and the study is underway, the CRA's responsibilities for grant activities are again variable. Some companies utilize the CRA in determining when grant monies should be paid, while others handle all grant payments in-house without the CRA's involvement. These companies usually pay either on a timed schedule, such as quarterly, or on the basis of CRFs received in-house or visits confirmed as completed in a sponsor system by the CRA during monitoring visits. Whatever the scheme, the CRA should understand it and be able to discuss it with the investigator.

Note that many companies will pay a small amount of the grant up front (maybe two subjects' worth), but will then apply this amount to the work being done. This allows the investigator to set up study procedures, pay for initial labs and other tests, etc., without having to use site funds.

Table 7: Grant amounts for one subject

Visit	1	2	3	4	5	6	7	8
Amount per visit	$937	$468	$468	$468	$937	$468	$468	$938
Cumulative amount	$937	$1,405	$1,837	$2,341	$3,278	$3,746	$4,214	$5,152

If grant payments are based on input from the CRA, the CRA will need to keep track of the work done and payments made. It is advisable not to pay in advance, with the exception of a possible up-front payment, just in case the site does not enroll any subjects at all. If an investigator is paid in advance and doesn't earn that amount, there is always the sticky business of trying to get the funds back. This is unpleasant for both the sponsor and the investigator, and even more so for the CRA, who is often caught in the middle.

Although some CRAs find it difficult to be involved in negotiating and paying grants, it does add stature in the eye of the investigator and gives the CRA more clout at the site. No matter how involved the CRA is, he or she should have a good understanding of both the process and the specifics for a site, to be able to discuss the grant with the investigator and to answer any site questions.

Contracts

A contract between the sponsor and the investigator will be signed before the trial begins at a site. This document usually contains the responsibilities of the investigator, including the number of subjects the site is expecting to enroll, timelines for enrollment, grant amounts and the regulatory requirements for the investigator. It also contains the responsibilities of the sponsor, including when and how grants will be paid, monitoring of the study and sponsor regulatory requirements. It will be signed by the appropriate company representative and by the investigator. (Note that in large institutions contracts may be signed by someone in the contract office rather than by the investigator.)

Contracts are rarely written, negotiated or signed by the CRA. The CRA may, however, be asked to take the contract to the investigator and/or collect the signed contract. The CRA will want to have a copy of the contract, if possible, to know what was agreed to for enrollment, timelines and payment schedules.

Key Takeaways

Study Documents

- There are a number of documents required before a study can begin at a site.
- Most sponsors will not ship the study drug until all required documents are collected.
- Copies of all documents must be kept in both the site's and the sponsor's study files.
- The CRA should keep track of the IRB approval process and letter, so the study is not unduly delayed.
- Shared databases and regulatory portals used for startup activities can reduce timelines and cost.

Financial Disclosure

- The purpose of financial disclosure is to identify any potential conflict of interest that could bias a clinical trial.
- Financial disclosure information must be gathered for all people listed on form 1572 and their immediate family members.
- These data are collected for the time period of the study and one year following.
- Financial disclosure information is reported to the FDA when the NDA is filed.

Investigator Meetings

- All investigators and coordinators, as well as relevant sponsor personnel, should attend the meeting.

- The meeting should be held at the time when most sites are ready to enroll.
- The purpose of an investigator meeting is to ensure that all sites have the same understanding of all protocol and administrative procedures.
- Sponsors should always have a full rehearsal before the meeting.
- CRAs should act as the host for their respective sites and ensure that site personnel meet the sponsor representatives.

Study Initiation Visit

- The purpose of an initiation meeting is to ensure that everyone at the site has a clear and accurate understanding of how the study is to be conducted.
- This meeting should be held after a site has all the study supplies, including the study drug, but before study personnel enroll any subjects.
- All relevant site personnel should be present for the meeting.
- The CRA is the SIV lead.
- The meeting should be documented in both the investigator's and sponsor's study files.

Investigator's Study Files

- Investigators are required to keep study records and documents during the trial and after the trial is closed.
- CRAs can help the investigator set up and organize these files and must check them regularly throughout the study.
- Maintaining files appropriately will ensure that they are in order for an audit.
- It is often simple to catch and correct problems with the files on an ongoing basis throughout the study. It may be impossible to correct the files once the study is over.
- More and more investigators are maintaining electronic study/regulatory files.

Grants and Contracts

- A CRA should be knowledgeable about grants and how they are calculated.

- If involved in payments, the CRA must track the study progress to keep abreast of money owed.
- Most grants are prorated by visit for each subject.
- Contracts between the sponsor and the investigator are signed before the study begins at the site.

CHAPTER 14

Study Monitoring

This chapter will discuss the CRA's main activity: study monitoring. Previous chapters discussed the importance of a good protocol, case report forms, investigator selection, investigator meetings and startup and initiation meetings in producing high-quality clinical trials. Without good study monitoring, however, the best preparation will not produce a high-quality study. Poor study monitoring is probably the largest single contributor to inferior study quality.

A good CRA can produce good studies under a variety of circumstances, with investigators and protocols of varying quality. On the other hand, a poor CRA will almost always generate a substandard study, regardless of the quality of the protocol and experience of the investigator. Good CRA site monitoring and management are essential for good studies.

The Monitoring Plan

The game plan used in athletics is a strategy that the coach and players develop before each game and includes what needs to be done to maximize the chance of winning. It changes for each game because the conditions, circumstances and opposition are different each time. So it is with monitoring. No two study sites are the same, even if they are following the same protocol. A CRA should spend some time putting together a good monitoring strategy including both general and specific information for each site.

The CRA's monitoring strategy should also include extensive prep work before and between onsite monitoring visits (which we cover in detail later in this chapter) that includes collecting/tracking statistics and data on the site status, (queries, EDC entry, new study subjects/screening and recruitment, follow up of protocol deviations and pending issues/items from previous remote or onsite monitoring visits, regulatory documents status, etc.). Monitoring should also include consistent communications with the remote monitor and clinical trials assistant on their site management activities to ensure all individuals involved are on the same page with site guidance and follow up. There is nothing worse than when study team members don't communicate about the sites they manage; and the sites suffer the most with duplicate contacts, conflicting information, etc.

Monitoring visits don't just start and end onsite. The activities completed before, during and after onsite monitoring visits are all critical to the success.

The study monitoring plan is essentially "the study game plan" for monitoring. It is usually created by the clinical trials manager or project manager for the study. If the sponsor has delegated the creation/completion of the monitoring plan to the CRO, then the monitoring plan has input from both sponsor and CRO clinical trials management. The monitoring plan details how the study will be monitored, how often it will be monitored (remote and onsite monitoring activities), specific monitoring activities to be completed during each respective monitoring visit type, and site communications (elements vary by sponsor/CRO and internal requirements). CRAs must be very familiar with the study monitoring plan, protocol, CRF guidelines, study manuals and study team internal documents relative to monitoring to ensure they are providing comprehensive site management and are in compliance with all required monitoring standards and activities at their sites.

How to Monitor

How to monitor a study in the field (meaning you must travel from your company/home office to the study site) requires considerable thought. Almost all field monitoring requires regular visits to the site by the CRA throughout the period of the study. On very rare occasions, an extremely simple, low-risk study might be monitored almost exclusively by telephone except for the start-up and closeout visits.

Over the past ten years, more sponsors/CROs have adopted a risk-based monitoring model for clinical trials conduct. The risk-based element targets critical study endpoints or influential visit data for review, based on risk analysis of the protocol and data. The risk-based model includes alternative monitoring practices as opposed to traditional, 100 percent onsite routine monitoring visits conducted at specific time intervals. These alternatives include centralized or remote monitoring of critical endpoints and data (via

EDC or some source documents/CRFs uploaded by site staff to a shared drive or transmitted electronically, and review of data analytics from other study data sources), and onsite review of targeted, critical visit data and source documents in lieu of 100 percent CRF/source document review (such as targeted review of drug administration and accountability data, inclusion/exclusion criteria, study endpoints and adverse event or safety reporting). This can occur in between or in lieu of some onsite monitoring visits.

Data is being more closely scrutinized to address trends and issues identified proactively instead of reactively and innovative technologies are a part of that analysis.

Alternative site management practices such as email correspondence, teleconference and video conference provide opportunities for consistent training, site management and dissemination of information to ensure better oversight of the investigational site study performance and data collection practices.

Section 5 of the FDA guidance document, "E6(R2) Good Clinical Practice: Integrated Addendum to ICH E6(R1)," recommends even more specific quality management practices:

> **5. SPONSOR**
>
> **ADDENDUM**
>
> **5.0 Quality Management**
>
> The sponsor should implement a system to manage quality throughout all stages of the trial process.
>
> Sponsors should focus on trial activities essential to ensuring human subject protection and the reliability of trial results. Quality management includes the design of efficient clinical trial protocols, tools, and procedures for data collection and processing, as well as the collection of information that is essential to decision making.
>
> The methods used to assure and control the quality of the trial should be proportionate to the risks inherent in the trial and the importance of the information collected. The sponsor should ensure that all aspects of the trial are operationally feasible and should avoid unnecessary complexity, procedures, and data collection. Protocols, case report forms, and other operational documents should be clear, concise, and consistent.

The quality management system should use a risk-based approach as described below.

5.0.1 *Critical Process and Data Identification*

During protocol development, the sponsor should identify those processes and data that are critical to ensure human subject protection and the reliability of trial results.

5.0.2 *Risk Identification*

The sponsor should identify risks to critical trial processes and data. Risks should be considered at both the system level (e.g., standard operating procedures, computerized systems, and personnel) and clinical trial level (e.g., trial design, data collection, and informed consent process).

5.0.3 *Risk Evaluation*

The sponsor should evaluate the identified risks, against existing risk controls by considering:

(a) The likelihood of errors occurring.

(b) The extent to which such errors would be detectable.

(c) The impact of such errors on human subject protection and reliability of trial results.

5.0.4 *Risk Control*

The sponsor should decide which risks to reduce and/or which risks to accept. The approach used to reduce risk to an acceptable level should be proportionate to the significance of the risk. Risk reduction activities may be incorporated in protocol design and implementation, monitoring plans, agreements between parties defining roles and responsibilities, systematic safeguards to ensure adherence to standard operating procedures, and training in processes and procedures.

Predefined quality tolerance limits should be established, taking into consideration the medical and statistical characteristics of the variables as well as the statistical design of the trial, to identify systematic issues that can impact subject safety or reliability of trial results. Detection of deviations from the predefined quality tolerance limits should trigger an evaluation to determine if action is needed.

5.0.5 Risk Communication

The sponsor should document quality management activities. The sponsor should communicate quality management activities to those who are involved in or affected by such activities, to facilitate risk review and continual improvement during clinical trial execution.

5.0.6 Risk Review

The sponsor should periodically review risk control measures to ascertain whether the implemented quality management activities remain effective and relevant, taking into account emerging knowledge and experience.

5.0.7 Risk Reporting

The sponsor should describe the quality management approach implemented in the trial and summarize important deviations from the predefined quality tolerance limits and remedial actions taken in the clinical study report (ICH E3, section 9.6 Data Quality Assurance).

Risk-based monitoring specific to central/remote monitoring of eCRFs and source documents will be reviewed later in this chapter.

A CRA must determine how to integrate telephone, email, text messaging, instant messaging and even fax communications into a monitoring strategy. This will differ depending on the program and site. It will depend on the technologies available, both sponsor and site SOPs, site capabilities and personal preferences at both the site and the sponsor companies. The CRA must also learn to understand the most effective and accepted face-to-face communications to use with site personnel during onsite monitoring visits.

In monitoring, like any business, many problems can be traced back to a lack of communication, inappropriate communication and/or unclear communication. Consistent and effective communication strategies should have a high priority in your monitoring strategy and the official study monitoring plan.

The intensity of monitoring will vary across studies and among sites. Must or should the CRA be present while the site is seeing study subjects? Will the CRA have any interaction with study subjects? In early phase I studies, the CRA may be required to be present during all or part of a subject's treatment. Therefore, the CRA must determine how long he or she will need to be there and make appropriate arrangements.

Sometimes a CRA is the sole monitor for a site, while at other times the CRA will co-monitor with other company CRAs. Establishing who will monitor requires consideration of the sponsor's SOPs for field monitoring, the complexity of the protocol, the condition being studied, the experience of the investigator and his or her staff and the training and experience of the CRA.

The study's overall monitoring plan should remain fairly consistent, with the exception of formal updates/amendments that will occur occasionally based on study requirements, different/additional monitoring strategies implemented, specific time points in the study or other factors. The CRAs monitoring strategy should remain consistent but adaptable, as individual site needs may change considerably during the course of the study, depending on many factors such as study conditions, protocol changes, site status and performance.

Frequency of Monitoring Visits

A key determination in a monitoring plan is the frequency with which the CRA will visit each site. There are a number of factors that must be considered in making this decision:

- Complexity of the protocol.
- Disease being evaluated.
- Experience of the investigator/staff.
- Number of study subjects enrolled at the site.
- Rate of screening/enrollment.
- Site performance (clean data vs. data discrepancies, timeliness of data entry, protocol deviations, noted findings during monitoring visits).
- CRA experience and effectiveness.
- Whether or not the study is using risk-based monitoring or 100% CRF/SDV review during routine onsite monitoring visits.

The protocol dictates the conduct of the study by establishing the procedures that subjects must undergo and their frequency. The more activities required during a study visit, the more monitoring will be required. The disease being studied also dictates the frequency of visits. For example, if the CRA is monitoring an infectious disease study, the course of therapy will probably be complete for each subject in about 10 days. This may mean a larger number of subjects must be monitored in a shorter amount of time. This requires a different frequency of visits than a cholesterol-lowering study with a treatment period of one or two years. Then you have oncology studies that have complicated monitoring requirements for calculating chemotherapy and drug doses, local and central lab results review, and parameters to calculate tumor growth, response and status. A number of oncology studies require 100 percent SDV/CRF review and multiday monitoring visits to sift through the endless varieties of source documents/medical records/assessments/calculations that have accumulated as a result of complicated study visits. Some studies require unblinded pharmacy staff to prepare the study drug for injection or infusion and blind the administration. In this case, there will be an additional monitoring plan; the unblinded monitoring plan for the unblinded CRA responsible for unblinded pharmacy monitoring at the site. Unblinded monitoring activities and frequency are different than blinded monitoring, but they are just as important a component of a monitoring visit.

All sites should be visited soon after the first subject or two are enrolled just to be sure the site understands and is correctly following protocol procedures. (Industry standard is that the first monitoring visit occurs within one to two weeks of the first study patient being enrolled at a site, but the remote monitor may be in contact with the site sooner after the first subject is enrolled to start the quality review/oversight discussions). Catching and solving problems early will save a lot of extra work as the study progresses. (See more about this in Chapter 18, Quality Management.) A critical benefit to central or remote monitoring of source documents or EDC is the ability for CRAs to review preliminary study visit data entry by sites early on in a trial, (before the first monitoring visit) to proactively determine site trends in protocol deviations, GCP non-compliance or eligibility/enrollment discrepancies. This expedites preventive action and can potentially lower incidence of corrective action. The rate of enrollment will also affect monitoring frequency. Generally speaking, the more subjects a site has, the more frequently the CRA will have to visit. The faster a site enrolls and the more data generated, the more frequently the site will need monitoring.

The CRA should visit a site regularly even though enrollment may be slow or non-existent. Slow subject enrollment may indicate a lack of enthusiasm on the part of site personnel regarding the study. In that case, a bit of CRA encouragement may help, which will probably involve visits. Site personnel often view frequent visits by the CRA as an indication of the importance of their study to the sponsor. Not only that, but seeing the CRA walk through the door reminds the site staff of their commitment to enroll subjects and complete the study on time. Call it encouragement or call it guilt—it generally works. Sometimes a few extra visits are all that is necessary to get a study back on track or to re-establish priorities at the site.

Some sponsors will build these extra visits, sometimes called "motivational visits" into the monitoring plan and study budget, which are essentially additional visits for the CRA to discuss enrollment/patient identification strategies with the site, what has worked, what has not worked, to have "lunch and learns" with the PI and Sub PIs, to further educate them on the study design or drug, to clarify what was misunderstood and/or perceived barriers to enrollment at the site (these are sometimes attended by the sponsor medical monitor or scientific personnel as a further show of support to the site), and to have the sponsor CRA or recruitment specialist accompany the site CRA to a visit as a show of support, motivation and to answer any questions the site has or even help the site strategize.

The frequency and amount of monitoring depend on whether they involve 100 percent SDV/CRF review or risk-based monitoring. Studies that use 100 percent SDV/CRF review will have consistent monitoring frequency intervals laid out in the monitoring plan (a common practice is every 6 weeks); whereas; risk-based monitoring models use targeted (and thus reduced) SDV/CRF review and this will dictate the frequency. The frequency and duration of monitoring visits will also vary from site to site depending on the experience of the investigator and the staff. A less experienced site may require more or longer monitoring visits, especially at the beginning of the study. Once the site has demonstrated the ability to do the study well, the CRA may be able to space the monitoring visits further apart.

The frequency of monitoring visits may change as the study progresses. Some sites will do a better job complying with GCPs than others and may need less frequent monitoring. Subject enrollment may complete or level off after a period of time, allowing for more time between monitoring visits. Subject visits may be spread out over the course of long-term studies and require less review; for example, weekly visits may be required initially, followed by monthly, and perhaps even quarterly visits as the study progresses. In short, a CRA must visit each site often enough to stay on top of the activities that are required for good monitoring. The more experienced the CRA, the easier it will be to make this determination.

Another factor that affects CRA visit frequency is the number and location of sites for which he or she has monitoring responsibility. There is always the chance that the CRA simply cannot physically visit the sites as often as he or she would like to or need to because of travel time and the actual number and location of sites. Here again, the CRA will have to spend some time integrating travel requirements with site experience and study complexity.

Another factor not often considered that can impact monitoring frequency at a site is the CRAs relationship with the investigator and site staff. If a CRA is organized and responsive to sites, professional and positive during monitoring visits, respectful of the study coordinator's time (keeping the established visit schedule, arriving on time to monitoring visits, sending timely confirmation letters and site reminders) and is proactive about scheduling visits in advance, that is the CRA who will get the desired monitoring visit days (Tuesday, Wednesday, Thursday), and locations onsite (conference room versus examination room). That is not the CRA who is consistently late to monitoring visits, frequently cancels visits and fails to schedule visits in a timely manner.

The CRA should schedule four hours, at the very least, for a site visit. With the complexity of protocols, regulatory requirements and good monitoring practice, the CRA will need to spend a day or more at most sites. Creative scheduling of your travel itinerary is a must. It helps to use the "loop method" for travel, in which the sites closest together are linked in your itinerary for a single trip. (See Appendix B for additional tips on traveling.)

As a general rule, a good CRA should be able to effectively monitor 12 to 18 sites. The number will change depending on the complexity of the study, site and CRA experience, site enrollment and locations. If the CRA is in a situation in which it is simply impossible to visit sites with the degree of frequency necessary for good monitoring, this should be discussed with his or her supervisor.

Planning the Amount of Time for a Monitoring Visit

Planning the amount of time you need to allow for a monitoring visit at a site is not always easy. Time management can be a difficult challenge, especially when you may also have to figure in schedules and other travel factors. When you are planning a visit, think of the activities you need to complete while you are there, which will include at least some, if not all, of the following:

- Meeting with the investigator.
- Meeting with the study coordinator.
- Review of study documents.
- Drug/device accountability, which may include meeting with the pharmacist/pharmacy depending on the site model.
- eCRF/CRF review and source document verification.
- Query resolution.
- SAE listing/review.
- Protocol deviation reporting/review.
- Training.
- Facilities reconfirmation.
- Addressing unresolved findings/issues from the previous visit.
- Review of the investigator site file.
- Review of staff GCP and training certificates.
- Any recruitment discussions for enrolling studies.

The most difficult amount of time for a CRA to estimate is often the eCRF/CRF review, including source document review/verification. When you start a new study, keep track of approximately how long it takes for you to review a subject visit (average). A subject's status in the study (screening versus randomization versus follow-up) will greatly determine the time for visit review. A good rule of thumb to remember is that a screening visit can take two to three times longer to review than a regular study visit. Once you have this information as a guide, you can estimate your total time for subject review by multiplying the number of visits you have to review by this amount of time. If you add the time you expect to need for the other activities you have planned, you will have a reasonable estimate of how much time you will need for your visit. You should then build in an extra hour for the unexpected that can arise (such as late study coordinators, internet/system issues).

A good tool for planning eCRF/CRF review is a monitoring log that shows the number of subjects enrolled and where each subject is in the study. Even if the study is using EDC and there is a means to electronically "check-off" a study visit or study patient record after review or even if the system reconciles your review automatically after completion or an IVRS/IWRS system tracks and generates updated subject enrollment/status data in real time, it is recommended you make and keep a monitoring log for all of your studies, as this will show you the progress of the study, and some system information is dependent on site data entry. Some CRAs maintain monitoring logs on Excel spreadsheets or OneNote or in Word documents or a handwritten monitoring log.

Table 1: Monitoring log—Protocol 1234-XYZ—Dr. J. Smith

Subject	Consent date	Baseline	Week 1	Week 2	Week 4	Final status	Comments
001 FGB	3-1-21	3-1-21	3-9-21			Drop-out	Dropped at Week 1—adverse events
002 KKO	4-12-21	4-12-21	4-20-21				
003 MKJ							

Above is an example of a monitoring log (Table 1). Note that the column headings are study-dependent. You can, of course, add other headings that might be useful, like a visit calculator to calculate when the study subject's visit should have occurred vs. when it occurred. In this example, the dates are the actual dates the subject completed each visit. You might want to put a check or highlight the visits when you have collected/reviewed the CRFs or add the date you collected/reviewed the CRFs for each visit (collected can mean electronic review and check off with an EDC system or physical collection of paper CRFs).

Let's say on your first monitoring trip, these are the subject visits that were completed. You added these dates to your log as you reviewed each subject.

Before you make your next monitoring visit, you add any new subjects enrolled to your log. You get this information from the weekly enrollment update by the site or from the eCRF or IVRS/IWRS database updates. Then you can pencil in any visits the subjects should have had since you were last there, count up these visits and have a pretty good idea about the time you will need to spend reviewing them.

Assume you will visit on May 25, 2021. How many visits might you expect to see? Pencil an "X" in these boxes and add them up. It looks like you may have nine new visits to review. If each one takes you approximately half an hour, you are looking at about four and a half hours for this activity. See this example of the updated monitoring log in Table 2.

Table 2: Monitoring log—Protocol 1234-XYZ—Dr. J. Smith

Subject	Consent date	Baseline	Week 1	Week 2	Week 4	Final status	Comments
001 FGB	3-1-21	3-1-21	3-9-21	X	X	Dropout	Dropped at Week 1—adverse events
002 KKO	4-12-21	4-12-21	4-20-21	X	X		
003 MKJ		4-30-21	X	X			
004 DDS		5-3-21	X	X			
005 RFD		5-15-21	X				

Add in the other tasks you have to complete at the visit and you will have a reasonable estimate of your time requirements.

Monitoring Activity

The CRA should have a general plan for what will be monitored at each site visit. Most sponsors have a site visit report or monitoring report that the CRA completes during and after a site visit. This report is a standard template within an electronic database or system, with questions about monitoring activities specific to that monitoring visit. The CRA will use this document for all field monitoring visits. It serves as both a checklist for the CRA and as documentation of the visit. However, the CRA must not view this as the only list of activities that must be completed.

To be successful as a CRA, it is important to develop a sense for what you should monitor at each site and how much attention should be given to each activity. Some CRAs develop source-document subject sheets that they maintain on study subjects (paper documents/notebooks, OneNote listings, Word documents or spreadsheets). These sheets note such items as date of consent, re-consenting, SAEs, protocol deviations, study status (visits completed), CRFs reviewed and other items of note to help keep themselves up to date.

It helps to be aware of where problems are most likely to arise during the conduct of a study. A good indication of potential problems is the list of activities that receive the most deficiencies during FDA audits. Some top deficiency categories for site inspections done by the FDA's Bioresearch Monitoring Program historically include:

- Failure to follow the investigational plan/agreement or regulations, or both.
- Protocol deviations.
- Failure to prepare or maintain adequate case histories/inadequate recordkeeping.
- Informed consent issues.
- Drug accountability/disposition issues for the study drug.

These areas, in addition to the items the sponsor wants to emphasize, should receive specific attention during monitoring visits. Sponsor expectations for studies are important. Independent CRAs and those employed by CROs need to review sponsor monitoring visit SOPs, familiarize themselves with the sponsor's data review requirements, know the study monitoring plan and pay attention during sponsor co-monitoring visits to ensure a clear understanding of those expectations.

A good practice in prioritization is to review the most critical data first, such as: informed consent forms, screening and randomization visits for newly enrolled patients, newly reported SAEs and accompanying information and impending subject efficacy or endpoint data for study patients. Interim or safety analysis during a study will drive priority in data review at sites. The interval of time between remote or onsite monitoring visits at a site will dictate priority of data review (how long unreviewed data has been sitting, how long has it been since the earliest enrolled patient data was reviewed).

It is always a good practice for a CRA to keep on top of activities such as reviewing the regulatory binder and completing drug accountability at every monitoring visit or every other monitoring visit. Putting aside even minimal time for these activities will help CRAs stay on top of trends and issues that may have gone unnoticed if the CRA got caught up with staying on top of data review and neglected these other important activities.

Many successful CRAs rely heavily on checklists that they have developed and refined over time. Basic checklists cover those things that should always be reviewed, regardless of the program, sponsor or site. This list can be modified as needed to fit each monitoring assignment. Sample checklists are in Appendix C. If a CRA thinks experience is a substitute for checklists, remember that all airline pilots use checklists every time they fly, regardless of how many hours of flying time they have. Which plane would you prefer to fly on: one whose pilot uses a checklist or one whose pilot thinks personal experience is enough to ensure the safety of the flight?

Author's Story

Checklists

I have trained new CRAs and CRA managers and I always impress upon these folks the importance of using a checklist, no matter how brief it is. Toward the end of my career as a CRA, I was training a new CRA in Pittsburgh. We were going to do site/investigator evaluations that day and I had told him to have a checklist for the various meetings. The first interview went fairly well, but he left out a few things. After the visit, we discussed the fact that he had not used a checklist. The second interview went the same as the first and the ensuing discussion was the same. It was the third interview that really gave me pause to wonder if he would make it as a CRA. Once again, no checklist was utilized. The new CRA seemed to have asked all the right questions, except for one: "How many patients do you have, doctor, who might qualify for this study?" I had to ask it for him. On our way back to the car, the young man looked at me and said, "I guess I should have used a checklist.

–A CRA

Preparing for a Monitoring Visit

Once the CRA has a good idea how to monitor, what to monitor and how frequently to monitor, it is time to prepare for the visit. There is a military saying: "Proper Preparation Prevents Poor Performance." Remembering the "5 Ps" will serve you well. A CRA should spend a considerable amount of time preparing for each site visit. In addition to a working knowledge of good clinical practice (GCP) and any state and/or local requirements, the CRA must know everything possible about the activity at the site, the protocol and the sponsor's monitoring SOPs/monitoring plan before arriving at the site. A CRA's preparation will be evident to the investigator and his or her staff; a lack of preparation can cause a loss of credibility.

Once a CRA has lost credibility, control of the site and the ability to generate a good study diminishes significantly. It takes an enormous amount of extra work to re-establish lost credibility, if it can be done at all. Remember that you only get one chance to create a good first impression. Establishing and maintaining a high level of credibility should be among a CRA's primary goals. The easiest way to achieve credibility is to be prepared.

Preparation for a monitoring visit includes tracking and collecting statistical data with respect to pending or completed EDC/eCRF entry, and queries pending from both onsite and remote monitoring activities (EDC/central lab/vendor queries). It also includes obtaining the status of regulatory documents (with input from the remote monitor or clinical trials assistants about what is pending submission, approval, or what is missing from the internal investigator file). And it involves tracking the resolution of pending issues from remote or onsite monitoring visits, such as reporting protocol deviations, correcting deficiencies noted during source document review (including consenting issues, eligibility issues, drug accountability or IP compliance), and following new subjects screened or enrolled and site recruiting efforts, etc.

Monitoring visits don't just start and end onsite. The activities completed before, during and after onsite monitoring visits are all critical to the success. One thing a CRA should do is set up site travel files for each site he or she monitors. Some CRAs are "old school" and prefer paper files for this purpose, which is fine. Other CRAs use such tools as One Note or Excel spreadsheets. Whatever method is used, these files should contain the items shown in Table 3.

Table 3: Travel file content

- Personal notes
- Copies of the last site visit report
- Study progress or enrollment logs
- Key site documents
  - Protocol
  - 1572
  - Latest drug shipment form(s)
- Pertinent correspondence
- Copies of any queries received
- Subject monitoring notes
- CRF guidelines
- SAE listings
- Essential document listings

There are so many portals and platforms that manage study activities and CRAs must have access to multiple programs to generate the tools for site files and monitoring visits. These include:

- Electronic trial master file to stay apprised of a site's regulatory documents in house and what is missing.
- EDC/eCRF systems to generate query reports and enrollment reports.
- Central vendor systems databases (imaging, labs) to track results, diagnostics.
- IVRS/IWRS systems to track study drug shipments, patient randomization and drug assignment.

It is also useful to have a monitoring bag or backpack containing UPS or FedEx mailers and labels, paper clips, pens, pencils, sticky notes, laptop (of course) and any printed materials like the protocol and monitoring plan. Some CRAs bring note pads and planners. All CRAs have their smart phones as these are issued by the sponsor/CRO. Your files should also contain any other items you think would be of value when you are at the site. These should be kept current. When preparing to leave for a monitoring trip, the CRA can simply pull/print or update the files on their computer for the sites to be visited. It also helps to have a generic travel file that includes checklists and a copy of the regulations. When leaving for a monitoring visit, the CRA can easily pack the generic file, the site-specific files and any other necessary supplies, and he or she is ready to go.

Prior to a site visit, the CRA should check with colleagues involved in the development program for the investigational drug, particularly the sponsor's medical monitor. This is especially important for CRAs who are based regionally and may not be aware of correspondence or other communications that have occurred between the site and the sponsor since the last visit (though they should be copied on all emails). The CRA should also check for any authorized protocol deviations or other changes in the conduct of the study at the site, as well as changes in enrollment or other study-related activity. For sponsor or CRO companies who utilize a clinical trials management system database, enrollment, protocol deviation and SAE listing, reports can be system generated by the CRA prior to the monitoring visit or during the monitoring visit for reference.

Some sponsors have in-house CRAs who oversee study activity, particularly error correction and data management, by monitoring incoming eCRFs/CRFs. Some of these in-house monitors have frequent contact with study site personnel. If a CRA is field-based, he or she should check with the in-house CRA to see what has transpired at a site since the last monitoring visit. The in-house CRA may also maintain some site performance, site communication or status logs; the CRA should review current copies of these documents prior to a site visit.

Before leaving for a monitoring visit, the CRA should contact the site by phone or email to confirm the visit. This serves a number of purposes. First, it reminds the site of the visit. Second, it confirms that the necessary site personnel will be there and available; if key people will not be available during the visit, it should probably be rescheduled. This call, or email, also allows the CRA to remind site personnel of expectations for the visit, any prior preparation that is needed (like source/eCRFs to retrieve, drug accountability logs, regulatory binders) and approximately how long the visit will last. Finally, it can help to avoid a wasted trip if the site is not prepared or if there has been a scheduling change or misunderstanding about the date.

Lastly, know where you are going. This may sound funny, but there are stories of CRAs who have become hopelessly lost on their first visit because they did not take the time to get the correct site directions or address for their GPS or smartphone. (There is more on travel in Appendix B.) As a hint, place the directions for finding each site in its travel file—including how to find the office within the hospital, etc. It's easy to forget when monitoring several sites and visiting only every six weeks or so.

With the advent of shared ride services like Lyft and Uber, transportation has become reasonable and convenient, especially in large cities where traffic is heavy and car rental is expensive and inconvenient. Using a shared ride service is especially beneficial when your investigative site is a large academic health center where parking is nonexistent or not centrally located to the investigative site.

If you are driving to the site, at the very least, ask the hotel staff how long it will take to get there as they have realistic predictions of traffic patterns and rush hour timeframes. You should not rely on GPS or map apps alone to predict how long it will take to get to the site.

If the CRA has prepared properly for a visit, the site will be expecting his or her arrival and will also have prepared for the visit.

Site Monitoring Visits

Professionalism

Before getting into the details of monitoring a site, it is important to focus briefly on conduct and appearance. Even in today's casual environment, it's important to look and act professional. CRAs can get off to a bad start because of the way they work and dress. The CRA should wear appropriate business attire and should always arrive at the site on time or a little early; remember to always call, email or text if you're not going to be on time, even when you are going to be just a few minutes late. The CRA must remember that he or she is an official representative of the sponsor and should always behave in an appropriate businesslike manner.

It is always important to regard a monitoring visit to an investigational site like a visit to an individual's home. You are their "guest" and must respect their policies for monitoring hours and conduct. Do not touch, move or "reorganize" anything (like regulatory binders) without permission. Do not leave your monitoring area a mess. Throw away trash, put things away or back in their respective places after use.

The respect you show to investigational site staff is reciprocal; often how a CRA is treated is a reflection of how he or she manages their sites. CRAs who manage by intimidation and criticism may have squeaky clean data but resentful site staff, who may complain to the sponsor and be uncooperative with interim analysis deadlines or last-minute monitoring visit needs. CRAs who take to heart the "site/CRA" team dynamic, who work with their sites, who impress with a positive influence, professionalism, education and mentoring will not only have credible data but also cooperative and happy site staff. A happy site is willing to help the CRA with almost anything and will strive for excellence in study conduct. They will also want to work with the sponsor/CRO again and again.

Monitoring requires a lot of unsupervised time "on the road;" consequently, CRAs must have excellent self-discipline. There are many temptations when traveling that can distract a CRA from work—shopping, museums, television or the latest bestseller. Although there may be some down time when in the field, the CRA can use this time to catch up on writing reports, reading protocols and other tasks. An employer deserves an honest day's work, whether the CRA is in the office or on the road. This should be balanced with making time to see the attractions in a city, have a nice dinner out, but after the tasks are complete.

Meeting with the Investigator

If possible, the CRA should spend a few minutes with the investigator at the start of the visit, so he or she knows you are there and what your activities will be while at the site. This is a good time to update the investigator on the overall progress of the study, including enrollment, timelines and any changes or other news from the sponsor.

Exit visits with the investigator should be routine. Since the investigator has ultimate responsibility for the study, the CRA should keep the investigator apprised of findings during the visit and how the study is going in general. The exit meeting is a good time to discuss how the study is progressing at the site, any corrective actions that need to be taken, grant or budget matters and any other items that need to be discussed with the investigator.

Investigators tend to be very busy and occasionally, after the study gets underway, they become less accessible. A CRA must make certain from the beginning that the investigator knows a short meeting is expected each time the site is visited. Good communication with the investigator is essential for a good study. If a CRA is having problems trying to meet with an investigator during an onsite monitoring visit, offer to have a telephone discussion. Though not as optimal as a face-to-face meeting, the willingness to work with busy investigators by having a discussion via teleconference will make them more amenable to future discussions.

If a CRA continues to encounter challenges with speaking to the investigator during monitoring visits, discuss this with the study project manager. The CRA must escalate and document all attempts to speak with the investigator to the study team. This may prompt the study team project manager to call the investigator themselves, or enlist the sponsor's assistance to contact the investigator. Often the sponsor's medical monitor can help, perhaps by calling the investigator personally—doctor-to-doctor contact sometimes works wonders.

Another aid for dealing with difficult investigators is to occasionally review the responsibilities that appear on the 1572 (Statement of Investigator) forms that they signed with them; specifically, section 9 of the 1572, investigator commitments. That can be a reminder that they agreed, in writing, to good study conduct, which includes good communication with the CRA. Sometimes nothing will work and an investigator will simply not meet with a CRA. In this case, the CRA must to do the best he or she can to keep the study on track. CRAs should always discuss these situations with their supervisors so that everyone is aware. Problems like these should also be documented in a visit report so that informed decisions can be made regarding future use or possible termination of the site.

Working with the Study Coordinator

For actual study conduct, the study coordinator or clinical research coordinator (CRC) is the most important person at the site. A CRA must establish a good working relationship with the coordinator. The coordinator can either make monitoring relatively easy and enjoyable or a nightmare, and the choice is usually dependent on the CRA.

A CRA needs to spend time developing a rapport with the coordinator and developing a monitoring routine that works well for both of them. Each should understand how the other works. The CRA should determine the best times and methods for routine communication with each coordinator and let the coordinator know his or her expectations as the field monitor.

Some CRAs have such a good relationship with their coordinators that all the materials to be reviewed at a visit are laid out and ready when the CRA arrives at the site. With others, the relationships are not as good, so study materials are not ready for review and monitoring becomes a challenge. A good relationship is worth nurturing; a bad one is costly.

Some CRAs simply have better interpersonal relationship skills than others. It's amazing what a smile and good manners will do and it's easy to develop a friendship over the course of a long study. Remember to always maintain a professional relationship, no matter how much you like the study coordinator. The CRA still must be able to enforce compliance if the study gets out of line. It is not easy to maintain your position of authority if the relationship becomes too friendly. It is important to establish best communication practices with the study coordinator (by email or telephone in between monitoring visits; in person and email or texting and email during monitoring visits). Some study coordinators like to be contacted several times during the day to address findings. Some study coordinators want the CRA to review things methodically at the end of a monitoring visit and have the CRA email them the findings pending and discussed at the end of the visit instead of leaving sticky notes. The CRA must work with the site and will probably have to swallow ego, suppress the need to be "right" and compromise more (but not on ethics) in order to maintain the relationship. It is more important to lose the battle and win the overall campaign than to win the small battle and lose sight of the end game and ultimate outcome.

Site Management

There are a number of general issues the CRA will want to be aware of when monitoring a site, including interpersonal relationships at the site, the stability of the staff, organization, how site personnel manage their time and an overall impression and feeling about the site. The atmosphere at a site affects the study. The better it is and the smoother things run, the better the study will progress.

Be observant when monitoring a site. Do people get along well with one another? Do they work together? Are there obvious antagonisms, one-upmanship, etc.? If one person is very busy, do others help out? If there are problems, the CRA may need to work around them in order to achieve monitoring objectives. At the same time, the CRA will need to be careful not to add to any bad situations; the CRA should always treat everyone well, be pleasant and smile. Stay out of site politics.

Look at the organization of the office. Are things running smoothly or are they always scattered? If they are scattered, the study will often run the same way, unless the CRA puts in additional time to help organize things for smoother operation. Do site people have enough time to do their usual jobs plus the study? Are things always late or done quickly but incorrectly? Were they prepared for the monitoring visit? Sometimes the CRA may need to put extra effort into helping site personnel organize and manage the study efficiently.

Another CRA responsibility is problem solving. Things rarely go exactly as planned and clinical trials are no exception. The CRA must be prepared for a variety of potential problems such as enrollment difficulties, personnel turnover, waning interest in the study by site personnel, poor conduct of the study and protocol violations. Experience, knowledge and good common sense are your best tools for problem solving.

A CRA needs to think about how to approach a site that does sloppy work. Some CRAs try to crack the whip right from the very start, while others adopt a more moderate approach. In general, a moderate approach is the best, using the minimum amount of pressure required to get the necessary results. It is important for a CRA to learn how to take care of site problems without alienating the investigator and site personnel. If the site staff are unhappy with the CRA, the study will languish and everyone loses.

If a problem arises that a CRA feels uncomfortable dealing with, or does not know how to solve, the CRA should speak with his or her supervisor or study project manager. Don't ignore problems; they seldom go away by themselves. If there are problems with site management, the CRA may have to monitor more often to ensure that the study is run properly and that things are done in a timely manner.

Monitoring Strategy

A CRA will need to develop an overall "hands on" monitoring strategy for site visits. In general, it is best to start with the most important activities, or at least the ones that must be done at each visit. This will ensure that if time runs short and everything cannot be completed, at least the most important things will have been reviewed.

One monitoring plan consists of the following activities, done in the order listed:

- Serious adverse event review.
- Informed consent review.
- New subject/subject screening visit review.
- Protocol adherence check.
- Review of delegation log/new staff conducting duties and training logs.
- eCRF/CRF review and source document review.
- Queries and error correction.
- Investigational product review and accountability.
- Review of previous findings from the last monitoring visit for resolution.
- Review of laboratory samples/lab queries.
- Study document file review.
- Review of supplies/inventory.

Of course, you will also want to spend some time with the investigator, the coordinator and, perhaps, other site personnel.

Some CRAs schedule additional time with study coordinators at the end of the monitoring visit to review and address findings generated during monitoring visits. Study coordinators do not appreciate a CRA generating a long list of findings and leaving it for the study coordinator to review without assistance. The extra time spent with the study coordinator will help ensure a greater level of study understanding and compliance. It will perpetuate a positive site dynamic.

Serious Adverse Event Review

One of the first things a CRA should do at each monitoring visit is ask the investigator and coordinator if there have been any serious adverse events since the last visit and, if there have been, if they were reported to the sponsor. Whether or not the serious events were reported to the sponsor, the CRA should examine the SAE transmittal form/EDC for information available about the events, including a review of the patient chart/eCRF and any supporting documentation.

If additional information about an SAE is available, but has not yet been sent to the sponsor, the CRA can collect it and ensure that it is submitted to the appropriate person at the sponsor in a timely manner. The CRA can also discuss with site personnel the need for any additional information necessary for complete reporting. (Serious adverse event reporting is discussed in detail in Chapter 15.)

Informed Consent Review

At each visit, the CRA should check the informed consents for each new subject enrolled since the last visit. Informed consent forms should be signed and dated by the subject or the subject's legally authorized representative. Check the dates (and times, if available) against the date/time the subject started the study; both should precede study entry. Others, such as a study subject, investigator or witness, should initial or sign the consent form, if required. The person signing the consent should also date it; site personnel must never date the subject's signature on a consent form.

The CRA should check how a site documents the informed consent process. Information pertaining to the appropriate documentation of the informed consent process was discussed in detail in Chapter 9.

The CRA should check to be sure the correct consent is being used, especially if the site is doing more than one study.

If the consent form for a study has changed (e.g., protocol amendment), the CRA must be sure all newly enrolled subjects sign the appropriate consent. Except for a file copy, any copies of the old, inappropriate consent should be destroyed so they are not used inadvertently. If subjects who signed the old consent are still part of the study, they should sign the new consent before continuing. The CRA should also check to be sure this was done.

It is a good idea to periodically go back and check all signed consents at the same time. One reason is to ensure they are all still there and available. It is also a good idea to flip through and look at all the signatures at once; they should vary, and it should be obvious that they were signed by different people.

If a site is using electronic informed consent, the CRA may be able to review the ICFs remotely, under the correct circumstances, ahead of the visit, which will help cut down the time and amount of activities to be completed during the monitoring visit.

Checking Protocol Adherence

CRAs should check protocol adherence when monitoring each subject's data. It is easy to become so involved in checking the eCRFs/ CRFs and source documents that the overall protocol adherence can be missed—it's the "not seeing the forest for the trees" syndrome. To ensure adherence, the CRA will want to check the following items:

- Subject Eligibility. Did the subject meet all the inclusion and exclusion criteria?
- Randomization. Was the subject randomized to the correct subject number and did he or she receive the appropriate IP assignment/kit?
- Medical History/Adverse Events/Concomitant Medications. Do concomitant medications match corresponding medical history or reported adverse events? Were concomitant medications given to treat adverse events captured in the source/CRFs? Does current medical history require treatment with a medication not listed in the source or CRF (diabetes, hypertension, thyroid disease, etc.)? A cross analysis of all three elements will help with accuracy in reconciliation.
- Protocol Activities. Were the correct activities done for or by the subject at each visit?
- Visit Schedule and Windows. The visit window is the number of days around the actual projected visit date when the subject can be seen. The window is usually the date plus and minus a number of days. For example, if the subject is due to be seen on May 6th and the window is plus and minus two days, the subject can be seen between May 4th and May 8th. Did the patient come in for each visit during the appropriate time period?
- Drug Dispensing. Was the subject given the appropriate drug and the appropriate amount at each visit? Did the subject return any unused study drug? Was enough study drug taken so that the subject met the rules for drug compliance?

CRAs often use the protocol and schedule of activities pulled right up on their computer or printed copies of the protocol and monitoring plan when they monitor to directly review eligibility criteria against screened subjects, to ensure sites are completing the required assessments within window, etc. CRAs also use visit calculators to ensure visit time windows are met.

eCRF/CRF and Source Document Review

Most of the CRA's monitoring time is spent on eCRF/CRF review and source document review (SDR). A suggested approach to this activity is the following:

- Start with new subjects, those enrolled since the last monitoring visit.
- Next, review the other currently enrolled subjects.
- Check all the eCRFs/CRFs for a subject before doing source document review.
- Then do SDR before checking the next subject's CRF.
- Finish one subject at a time.

The reason for starting with new subjects is that the CRA will want to be sure they qualify for the study. If the subject does not qualify or if other mistakes are being made, it is best to catch them soon after the subject is enrolled, rather than later.

CRF review and SDR require a different focus. It is easier to review the CRFs before looking at the source document. We will look at each of these activities in more detail. Finishing one subject at a time is simply a good organizational tool. When the CRA has finished with the activities for a subject, put those items away. It is too easy to get mixed up when trying to review multiple subjects at the same time.

eCRF/CRF Review

When reviewing the CRFs for a subject, first check each single page or eCRF field. The CRA should check for completeness to ensure that each item has been completed and each blank is filled in. Are the answers within range? Is the header complete and correct? (The header is the top part of each form that lists the subject and study identifiers.) Is the form signed/checked off/validated, if appropriate, and by the correct person? Are the format/forms legible and all fields complete? If the CRA has trouble interpreting what has been recorded, the data entry person may also have trouble reading what has been recorded.

Next, check all of the pages/fields for a single visit. Check for completeness and correct dates. Is the visit within the window allowed? Check to be sure the timing of procedures was appropriate. If, for example, there was to be a blood draw followed by another activity, the blood draw should have been done first, and the times should reflect this. Any time there is a specific order to be followed for activities, that order must be followed. Check for consistency across forms/fields. If the subject is getting better according to various ratings, then the overall rating should reflect an improvement. If a form says there was a concomitant medication administered for an adverse event, then the medication should be listed on the concomitant medication form/field and the adverse event entered on the adverse event eCRF/ CRF. In addition, the CRA should think about what appears on the forms and whether it makes sense, given the subject condition and the study activities. If something does not make sense, the CRA should discuss it with the study coordinator and/ or investigator.

The CRA should also check across visits. Are the data consistent from visit to visit? Is the timing of procedures appropriate? Do the data match where necessary? Are the visit windows correct over time? Usually each visit window is calculated by going back to the starting or baseline date, not from the previous visit. The reason is if a subject is always two days late, and if the window is always calculated from the last visit, you are adding two days and two more days and two more days and so forth. After a while, there is not enough study drug for the subject to finish all the visits specified by the protocol.

The CRA should look for data trends and inconsistencies to ensure the data is authentic across subjects at a site.

Lastly, be sure it is the same subject at each visit, with the same initials, number and other identifier. It is always better to straighten out any problems while reviewing CRFs at the site, as opposed to having the forms sent in and making corrections later. After completing the case report form review, it is time to do the source document review. Error correction will be discussed following the source document review section.

The above details on CRF review may or may not apply to EDC/eCRF systems so we kept it general to address both situations. With eCRF/EDC systems the CRA will not need to do all of this kind of CRF review as most basic edits will be done automatically by the EDC programmer in house, by the sponsor's data management group or by remote monitor. The CRA will still need to work with the site on data queries. More discussion of this can be found in the EDC section of Chapter 11.

Source Document Review

Source document review/verification, involves checking the data recorded in the eCRFs/CRFs against data found in available source documents, including the patient's medical chart, electronic medical record (EMR) data, electronic source (eSource), laboratory reports, radiology reports, hospitalizations and other supporting documents. A source document is any document on which the data are first recorded and can range from a patient's blood pressure recorded on a sticky note to a physician's note to a dictated X-ray report.

The purpose of source documentation is twofold: first, to verify that the subjects exist, and second, to verify that data in the eCRF/CRF are consistent with the information found in the source documents, which verifies the integrity of the data.

One would expect to see basic demographic information in an office medical chart for a patient, including name, address, phone number, insurance information, etc. The CRA is not interested in the particulars of this information, but only that it exists. The usual office medical chart will also contain lab reports or reports of other diagnostic or confirmatory medical tests. The name and identifying information should match the other information in the chart. This information is indicative that the person entered in the trial actually exists.

Many hospitals, health organizations and physician/medical practices are transitioning or have transitioned to an electronic medical record (EMR) system for patient medical record data. Historically paper-based EMRs have been implemented to comply with the mandate that healthcare providers and other eligible professionals (EP) must demonstrate "meaningful use" of EMRs in order to maintain current Medicaid and Medicare reimbursement levels.

The transition to a patient EMR system (at investigational sites) has forced the classification of EMR data as "source." A patient's original medical record has always been considered a part of source documents, of course, to varying degrees dependent on site data collection practices. Some sites only class the medical record as study source for the accompanying demographic, diagnostic, medical history, medication information that is recorded in the study patient's CRF and confirmed by CRAs during monitoring visits; they use paper source documents for capture of specific study visit or procedures data. Some investigational sites record study-specific data in the patient's medical record or typically use standard-of-care information or patient visits as part of study data. Regardless of site process, with the transition to an EMR system, the patient's EMR is also a source document.

There are numerous EMR programs being utilized. Some sites use systems that require direct entry of notes made by physicians or nurses or patient medical information into the system. Other sites complete progress notes or charting on paper forms and scan/upload them in the EMR system.

Monitoring practices have adapted to include electronic record review.

There are several means by which investigational sites will provide CRAs with access to a study patient's EMR for review:

- A printed EMR.
  - Site staff will print a study patient's EMR and place it in a subject study folder for CRA review during monitoring visits. The site staff will be requested to confirm that the EMR printout is consistent with the actual patient EMR and that everything applicable has been printed as far as patient visits and medical data. They should also "certify" the printout. The person tasked with printing out the EMR should initial and date the document. Sites provide EMR printouts because they do not have the capability to provide the CRA access to the EMR for review of study patient data or they are not permitted to provide the CRA access to the EMR due to institutional HIPAA or data privacy rules.
- Review of a study patient's EMR with the study coordinator or site staff.
  - The study coordinator or site staff member is logged in to view the EMR and the CRA sits with them to review the required portions of the study patient's EMR. This usually happens when a site does not have the technological means to provide the CRA direct EMR access to review study patient data.
- Direct, read-only review of a study patient's EMR.
  - Sites will provide CRAs with "read-only" access to study patient's EMR data. The CRA's review is limited to designated study patients; they cannot access other data in the system.

- CRAs are provided with their own unique username and password to log into the system.

How a CRA is provided a study patient's EMR for review varies per investigational site model and technology practices. Most small single-investigator practices will only have the means to provide the CRA with printed copies of the study patient's EMR for review. Either their EMR system does not have the capability to provide read-only access to only a study patient's EMR or they don't have a staff member who can sit with a CRA for several hours during a monitoring visit to allow the CRA to review study patients' EMR data (with the staff member logged into the EMR and observing the CRA). These sites may allow the CRA to "spot check" the EMR system with the printed EMR by providing a site staff member who is logged into the EMR to show the CRA that the printed sections match those in the EMR.

Larger health organizations or academic institutions may have the IT infrastructure and technology to provide CRAs with read-only access to the study patient's data they need to review at specific monitoring visits. They may also have extra staff sit with the CRA for a few hours during monitoring visits for the purpose of study patient EMR review, as noted above. The CRA may have to sign a confidentiality agreement to obtain username/password access to the institutional EMR, but it is critical that the CRA have his or her manager review the confidentiality agreement for appropriateness before signing anything. Remember that investigational sites may need several weeks' notice to obtain the CRA's login credentials for the EMR system. Providing site staff advance notice of this is important. In this age of technologically driven data review, the only investigational site model almost completely exempt from EMR system integration of data is dedicated research sites. As they are not a fee-for-service medical practice and historically treat only research subjects during study conduct, research sites do not maintain traditional medical records. Most dedicated research sites maintain paper source documents to note a patient's medical history, demographics, medication and study-related data. Research staff may have requested and successfully obtained a copy of a study patient's medical record from their primary physician, but it was a paper-based printout or copy of the patient's electronic medical record. Research sites are one of the few investigational site models that use primarily paper records (besides some investigator physician medical practices). However, this trend is slowly changing as dedicated research sites are transitioning to electronic source (eSource) systems. eSource systems allow source documents to be created within a database for study patient visits, medications, adverse events, drug accountability logs, etc. These systems allow unique username/password access; they are validated and the systems are backed up, similar to EMR systems. eSource systems allow paper documents with wet ink signatures to be uploaded and also allow physicians and staff to electronically sign documents. eSource systems can accommodate CRA log in and use to review data with log on credentials required much the same as EMR systems.

During site selection, sponsors need to ensure the integrity of a site EMR system/eSource system by ensuring it meets all or the integral elements of 21CFR11: unique username/password access, audit trail with data changes, system validation and system backup. This can be confirmed with the site IT representative or EMR users (study coordinators, data managers, etc.).

During the COVID pandemic, EMR systems and eSource were critical for successful remote monitoring visits. CRAs were provided access to these systems to facilitate data review. Some EMR systems allowed for source documents to be uploaded for review; sites that used EMR systems would also maintain a cloud-based system for uploading regulatory and source documents for CRA review. This allowed for full monitoring during the pandemic when onsite visits were curtailed. Some sponsors even provided sites with systems with which to upload source documents for remote monitoring, as some sites did not have these capabilities or systems.

When the data in the case report forms are in agreement with data contained in source documents, it is an indicator of the quality and veracity of the information being gathered for the study. It is not necessary for every entry in a CRF to have a matching entry in a source document; but where the data do appear in both, they should agree. Neither ICH GCPs nor FDA regulations require that source documents be kept for all entries on case report forms. Under 21 CFR 312.62(b), "An investigator is required to prepare and maintain adequate and accurate case histories that record all observations and other data pertinent to the investigation.... Case histories include the case report forms and supporting data including, for example, signed and dated consent forms, progress notes of the physician...hospital chart(s) and nurse's notes."

ICH GCPs say only that the study monitor shall verify that "the data required by the protocol are reported accurately on the CRFs and are consistent with the source data/documents." Despite the lack of any regulatory requirement, many companies require a matching source document for nearly every CRF entry. Whether or not this is the case, the CRA should verify that, where matching data do exist in source records, they are consistent with the CRFs.

On occasion, the original collection of data may be done directly on the case report form; in effect, the case report form becomes a source document. This is frequently seen in rating scales, such as the Hamilton Depression Rating Scale, because it is easier to collect the information directly on the CRF as opposed to transcribing it later. It is not wrong to do this, but a note should be made to the investigator's study file that this is being done. The sponsor may request/require this to be done.

What happens if there is a discrepancy between the case report form and the source document? Usually the source document takes precedence, but the CRA should always ask the investigator or coordinator to determine which one is correct and to make the appropriate corrections. If the source document is corrected, the site staffer making the change should sign and date the document, including an explanation, as appropriate. CRAs should not make changes on either the source documents or the case report forms; this is the responsibility of site personnel. The CRA must remember that even one change on a CRF can have an impact on other data. Be sure to check this, both within the visit and across visits.

There are significant differences among sponsors with respect to the amount of source document review a CRA must do. Some companies require "100 percent source document review," but the definitions of 100 percent source document review also vary, from the expectation of a source document for every data point for every subject to 100 percent verification of the data insofar as it exists in source documents. Other sponsors have a sampling scheme, and these also vary considerably. Whatever the scheme, however, a majority of the subjects' case report forms are normally reviewed for critical information, such as inclusion and exclusion criteria, a signed consent, adverse events and critical study-specific parameters.

Some source document review sampling scheme examples are:

- 10 percent of the subjects are done.
- The first subject and then every other subject thereafter are done.

- The first two subjects are done. If there are no problems, every fourth subject thereafter is done. If problems are found, do two more subjects. Iterate as needed.
- All subjects, but only certain variables, are done.

Risk-based monitoring involves reduced or targeted SDV/CRF review and the endpoints and sampling vary by sponsor and study.

No matter how much source document review/verification is done, it will never replace common sense. A CRA must think about what is being seen on the CRFs (paper or electronic) and in the source documents and determine if it makes sense in terms of both the study and good medical practice and if the practices support credible data and patient safety.

The acronym, ALCOA is an industry standard for appropriate source document content and standards, and must be considered during review of study/patient source documents.

A-attributable
L-legible
C-contemporaneous
O-original
A-accurate

There are four additional letters that support ALCOA—CCEA (complete, consistent, enduring and available).

Author's Story

The wrong consent form

I was monitoring with a CRA and decided to check all the consents while he was doing the case report form and source document review. The site was a busy one, doing a number of studies. As I looked through the consents, I noticed one that was different—in fact, it was not for our study at all. It was for a very similar study, but one being done for a different sponsor. It was interesting reading, but not the right consent.

The study coordinator was chagrined, as was the CRA. The subject was, in fact, in our study, the correct CRF was being used and the correct activities were being done. The coordinator had just inadvertently grabbed the wrong consent for him to sign.

To remedy this situation, the investigator contacted the subject, explained the problem and asked him to sign a new, correct consent form. The situation was documented in the site's study file, including the changes they made to their procedures to ensure that it would not happen again. From then on, consents for each study were placed in a separate folder, clearly marked and stored in separate locations, rather than together in one file.

—A CRA

Electronic Source

The FDA has a guidance document for electronic source data that came out in September 2013, entitled "Guidance for Industry: Electronic Source Data in Clinical Investigations." As noted in the introduction section of the guidance, page 1:

> This guidance provides recommendations to sponsors, Contract Research Organizations (CROs), clinical investigators, and others involved in the capture, review and retention of electronic source data in FDA-regulated clinical investigations. In an effort to streamline and modernize clinical investigations, this guidance promotes capturing source data in electronic form. It is intended to assist in ensuring the reliability, quality, integrity and traceability of data from electronic source to electronic regulatory submission.
>
> This guidance addresses source data in clinical investigations used to fill the predefined fields in an electronic case report form (eCRF), according to the protocol. The guidance discusses the following topics related to electronic source data:
>
> - Identification and specification of authorized source data originators.
> - Creation of data element identifiers to facilitate examination of the audit trail by sponsors, the FDA and other authorized parties.
> - Ways to capture source data into the eCRF using either manual or electronic methods.
> - Clinical investigator(s) responsibilities with respect to reviewing and retaining electronic data.

- Use and description of computerized systems in clinical investigations.

This guidance is intended to be used together with the FDA guidance for industry on Computerized Systems Used in Clinical Investigations (the computerized systems guidance) and FDA regulation on Electronic Records and Electronic Signatures. Electronic structures and standards related to electronic submissions are out of scope for this guidance.

The background section, page 2, describes what the FDA considers electronic records and source data.

With the use of computerized systems for capturing clinical investigation data, it is common to find at least some source data recorded electronically. Common examples include, but are not limited to, clinical data initially recorded in electronic health records maintained by healthcare providers and institutions, electronic laboratory reports, digital medical images from devices and electronic diaries completed by study subjects.

FDA regulations define an electronic record as any combination of text, graphics, data, audio, pictorial or other information represented in digital form that is created, modified, maintained, archived, retrieved or distributed by a computer system. An eCRF is an example of an electronic record.

The eCRF is an auditable electronic record of information that generally is reported to the sponsor on each trial subject, according to a clinical investigation protocol.

The eCRF enables clinical investigation data to be systematically captured, reviewed, managed, stored, analyzed and reported.

Source data includes all information in original records and certified copies of original records of clinical findings, observations, or other activities in a clinical investigation used for reconstructing and evaluating the investigation. Access to source data is critical to the review and inspections of clinical investigations. The review of source data by both the FDA and sponsor is important to ensure adequate protection of the rights, welfare and safety of human subjects and the quality and integrity of the clinical investigation data. Source data should be attributable, legible, contemporaneous, original and accurate (ALCOA) and must meet the regulatory requirements for recordkeeping.

Capturing source data electronically and transmitting it to the eCRF should:

- Eliminate unnecessary duplication of data
- Reduce the possibility for transcription errors
- Encourage entering source data during a subject's visit, where appropriate
- Eliminate transcription of source data prior to entry into an eCRF
- Facilitate remote monitoring of data
- Promote real-time access for data review
- Facilitate the collection of accurate and complete data

Electronic source data origination is further clarified on page 3.

Electronic source data are data initially recorded in electronic format. They can include information in original records and certified copies of original records of clinical findings, observations or other activities captured prior to or during a clinical investigation used for reconstructing and evaluating the investigation.

The guidance gives further examples of data elements on page 3:

A data element in an eCRF represents the smallest unit of observation captured for a subject in a clinical investigation. Examples of data elements include race, white blood cell count, pain severity measurement or other clinical observations made and documented during a study. Each data element is associated with an authorized data originator. Examples of data originators include:

- Clinical investigator(s) and delegated clinical study staff
- Clinical investigation subjects or their legally authorized representatives
- Consulting services (e.g., a radiologist reporting on a computed tomography (CT) scan)
- Medical devices (e.g., electrocardiograph (ECG) machine and other medical instruments such as a blood pressure machine)
- Electronic health records (EHRs)

- Automated laboratory reporting systems (e.g., from central laboratories)
- Other technology

A list of all authorized data originators (i.e., persons, systems, devices and instruments) should be developed and maintained by the sponsor and made available at each clinical site. In the case of electronic, patient-reported outcome measures, the subject (e.g., unique subject identifier) should be listed as the originator.

When identification of data originators relies on identification (logon) codes and unique passwords, controls must be employed to ensure the security and integrity of the authorized user names and passwords. When electronic thumbprints or other biometric identifiers are used in place of an electronic login/password, controls should be designed to ensure that they cannot be used by anyone other than their original owner.

When a system, device or instrument automatically populates a data element field in the eCRF, a data element identifier... should be created that automatically identifies the particular system, device or instrument (e.g., name and type) as the originator of the data element. For example, if an ECG machine automatically transmits to the eCRF, a data element identifier should be generated that identifies the ECG machine as the originator.

Risk-Based Monitoring: Remote and Central Monitoring Practices

The FDA has two guidance documents for risk-based monitoring that are relevant to the premise and methods that support this quality process, listed below in chronological order. The first guidance referenced below came out in 2013. The second is an April 2023 final guidance that supports the first guidance but adds more measures.

The August 2013 risk-based monitoring guidance, titled Guidance for Industry: Oversight of Clinical Investigations—A Risk-Based Approach to Monitoring, aims to assist sponsors of clinical investigations in:

> ... developing risk-based monitoring strategies and plans for investigational studies of medical products, including human drug and biological products, medical devices and combinations thereof. The overarching goal of this guidance is to enhance human subject protection and the quality of clinical trial data by focusing sponsor oversight on the most important aspects of study conduct and reporting.
>
> This guidance makes clear that sponsors can use a variety of approaches to fulfill their responsibilities for monitoring clinical investigator (CI) conduct and performance in investigational new drug (IND) studies conducted under 21 CFR part 312 or investigational device exemption (IDE) studies conducted under 21 CFR part 812. The guidance describes strategies for monitoring activities that reflect a modern, risk-based approach that focuses on critical study parameters and relies on a combination of monitoring activities to oversee a study effectively. For example, the guidance specifically encourages greater use of centralized monitoring methods where appropriate.

The dynamic of traditional onsite monitoring and data review practices has shifted with the advent of internet/cloud-based programs that adequately support real-time, remote data review. Central or remote monitoring practices allow sponsors faster and more efficient access to critical study data points via electronic data capture systems, data analytics systems or shared research drives for CRF/source document uploading. This provides an additional level of oversight and serves as one indicator of site compliance to study conduct and patient safety.

Over the past several years, some CROs/pharma/biotech companies have adopted a risk-based/remote monitoring program, replacing the frequency and intensity of onsite monitoring visits that focused on 100% source/CRF review with a hybrid of remote data review and onsite targeted monitoring of source documents/CRFs. The complexity of a study, treatment and procedures dictate the ability to perform a portion of remote or onsite monitoring. A thorough risk assessment of the protocol and investigational sites is required. Targeted review of critical endpoint data to assess trends in noncompliance, protocol deviations and data errors onsite will also determine the need and frequency of onsite versus remote monitoring visits. Those sites with higher instances of data errors or protocol non-compliance will require more frequent onsite monitoring visits, not just for the purpose of additional source document/CRF review but also for the purposes of site auditing, training and CAPA.

There are several means of remote/central monitoring practices, including:

- Data management, remote monitor or CRA staff review EDC data from a central or remote location to pinpoint critical study visit discrepancies and trends.
- CRAs review EDC and source documents during "remote" or onsite monitoring visits; targeted data review of such things as informed consent forms, eligibility criteria, safety or critical data points, drug accountability logs, regulatory documents, medication logs, SAEs, endpoint of efficacy data—anything identified during a risk assessment as critical. Investigational site staff transmit study source documents to accompany the EDC or source documents and CRFs are uploaded to a shared drive for this review purpose if not onsite.
- Email/telephone/videoconferencing occurs to discuss discrepancies, retraining or corrective action. The investigator may need to be present for some of these telephone calls.
- Onsite monitoring of data also occurs.

It is a challenging transition for investigational sites to accept the dynamic of remote and onsite monitoring plans, although this has become a standard practice in recent years.

The guidance explains, however:

> During the past two decades, the number and complexity of clinical trials have grown dramatically. These changes create new challenges to clinical trial oversight, particularly increased variability in clinical investigator experience, site infrastructure, treatment choices and standards of healthcare, as well as challenges related to geographic dispersion.
>
> At the same time, increasing use of electronic systems and records and improvements in statistical assessments, present opportunities for alternative monitoring approaches (e.g., centralized monitoring) that can improve the quality and efficiency of sponsor oversight of clinical investigations.
>
> The FDA encourages sponsors to develop monitoring plans that manage important risks to human subjects and data quality and address the challenges of oversight in part by taking advantage of the innovations in modern clinical trials. A risk-based approach to monitoring does not suggest any less vigilance in oversight of clinical investigations. Rather, it focuses

> sponsor oversight activities on preventing or mitigating important and likely risks to data quality and to processes critical to human subject protection and trial integrity.
>
> Moreover, a risk-based approach is dynamic, more readily facilitating continual improvement in trial conduct and oversight. For example, monitoring findings should be evaluated to determine whether additional actions (e.g., training of clinical investigator and site staff, clarification of protocol requirements) are necessary to ensure human subject protection and data quality across sites.

CRAs who are not already comfortable with the use of internet or web-based programs for the purposes of remote monitoring will need to quickly orient to computerized review of study data to stay current with technology-driven data collection practices.

The FDA's April 2023 guidance on risk-based monitoring, titled "A Risk-Based Approach to Monitoring of Clinical Investigations," notes in Section 1 that the document expands on the agency's August 2013 guidance to provide:

> … information on risk-based approaches to monitoring the conduct of clinical investigations of human drug and biological products, medical devices, and combination products. Clinical investigation monitoring is a quality control tool for determining whether investigation activities are being carried out as planned. This guidance contains recommendations on planning a monitoring approach, developing the content of a monitoring plan and addressing and communicating monitoring results. This guidance expands on the guidance for industry Oversight of Clinical Investigations – A Risk-Based Approach to Monitoring (August 2013) (the 2013 RBM guidance) by providing additional information to facilitate sponsors' implementation of risk-based monitoring.

In Section 2, the guidance describes a system to manage the quality of the investigation that should include a risk-based approach to monitoring:

> Sponsors of clinical investigations involving human drugs, biological products, medical devices, and combination products are required to provide oversight, including ensuring proper monitoring of the investigation. Such oversight helps to ensure adequate protection of the rights, safety, and welfare of participants in the clinical investigation and the integrity of the

data submitted to FDA. Therefore, sponsors should implement a system to manage, throughout all stages of the clinical investigation, both risks to participants (e.g., a safety problem) and to data integrity (e.g., incomplete and/or inaccurate data).

This system to manage the quality of the investigation should help ensure data integrity while safeguarding the rights, safety, and welfare of trial participants, for example, by focusing on the design of efficient clinical trial protocols, tools for identifying and tracking potential risks, and procedures for data collection and processing. This system should include a risk-based approach to monitoring tailored to the potential risks for the specific clinical investigation. Effective implementation of risk-based monitoring, including the prioritization of monitoring and other oversight activities directed at processes and procedures critical for human subject protection and maintaining data integrity, should help maximize the quality of a clinical investigation.

Although FDA's regulations require sponsors to monitor the conduct and progress of theirclinical investigations, FDA regulations are not specific about how sponsors are to conduct monitoring. FDA recommends that sponsors use a risk-based approach to develop theirmonitoring plans and to revise their monitoring plans, if needed, as the clinical investigation proceeds. This risk-based approach should be informed by the sponsor's overarching quality management activities undertaken in the development of the protocol and associated investigational plans and should be adjusted throughout the conduct of the investigation as needed.

As described in the 2013 RBM guidance, FDA recommends that at the protocol design stage, sponsors identify the critical data and processes necessary for human subject protection and maintaining data integrity for the investigation. Once these are identified, sponsors should perform a risk assessment and determine whether risks to critical data and processes may be mitigated through revisions to the protocol and investigational plans. When risks cannot be resolved through such revisions, sponsors should determine how remaining critical risks will be identified, tracked, and managed via the sponsors' monitoring plan or related study oversight plans during the conduct of the investigation. Such efforts to build quality into the design and execution of clinical investigations should be informed by representative study team members involved with conduct, monitoring, and/or reporting of the investigation. Perspectives from patients within the target population to be recruited for a clinical investigation would also be valuable.

Monitoring should be conducted per the pre-established monitoring plan, and important issues identified through monitoring should be addressed as they are identified. Monitoring plans should also include directions for when and to whom important issues identified during monitoring should be escalated. In addition, FDA recommends that monitoring plans provide guidance on when and how to adjust monitoring activities based on observed monitoring findings. For example, when important issues are identified during monitoring of a clinical site, there may be a need to increase the duration or frequency of on-site visits at that site...

The study-level monitoring plan and associated monitoring activities are among the elements utilized by sponsors in their overall risk-based quality management approach to product development; they are important tools to facilitate sponsors identifying and addressing issues during the conduct of clinical investigations. The 2013 RBM guidance outlines factors that sponsors should consider in developing a monitoring plan and tailoring monitoring plans to the needs of the investigation and provides examples of monitoring methods and techniques. Since finalizing the 2013 RBM guidance, FDA has concluded that additional guidance may be beneficial regarding its recommendations for planning a monitoring approach, developing the content of monitoring plans, and addressing and communicating monitoring results.

The guidance also includes several questions and answers to assist sponsors in planning and conducting risk-based approaches to monitoring, such as:

Section A, Monitoring Approach

Q3. What factors should sponsors consider when determining the timing, types, frequency, and extent of monitoring activities?

As described in detail in the 2013 RBM guidance, during the risk assessment, sponsors should consider a range of factors to inform the development of the monitoring plan. While some factors described below (see bulleted factors) relate to the investigation overall, other factors relate to specific clinical sites; therefore, FDA recommends that the monitoring plan be organized to account for both the overall investigation and site-specific risks, recognizing that some mitigating activities may not be relevant for all sites.

Sponsors should consider:

- How well established the clinical investigation infrastructures are at different clinical sites
- Relative experience of the clinical investigator and of the sponsor with the clinical investigator
- Electronic data capture to be utilized
  - Use of electronic data capture (EDC) systems with the capability to assess quality metrics (e.g., missing data, data error rates, protocol violations) in real time could help identify potentially higher risk sites for the purpose of targeting sites in need of more intensive monitoring.
- Stage of the study (e.g., for a complex study, more intensive and on-site monitoring might be warranted early, but once procedures are established, less intensive monitoring might suffice)
- Quantity, extent, complexity, and criticality of data to be collected

When developing the monitoring plan, sponsors should determine the types and intensity of monitoring activities best suited to address the identified risks while also facilitating identification of unanticipated risks. When suitable, statistical and analytical methods to monitor critical data in a centralized manner may be particularly advantageous. Monitoring activities should evolve based on additional issues and risks that may be identified during the conduct of the investigation. The types and intensity of monitoring activities also should be proportionate to the risks to participants' rights, safety, and welfare and to data integrity inherent in the investigation.

While source data verification (SDV) may be a part of a risk-based monitoring approach, the extent to which SDV is used should be guided by the sponsor's risk assessment process and focused on critical study data and processes. Focusing more monitoring activities on risks to the most critical data elements and processes should enable sponsors to achieve the objective of conducting a quality clinical investigation, including human subject protection and data integrity, without necessarily having to conduct frequent routine visits to all clinical sites and extensive SDV.

FDA also recommends that sponsors consider the following additional factors:

- Adequate staffing to support the clinical investigation. Specific considerations include relevant study-specific trainings of site staff, the experience and qualifications of the research coordinator and specialized research professionals working with and under the direction of the clinical investigator, and turnover of personnel at the investigational site or among monitoring staff.
- Location where participants will be seen and whether they will be seen at more than one location to complete investigation procedures (for example, data collection at the imaging center, at a local physician's office, or at the participant's home), including when all activities take place at locations remote from the investigator without the need for a physical clinical site.
  - When designing the monitoring plan, sponsors should take into consideration where and how the data are going to be collected in the investigation relative to where the sponsor oversight activities will be conducted (for example, to confirm that appropriate controls, instructions, and training tools are in place).
- Benefit of an early monitoring visit or other early monitoring activities
  - By scheduling an early monitoring visit (for example, soon after the first few trial participants enroll in the investigation) or by carrying out other early monitoring activities, sponsors can help ensure early in the investigation that the protocol is being followed and procedures are being performed correctly at clinical sites. Additionally, if early monitoring identifies issues, such as a number of protocol deviations, corrective actions can be implemented sooner. For complex studies, early and more intensive on-site monitoring might be warranted

Q4. How can a risk-based approach to monitoring that includes centralized monitoring help minimize missing data or protocol deviations?

Centralized monitoring is a systematic analytical evaluation of study conduct across multiple clinical sites, carried out by sponsor personnel or representatives (e.g., clinical monitors, data management personnel, or statisticians). Centralized monitoring may allow sponsors to (1) review study-wide data for inconsistencies or omissions; (2) perform activities such as data checks, for completeness and consistency; (3) verify source data; (4) ensure that institutional review board and informed consent documents are current; and (5) determine which clinical sites need on-site review.

Depending on how centralized monitoring is used, incorporating centralized monitoring as a part of a risk-based approach to monitoring may help ensure the quality of a clinical investigation by allowing sponsors to aggregate and compare site data and detect potential anomalies more quickly. By reviewing study data and metadata in real time across clinical sites, sponsors may be able to identify quality issues, such as delays in entering data or incomplete entries, earlier than when relying on on-site monitoring alone. Sites with multiple issues detected through centralized monitoring, such as delays in assessments or missing assessments, may also provide an early signal that the sponsor should promptly determine whether there is a need for a site visit and corrective actions to minimize the likelihood of similar issues occurring during the remainder of the clinical investigation.

Section B. Monitoring Plan Content

Q6. What elements should sponsors include in monitoring plans?

Monitoring plans should be developed for each investigation based on the risk assessment for that investigation. Monitoring plans should address both study-specific and site-specific risks.Monitoring plans also should be designed to enable the management of anticipated and unanticipated risks. As stated earlier, sponsors are encouraged to develop risk-based monitoring plans that emphasize critical risks with the greatest potential to adversely affect investigation quality, including (1) the rights, safety, and welfare of participants in a clinical investigation; and(2) the collection or analysis of critical clinical data such as safety and efficacy/effectiveness endpoints. Section IV.D of the 2013 RBM guidance discusses in detail the recommended components of a monitoring plan. Sponsors also may reference in the monitoring plan other clinical trial management plans used for risk management (e.g., a data management plan) that address the components recommended in the 2013 RBM guidance rather than repeat the same information in the monitoring plan.

In addition to the components recommended in the 2013 RBM guidance, FDA recommends that monitoring plans also include the following components, which will help explain how the sponsor intends to address the risks that could affect the clinical investigation:

- A description of the investigation design, including the blinding and randomization procedures, if applicable
- Processes for confirming that randomization is performed according to the protocol and investigational plan or plans
- The sampling plan or plans that will be used to identify the specific records and data that will be monitored, including (1) the rationale for how the sampling plan provides a representative picture of the overall information; and (2) how the sampling plan will be implemented
- A description of the types of issues identified through monitoring that would trigger immediate issue escalation
- An approach for determining whether (1) an important issue that is detected at a clinical site may also be present at other clinical sites; and (2) the finding suggests a systemic problem with the protocol or associated investigational plans that requires remediation.

Section C. Follow-Up and Communication of Monitoring Results

Q7. How should sponsors follow up on significant issues identified through monitoring, including communication of such issues?

Significant issues should be thoroughly evaluated in a timely manner at the appropriate levels (for example, sponsor, clinical sites) as described in the monitoring plan. A root cause analysis followed by appropriate corrective and preventive actions should be undertaken promptly to reduce the impact of the identified issue on the rights, safety, and welfare of participants in the clinical investigation and/or the integrity of the data. Additionally, the risk assessment and monitoring plan should be reviewed and revised, as needed, to help ensure the risk of recurrence is decreased, or if possible, eliminated. In instances in which corrective actions modify study processes, the protocol and/or associated investigational plans should be amended to reflect changed processes. Related systemic issues should be identified and resolved promptly to help ensure that investigation quality, including the rights, safety, and welfare of investigation participants and data integrity, is maintained.

Examples of preventive and corrective actions that may be warranted include but are not limited to (1) improved training for the clinical investigator and site staff; (2) halting enrollment at a clinical site pending resolution of identified issues; (3) clarifying or revising the protocol and/or other related investigational plans and documents; and/or (4) modifying vendor service agreements to ensure adequate trial support.

Significant issues identified through monitoring and oversight activities and the actions to be taken should be documented and communicated to the appropriate parties, which may include, but are not limited to (1) sponsor management; (2) sponsor teams; (3) clinical sites; (4) institutional review boards; (5) other relevant parties (for example, DMCs and relevant contract research organizations); and (6) applicable regulatory agencies, including FDA, when appropriate.

See the 2013 RBM guidance for additional recommendations regarding follow-up and communication of significant issues identified via monitoring.

Q8. How should monitoring activities and the results of these activities be documented and shared with those involved in the investigation?

As described in the 2013 RBM guidance, documentation of monitoring activities should generally include the following: (1) the date of the activity; (2) the individuals conducting and participating in the activity; (3) a summary of the data or activities reviewed; (4) a description of any noncompliance, potential noncompliance, data irregularities, and/or other deficiencies identified; and (5) a description of any actions taken, to be taken, or recommended (see section V of the 2013 RBM guidance for additional information). Such documentation should include the results of monitoring activities in sufficient detail to allow verification of adherence to the monitoring plan describing those activities. Monitoring activities to be documented should include on-site and remote monitoring of clinical sites and centralized monitoring across clinical sites.

> Reports of monitoring activities should be provided to appropriate management (including sponsor staff responsible for the conduct and oversight of the clinical investigation) in a timely manner for review and follow-up. In addition, sponsors should inform the clinical investigator of monitoring findings from monitoring activities that are relevant to the clinical investigator's activities.

Errors, Queries and Corrections

Perhaps the most important errors a CRA might find are those that result in protocol violations. These include such things as a subject not meeting the inclusion/exclusion criteria, a wrong diagnosis, a subject taking disallowed medications, problems with visit windows, unreported or late reported SAEs and others. Often these are found during source document review. Other errors are also found during source document review and run the gamut from incorrectly transcribed data to things that are just plain wrong. Then there are the CRF errors discussed earlier, such as missing data or out-of-range values.

Correcting errors is easier if the CRA has an effective procedure for dealing with them. It is helpful to have an Error Query/Correction form that is simple and easy to work with. A sample of this form is in Appendix C. Some CRAs rely heavily on sticky notes. Although they are good reminders and mark CRFs nicely, they can fall off and get lost; plus, they do not generate an audit trail. A written correction form/log is more effective overall.

When potential errors are found, the CRA should note them in the corrections/questions log and discuss them with the study coordinator. When they are resolved, the coordinator should make the necessary corrections to the CRFs and sign/date the correction form/log; CRAs do not make the corrections. Corrections are made by drawing a line through the incorrect entry, making the correct entry and dating and initialing it. If the reason for the change is not clear, a reason should also be added to the form. It is never acceptable to use whiteout or to erase a wrong entry before correcting it; anyone reviewing the forms must be able to see what was changed, when and why. Write-overs are also unacceptable. See the example below for a change made correctly.

Date 01/16/~~08~~ 09 JAK 2/5/09

It is in the CRA's best interest to find and have the coordinator correct errors at the site before verifying the eCRF/CRF. Despite everyone's best efforts, additional errors are usually found when the CRFs go to data entry. Computer-generated errors will be sent back to the site and/or to the CRA. These are usually called queries. Different sponsors have different methods of conducting queries, but usually there is a query form sent to the site; it lists the errors and where they are located on the CRF and asks for a correction or explanation to be made and sent in. Sometimes the CRA is involved in the correction process; sometimes it is solely between the site and data management.

EDC or eCRF systems require electronic review and generation of queries for questions/discrepancies on eCRF data. They can be user or system generated. They are worded in the same manner as handwritten queries on correction forms/logs. The user generating the query (CRA or data management staff) and the individual resolving the query and related activity (study coordinator or data manager) are recorded electronically, including further clarification and resolution. There is an electronic audit trail for query creation and resolution. This is detailed in Chapter 11, "Preparing for a Study: Protocols, Case Report Forms and Electronic Data Capture."

Whether errors are found by the CRA or come in the form of queries, they should be used as training tools by a CRA. The CRA should explain to the site personnel why each one is an error and how it can be avoided in the future. It is important to review and enter the forms for the first few subjects as early as possible in order to give timely feedback to the site, with the goal of eliminating similar errors in the future. This is especially important in the case of consistent errors, which are usually due to misunderstanding. Most study coordinators want to do the job correctly and will be pleased to have feedback if it is friendly and constructive.

Error rates should decrease as the study progresses, due to feedback and training by the CRA and data management, as well as to experience on the part of site personnel. If a site continues to have a high error rate due to carelessness, the CRA will need to discuss this with both the investigator and coordinator.

Errors are very costly, both in terms of money and people hours to correct. Although most of the cost is borne by the sponsor, about one-third of the cost is borne by the site.

Good, High-Quality Data

We talk a lot in this business about "good, high-quality data," but this term isn't usually defined. By asking a number of people how they would define good, high-quality data, the following list of characteristics was generated. The general characteristics for good data are:

- They can be evaluated and analyzed.
- They allow valid conclusions to be drawn.
- They are complete and accurate.
- They do not need to be queried.
- They are consistent across subjects and sites.

More specific characteristics are:

- Subjects meet the entry criteria.
- All fields are complete.
- Entries are legible and understandable.
- Values are within range.
- Entries make logical sense.
- The units (for measurements) are correct.
- There are no extraneous comments.

If these characteristics are met, the data should lead to valid conclusions and results that are reproducible. This is the goal for clinical studies.

There are a number of steps sponsors can take to help eliminate errors and generate good, usable data. First, the sponsor should develop a good CRF or EDC system that is readable, easy for sites to use, intuitive and has clear directions. Second, don't ask for the same information more than once in the CRF/EDC system; when this happens, the data frequently do not match. (See the section on case report form development in Chapter 11.)

Clear, detailed instructions and good training are also instrumental in minimizing errors. Most errors are due to misunderstandings and these misunderstandings can be eliminated with training. CRA monitoring soon after the first few subjects are enrolled is a big help in clearing up misunderstandings. Fast turn-around on edits and queries will eliminate repeat errors, as well as cross-form edits of which the site was not aware. All of these items will help the site achieve lower error rates, with big cost savings in terms of both time and money for both the site and the sponsor.

Investigational Product (Drug, Biologic, Device)

Both the sponsor and the investigator have a number of responsibilities when it comes to the investigative drug/device. Sponsor responsibilities include:

- Keeping records showing the receipt and shipment, including the:
  - Name of the investigator to whom the drug was shipped.
  - Date, quantity and lot number shipped.
- Retaining accountability records as per regulations.
- Retaining drug samples and reference standards.
- Discontinuing shipments to investigators who fail to maintain proper records or make them available.
- Assuring the return, or destruction, of all unused drug.

Investigator responsibilities for drug accountability include:

- Maintaining control of drugs under investigation.
- Assuring that the administration of the drug (or device) is under his/her (or a sub-investigator's) supervision.
- Administering the drug/device only to those authorized to receive it.
- Maintaining records of the drug distribution, including dates, quantities and use by subjects.
- Returning unused drug to sponsor or destroying it upon sponsor authorization.

These responsibilities are found in regulations 21 CFR 312.57, 312.58, 321.59, 312.61 and 312.62.

In addition, industry practice is that study drugs are stored in secure, limited access areas (locked cabinet, locked room, locked refrigerator).

The CRA is the sponsor representative most likely to be involved with ensuring that the drug/device is being handled correctly at a clinical site, including both storage and accountability. Consequently, the CRA will want to check on the investigational drug or other product at each monitoring visit.

During the site visit, the CRA will want to check that the drug is being used properly and distributed correctly to study subjects, according to the protocol and the randomization scheme.

The CRA should check, at a minimum:

- Master- and subject-specific drug accountability logs for drug shipment receipt and drug inventory notations, as well as subject-specific drug dispensation and return entries.
- Source documents for subject-specific drug compliance counts by the study coordinator and that they reconcile with the drug accountability log.
- Sponsors are almost all using some type of interactive response technology (databases/systems/portals that are internet based) that uses Interactive Voice Response Systems (IVRS) or Interactive Web Response Systems (IWRS) to manage drug shipment and tracking centrally, that electronically maintain listings of study drug assignments, study drug inventory, etc. This needs to be crossed checked with the site master and subject-specific drug accountability logs, source documents, IVRS/IWRS receipts, diaries, EDC systems—whatever is applicable for the study.

The CRA should cross-check study drug randomization documentation/kit assignment against drug accountability logs to ensure accuracy. The CRA should review patient drug diary entries to ensure the data reconciles with site source/drug accountability counts.

Some sites are using electronic drug accountability systems to document all IP shipments, dispensation, return, high-level inventory, subject compliance counts and all drug accountability in lieu of the traditional paper drug accountability logs. The CRAs are either given direct access to these systems to review drug accountability during monitoring visits or the drug accountability logs are printed out from the electronic system during monitoring visits for CRAs to review. Regardless, CRAs need to be flexible with the drug accountability logs/systems used by a site as long as the systems are study compliant and the sponsor approves their use.

The CRA should also be sure that the drug is being stored properly, in a secure manner and that any special conditions, such as refrigeration, are being met. The CRA should check study drug temperature monitoring and documentation to ensure study drug is being stored in the required temperature parameters. Sites will use min/max thermometers or web-based, 24-hour temperature monitoring systems with the ability to print temperature ranges for a specific time period for CRA review.

If sufficient supply of the study drug has not been sent to complete the entire study and additional shipments are required, find out where the shipments are received, who receives them and when the receiving area is staffed. Avoid having drug shipments delivered when they might end up sitting on a receiving dock over a weekend or holiday. Not only is loss a concern, but it is also not a good idea for a product to be exposed to heat or freezing temperatures for very long. Know how long it takes a drug shipment to arrive at the site after an order is placed, and be sure that whoever is responsible for requesting shipments is aware of when new shipments to a site will be necessary. Whatever method of shipment is being used for investigational supplies, it should require a signature upon receipt. This significantly reduces lost or improperly handled study drugs and provides an audit trail for the receipt of the product.

It is important to verify that the study coordinator is accounting for the study drug (product) on a regular basis as the study progresses. It does not work to wait until the end of the study and then try to reconcile how much study drug is left with how much study drug is supposed to be left; it is much more successful to do this on a continuing basis. The concept of drug accountability is pretty simple: the amount of study drug shipped to the site minus the amount of study drug used by the subjects should equal what is left at the end of the study. The problem is, it never seems to work out like this. It depends on how well the site manages the study drug. It is often better if the drug is stored and dispensed by a pharmacy; it tends to do a better job of accounting for it and maintaining records, since that is its primary responsibility. A sample drug accountability form is in Appendix C.

Some sponsors require that the unused study drug be returned. In general, this is a CRA responsibility. On a periodic basis, the CRA will inventory and return to the sponsor the amount of study drug that was unused and returned by subjects, or not used at all because of early discontinuations. After it has been inventoried and packed by the CRA, the site can contact a shipper to pick it up for return. Again, it is usually better to do this periodically throughout the study rather than once at the end. It is easier to keep records straight, and it gets the unnecessary containers out of the way at the site or pharmacy.

Some sponsors will approve of sites destroying unused or used drug, provided the site has an appropriate and documented destruction process or utilizes a third party with appropriate and documented destruction methods. CRAs will need to review the site's drug destruction process and/or have the sponsor review the site's drug destruction process before allowing a site to destroy used or unused drug during the course of a study.

Use of an External Pharmacy

Some investigators may need to outsource the responsibility of study drug storage and preparation if they do not have appropriate equipment or capabilities at their own site. This can happen with complicated therapeutic indications and/or study designs that require specific study drug preparation and calculation for dosing, frequency of dosing and extensive dosing timeframes (e.g., a two-hour infusion every six hours).

The author has seen firsthand the 483 findings issued by the FDA to an investigator (who used an outside pharmacy) regarding inappropriate study drug dosing, timeframes, storage and transport because they did not ensure adequate training and oversight of third-party pharmacists/staff used in study conduct.

Investigators should ensure that all pharmacy staff involved with study drug storage, preparation and dosing attend the site initiation visit and receive specific training on study drug and pharmacy manuals. The investigator may want to visit the pharmacy in person or send a trusted staff member at consistent intervals during the study to confirm that drug preparation, dosing and dispensation/return documentation is being completed accurately. Investigator responsibility extends to all third-party or external vendors they involve in study conduct.

Unblinded Pharmacy Monitoring

A number of trial designs include a placebo arm, which may warrant the need for key unblinded personnel to help preserve the integrity of the Investigational Medicinal Product (IMP) blind. This is required when placebo differ in size, appearance, preparation or storage requirements as compared to the IMP.

The investigator/site personnel would be exposed to the identity of IMP assignment, should they be involved in the preparation or accountability of said IMP/placebo. They must therefore remain "blinded" to all components of IMP identification and designate an appropriate individual to serve as an unblinded pharmacist (e.g., the individual to receive, document, prepare and sometimes administer the IMP in lieu of blinded site personnel).

This can also occur when a comparator drug has a different appearance than the actual study drug after preparation and unblinded staff are required to prepare the study drug and comparator and blind the vehicle for administration (e.g., injection or infusion and masking the syringe or infusion bags/lines).

Though the circumstances vary according to trial requirements, the "unblinded pharmacist" typically is the only member of the site staff privy to the IMP assignment, preparation and storage process and is responsible for maintaining appropriate IMP storage, accountability logs and drug assignments from the IVRS or IWRS vendor not accessible by blinded site personnel. He or she also is tasked with conducting unblinded pharmacy monitoring visits with the unblinded pharmacy monitor.

The individual serving as the unblinded pharmacist is not required to be a licensed pharmacist, nor is he or she necessarily required to have research experience, though this is optimal. He or she should be appropriately trained/experienced/licensed (as required) with the storage and preparation of most forms of medication and accompanying administration (oral, parenteral, patches, buccal, etc.). Investigative sites typically utilize licensed personnel or personnel involved in medication administration for this task, such as nurses, respiratory therapists, pharmacy technicians, etc. It varies by state law and the delegation parameters of the investigator and sites must ensure they comply with state law, sponsor and regulatory requirements. The most important thing is that the identity of a patient's IMP assignment is preserved and that the assignment is prepared and dispensed correctly.

The CRO or pharmaceutical company responsible for managing all aspects of trial monitoring must also assign an appropriate unblinded pharmacy monitor to review subject IMP dosing and administration information and perform IMP accountability. Unblinded pharmacy monitoring is conducted exclusively with the unblinded site pharmacist and never with blinded site personnel.

The responsibilities of an unblinded pharmacy monitor include counting pills or measuring unused/used IMP vials to ensure appropriate subject dosing. The unblinded pharmacy monitor will review and cross reference IVRS or IWRS randomization and IMP assignments with source documents, diaries and drug accountability logs to ensure accuracy of IMP assignment, dispensation, dosing, compliance and documentation. The unblinded pharmacy monitor schedules unblinded drug accountability visits and works with site unblinded pharmacy staff. They may train unblinded pharmacy staff on IMP preparation, dispensation and provision to blinded staff. They provide secure and appropriate correspondence regarding drug assignment and dosing and giving the investigator timely IMP accountability status. They review unblinded pharmacy documents and correspondence and ensure a clear separation of blinded and unblinded monitoring activities.

Clear instruction regarding unblinded pharmacy activities, monitoring, communication and documentation practices will ensure the integrity of the IMP blind and that IMP preparation and administration is conducted in compliance with the protocol and the best safety practices for clinical trial participants. This is noted in the unblinded monitoring plan.

The unblinded CRA or team at the sponsor will help create an unblinded pharmacy monitoring plan that includes a communication plan between key unblinded personnel, specific timelines for monitoring frequency and appropriate confirmation, report and follow-up letter templates. It should also include the means by which unblinded pharmacy monitoring is conducted—a decided number of onsite visits or one onsite visit per site with subsequent review of subject drug accountability data performed remotely.

The blinded and unblinded CRAs for a study should not schedule monitoring visits on the same days to ensure all means are employed to prevent unblinding study/site personnel.

Sample Collection

If blood or other samples are to be collected during the study, the CRA should ensure that this is being done and is being done properly. The timing should be checked to verify that the collection is being done in accordance with protocol requirements. If the samples are stored and batched for shipping, the CRA should verify that storage conditions are appropriate and that sample collection, storage and shipment is documented.

The shipping must be done properly and according to all applicable laws and regulations. There are significant fines for not following appropriate packing and shipping procedures. Proper shipment of dangerous material protects the shipper from exposure to these risks. To verify potential exposure, refer to 49 CFR 107.301-107.339 (hazardous material transportation regulations).

Reports generated on the samples should be communicated and kept according to instructions.

Large central labs have portals or vendors with study training on sample shipment, listings of results and logs of samples received, etc. CRAs reference these portals during monitoring activities.

Study Document Review

Another monitoring task is checking the investigator's study document file. It is recommended that the CRA check this file at the first monitoring visit after the study starts to ensure that copies of all pertinent documents are available and filed. If something is missing, it should be relatively easy to get a copy of it early in the study. The CRA may have a copy in his or her file, or the sponsor will have it. Having everything present and accounted for is a good way to start the study.

The CRA should be able to cross-check the investigator study document file with the Electronic Trial Master File (eTMF) at the sponsor/CRO company. The eTMF is an electronic filing/storage system (a structured means of storing essential and other study documents and other digital content for clinical trials that are required to comply with regulatory agency requirements and institutional requirements). The eTMF will house each study investigator's study/essential documents in one section, as well as maintain other eTMF sections for country specific documents, sponsor internal documents, master ICF and other templates, etc. The investigator section of the eTMF at the sponsor/CRO should be a mirror image of the site regulatory file, and the CRA should cross review both files at each monitoring visit to ensure the appropriate documents are file/stored.

The CRA will not need to check the investigator's document file at every visit, unless the sponsor requires it. However, it should be checked periodically, especially if the CRA is aware of changes or when new documents have been added. It is also critical to check it at the end of the study, before it is filed for long-term storage.

Here are some hints for a CRA when checking study documents. Use a checklist for this activity, as it is easy to miss something without a list; a sample checklist can be found in Appendix C. Be sure that the current versions of documents, primarily the protocol and consent, are being used. Earlier versions should be retained in the file for reference only.

Copies of form 1572, IRB approvals and drug shipment invoices (the most common missing documents) should be retrieved from the eTMF during monitoring visits so that you can provide these to the site if they are missing. You can also email the in-house CRA or remote monitor and request the document, which will probably be sent to you during the course of your monitoring visit.

Investigator and sponsor document files are now maintained electronically, and reconciliation and provision of missing investigator study documents have become more efficient; reconciliation and identification of missing study documents can be completed remotely, which saves time during onsite monitoring visits.

Author's Story

Great study, wrong protocol

Once, while doing an antihypertension study in a physician's office in North Carolina, we discovered an unusual amount of errors in the case report forms. We reviewed the study requirements and then corrected the errors properly; yet, something did not seem quite right. Our in-house folks checked their records and I, as the field CRA, checked the investigator. We discovered that the physician had inadvertently been sent a different protocol than he had signed up for. But ... he had done the wrong protocol correctly! He had used the CRFs from the study he had signed up for, but performed an entirely different protocol! We never truly discovered how it happened and we submitted appropriate documents to fix the problem. A CRA truth learned the hard way: never assume the investigator has the correct protocol. Check the files and make sure the proper and current protocol is the one being done. Make sure the CRFs are for the correct protocol.

—Senior CRA

Confidentiality

During all monitoring activities, the CRA must be attentive to confidentiality. No study record, other than the consent form, should identify the subject. The CRA has an obligation to help protect the confidentiality of all study subjects. The study documents are also confidential. During site visits, sometimes CRAs have seen competitor's protocols lying around unprotected. All one needs to see is the protocol cover page to know the name of the drug and phase of development. The CRA should periodically remind the investigator and coordinator of the confidentiality of these documents, and ensure that they are kept in a secure location.

Monitoring Locations and Preservation of Confidentiality

Appropriate monitoring space is an ongoing challenge with investigational sites. There is sometimes barely enough room to accommodate investigational site staff, let alone several CRAs during a monitoring visit. The most important thing to ensure during monitoring visits is that the CRA is in a location that ensures a level of privacy and prevention of outside review of confidential study files. CRAs from different sponsor or CRO organizations should never be placed at the same desk/table area to monitor. A large, dedicated monitoring area with individual cubicles and space between cubicles, or a room with separately placed desks, or individual monitoring rooms/exam rooms are most appropriate. Conversations between monitoring colleagues from the same company working in a shared area should occur outside of the shared room or in a manner so that other CRAs do not hear or understand the content. Telephone calls to or from the headquarters or the home office should occur in a private area. Confidentiality should be preserved and maintained at all times.

The Health Insurance Portability and Accountability Act

The purpose of the Health Insurance Portability and Accountability Act (HIPAA) is to improve the efficiency and effectiveness of the healthcare system by encouraging the development of healthcare information systems using electronic data interchange for health-related administrative and financial transactions. In addition, HIPAA seeks to establish the required use of national transaction standards while maintaining patient privacy when business and patient information is transmitted electronically between organizations.

All vendors of electronic medical record (EMR) systems must conform to the standards in the Administrative Simplification component of HIPAA. This component encompasses four standards:

1. Electronic transactions and code sets.
2. Privacy of individually identifiable health information.
3. Security to preserve patient confidentiality.
4. Creation of unique health identifiers for patients, health plans, providers and employers.

The fourth standard is one part of HIPAA that will directly affect clinical research. It addresses standards by which unique patient-identifying information can be transmitted electronically, possibly over the internet.

The final HIPAA rule came into effect in 2003. Specific areas of the final regulation affecting researchers are: de-identification of patient health information, as mentioned above; single authorization from the patient required for all uses and disclosures of patient health information; the combining of patient authorization forms with the informed consent document; and the elimination of an expiration date or event for research authorization. The final regulation also has one set of transition provisions for all forms of research regardless of whether they involve treatment or not. The full text of the final HIPAA rule and an explanation of modifications can be found at hhs.gov/ocr/hipaa.

The End of the Visit

Before concluding a monitoring visit, there are some miscellaneous items to attend to. It is important to check the last site visit report for any noted problems or unresolved issues. These items should be followed up on until they are resolved, and the site visit reports must show how they were followed up. This is something an auditor will look for if the site is inspected later, plus it is good monitoring practice.

The CRA will also want to see if more study supplies need to be ordered, including drug/product, case report forms, lab kits and anything else that may be necessary for the study. If so, ordering should be done before the CRA leaves the site.

If the CRA is involved in grant requests, this should be discussed with the investigator and, if appropriate, a grant request should be submitted.

Before leaving, plan ahead for the next monitoring visit. Explain what materials should be ready for review. If there are scheduled enrollment updates planned, remind the coordinator. The CRA should always schedule the next visit before leaving the site, while both the CRA and the coordinator have their calendars available.

If possible, it is good to write the CRA visit report before leaving the site. If not, write it as soon as possible after leaving, while the details are still fresh in your mind. Before leaving, be sure you have everything you need to take with you and that it is organized. The investigator and the CRC should have been debriefed about monitoring findings and the status of the study. Before leaving, the CRA should thank everyone for his or her time and efforts during the visit.

If the CRA has told site personnel that he or she will find out any particular information for them, be sure this is done and reported back. It is also nice to follow the visit with a letter recapping any pertinent information, thanking the site personnel for the work they have done and verifying the date of the next monitoring visit.

Monitoring Visit Reports

Most sponsors have a standard monitoring visit report form used to document visits to investigative sites. If a sponsor does not have one, the CRA will want to devise a form to use for this purpose; there is an example of a monitoring report in Appendix C.

The purpose of the monitoring visit report is to document the findings from the monitoring visit. The CRA should use this form to summarize what was done at the investigative site, including CRFs/eCRFs and source documents reviewed and verified. This is also where problems must be documented, including what was done to solve them or the recommended action items for the next visit.

It is important to remember that the visit report is a business document and can be accessed by the FDA in case of a sponsor inspection. The language used should be businesslike and factual; this is not the place to vent frustrations with a site. If the monitoring visit was not as successful as the CRA had hoped, these frustrations can find their way into the report; this is not appropriate. Here are some examples of unacceptable and acceptable language for a visit report:

- Unacceptable: "Coordinator doing sloppy work!!! She is the worst coordinator I have ever seen."
- Acceptable: "CRFs incomplete and needed many corrections. Coordinator was instructed in the proper way to fill in the forms."
- Unacceptable: "Investigator shows no interest in the study. He is never available to meet with me and probably doesn't even know what is going on in the study."
- Acceptable: "Investigator not available during this visit. Time with him was scheduled for my next visit, and a letter will be sent verifying the appointment time."
- Unacceptable: "This study is so screwed up nobody can tell what's going on. We should close it and never let them do studies again. This is a really terrible site. The coordinator is a dunce, and the investigator thinks he walks on water."
- Acceptable: "There are many aspects of this study that need clarification and correction. It is recommended that someone from our compliance department visit the site with me within the next two weeks so that we can determine what needs to be done to ensure that the study is brought into compliance with good clinical practices. After this visit, we will recommend any further actions that appear necessary."

Remember that monitoring visit reports are the official record of CRA visits and will stay in the sponsor trial file for many years. They should reflect what took place at the visit, what was transmitted to the sponsor and problems that were found, plus potential solutions. The ICH E6 Guidelines for Good Clinical Practice summarize monitoring reports very well:

- The monitor should submit a written report after each monitoring visit.
- Reports should include the date, investigative site, name of the monitor, name of the investigator and any other individual(s) contacted.
- Reports should contain a summary of what was reviewed and statements concerning significant findings/facts, deviations and deficiencies, conclusions, actions taken or to be taken and/or actions recommended to secure compliance.

Follow-up Letter to the Investigator

It is a good practice for the CRA to send a follow-up letter to the investigative site after a monitoring visit. In this letter, the CRA should thank the site for its time and recap the findings from the monitoring visit. If there are things the site must do, or correct, before the next visit, they should be listed. If there were any questions the CRA could not answer while there, they should be addressed in the letter. A good way to end the letter is to give the date of the next monitoring visit and say you are looking forward to seeing them. For example:

I'm looking forward to seeing you again at my next monitoring visit, August 17, 2019. I will be in touch with (Study Coordinator) a few days before the visit.

Keep your letter friendly, but very professional. These letters are usually kept by the site and become part of its study document file.

Author's Story

When I was a brand-new study coordinator, I noticed that the monitors would send nice letters after each monitoring visit summarizing what they accomplished and what was still outstanding for resolution. What I did not realize was that the list of pending items in the follow-up letter was meant as a "to do" list for me to start working on between monitoring visits. I thought it was a list of activities for me to accomplish at the next monitoring visit, with the monitor. No wonder my first monitors kept asking me why I waited until they arrived to work on things. They must have thought me lazy. The truth was, I was so overwhelmed and busy learning how to be a study coordinator—reviewing protocols, regulatory binders and case report forms left by my predecessor—that I did not have time to address the items until the monitor came back to remind/help me. The lesson learned by all; Never presume an inexperienced study coordinator knows what to do with a monitoring visit follow-up letter.

–Elizabeth

Performance Evaluation Monitoring Visits/CRA Sign-off Visits

It is important for CRAs of all experience levels to be aware of the performance evaluation monitoring visit/CRA sign-off visit process. The appropriate preparation for and proficiency demonstrated during this process will positively impact a CRAs job performance, whether as a new CRA being signed off for the first time to independently conduct the monitoring visit types or an experienced CRA having continuing proficiency confirmed.

Even if deficits are noted in the performance of the CRA being evaluated, the manner in which the deficiencies are communicated can transform perceived criticism into a positive learning opportunity that will exponentially improve performance.

The performance evaluation monitoring visit is the process of assessing appropriate monitoring visit conduct and confirmation of monitoring task completion by field CRAs. This process includes confirming the performance of new CRAs to independently conduct monitoring visits, also known as the "sign-off visit," assessing the conduct of experienced CRAs in job performance, and ad hoc evaluation of CRAs with suspected performance or quality issues.

The very nature of the field CRA's position working autonomously at investigational sites (away from the CRO/sponsor company office) creates an important need to physically evaluate the CRA's conduct of interim monitoring visits at these very same institutions.

Research organizations historically require annual performance evaluation visits for established CRAs, to confirm continuing proficiency or areas of improvement, and "sign-off visits" as required for CRAs new to an organization or new to the CRA role.

The individuals qualified to evaluate and sign off CRAs are experienced or Senior CRAs and/or clinical team managers, CRA managers, or others in a management role experienced with monitoring. There is a specific training process and qualification process for sign-off visit leaders that requires periodic refresher training.

The sign-off visit process for new CRAs involves observation of the intended monitoring visit type, prior to the new CRA being evaluated on the conduct of said monitoring visit type. CRAs participating in having their monitoring visit observed (by the new CRA trainee) do not necessarily need to be sign-off visit leaders, but at the very least, competent CRAs in good standing. CRAs conducting performance evaluations should be mindful of the fact that their behavior during the observation of the monitoring visit is almost as important as their performance during the sign-off visit. They must communicate with the CRAs they are observing to obtain the investigational site location and the tools used in the conduct of the monitoring visit, such as protocols, checklists and study manuals. They should be punctual, professional and never interfere in any aspect of the monitoring visit as they are only there to observe.

The new CRA being signed off (after the observation monitoring visit, during their own official monitoring visit) must show competence in the activities and tasks required to conduct a successful monitoring visit (meeting with the investigator and staff, drug accountability, source/CRF review and regulatory binder review). The individual evaluating the CRA is making a subjective assessment of their performance based on their own experience with the role and responsibilities of a field CRA. However, it is important for the evaluator to remember that the new CRA needs to show competence, not expertise. A new CRA during a sign-off visit may show uncertainty in an element of monitoring visit completion, but that should not dissuade the evaluator from approving them for independent visit conduct as the entire picture of performance must be assessed.

Evaluating experienced CRAs can be challenging, as those being evaluated may presume their experience alone will validate performance, and they may be unresponsive to recommended areas of improvement.

The CRA being evaluated must remember three vital points during the evaluation process:

- Prepare for the performance evaluation visit by reviewing the protocol, checklist, study tools and anything that will keep skills sharp.
- Communicate with the evaluators throughout the process, informing them of a plan to prioritize and complete tasks onsite, scheduling times to speak with the investigator and study coordinator, pointing out important study changes or areas of focus, and helping the evaluator identify appropriate data to review to complete the evaluation.
- Follow through with required actions and correspondence with investigational site staff and the evaluator (whomever appropriate to ensure transparency).

The evaluator must request and review all required study tools to be knowledgeable enough to adequately evaluate the CRA. The evaluator should review source/CRF data already reviewed by the CRA to ensure the data was reviewed/retrieved adequately. The evaluator must be punctual, professional and not overly interfere with monitoring visit conduct. They are there to assess, and not conduct, the monitoring visit.

The tools utilized for CRA evaluation differ by organization but include a checklist for the evaluator during the monitoring visit and a report that is completed (after the visit) and provided to the CRA's line manager regarding specific performance and areas of strength or deficiency.

Deficits identified will guide the level of retraining, or additional evaluation, as required. This process is communicated in a professional, effective manner at the visit's conclusion. The delivery of the message is most critical to the recipient's understanding and acceptance of corrective action. Comments regarding the evaluation should never be made in front of or in ear shot of investigational staff. It would undermine the CRA and could weaken the site's confidence in the CRAs performance.

Someone who does not initially "pass" the evaluation visit would naturally be disappointed, or even devastated, as it negatively reflects professional diligence and performance (to them). However, it is important to understand that failure to pass the evaluation can also be a result of poor training or management. Each situation must be considered separately.

What is of paramount importance is that, once a deficiency is identified, it is corrected with retraining to educate and prevent future error. The site, the study and, most importantly, the CRA benefit from the process.

An example of a performance evaluation monitoring visit report is included in in Appendix C.

Conclusion

Successful monitoring is the result of experience; knowledge of the protocol, CRFs, the study drug, therapeutic area, regulations and SOPs; people skills and management ability. It is not easy, but can be fun and rewarding when done well.

To close this chapter, here is a story from a CRA friend that's a great example of the strange things a CRA experiences.

The most fruitless trip for no real reason

Our company was doing a very large phase 4 study to support changing a prescription drug to an over-the-counter drug. Subjects were recruited through pharmacies and received a quarterly telephone call to check on their status. If subjects reported that they had been hospitalized, we physically went to their location to investigate the case.

I received notification to investigate a case of a person who had been hospitalized with "AH Blood Poisoning." This was a very unusual report because no one had ever heard of such a thing. Besides being an unusual case, the person and his physician lived in Star Lake, N.Y.

It was January, and Star Lake is located in upstate New York between Watertown and Lake Placid. The snow was about two feet deep, and I arrived late. The hotel was old, with one telephone and a bar, whose elderly keeper was also the hotel room clerk. If one asked politely, he would make you a burger for dinner. The next morning, breakfast was at the local grocery store because there were no restaurants.

The hospital was very small and the physician's office was next door in a small building. The physician was pleasant and most helpful; but he, too, had no clue what "AH Blood Poisoning" was. He told me the man had an infection in his arm because his pet cockatoo had bitten him and this resulted in cellulitis. The man recovered after a course of antibiotics. I reported the cellulitis to our in-house study coordinator and apologized for not being able to ascertain exactly what "AH Blood Poisoning" was. A few days later, he called me back and said, "I think I know what happened. The telephone operators who interviews subjects takes down whatever they say verbatim. I checked with the interview service and confirmed that the man had answered the question about whether anything untoward had happened with, 'I had, ah, (AH) blood poisoning.'" And that was the end of the great "AH Blood Poisoning" mystery!

–A CRA

Key Takeaways

- A CRA should develop a plan for monitoring each investigative site.
- The frequency and timing of monitoring visits depend on the complexity of the study, the rate of enrollment, and site experience and performance.
- Investigative sites should be visited soon after the first subject or two are enrolled.
- CRAs should use checklists for various monitoring activities.
- CRAs should maintain a file for each investigative site.
- CRAs should confirm each scheduled site visit before leaving on a trip.
- CRAs should spend some time with the investigator and the coordinator at each monitoring visit.
- Serious adverse events should be checked at each visit.
- Informed consents must be checked for all study subjects.
- The bulk of CRA monitoring time is spent on case report form review and source document review.
- The purpose of source document review is to verify that the subjects exist and the integrity of the data.
- Risk-based monitoring programs/plans are being implemented more regularly.
- Quick feedback and explanation of errors and queries will help reduce the number of corrections needed in the future.
- CRAs must never correct or modify source documents or case report forms themselves. Corrections can be done only by site personnel.
- Drug accountability should be done throughout the study.
- Study documents need to be checked at the beginning and at the end of the study, and periodically throughout the study.
- The monitoring visit report should summarize the activities that took place during the visit, including what was reviewed, what was sent to the sponsor and any problems that were found, along with solutions.

- A follow-up letter should be sent to the site after each monitoring visit.
- The performance evaluation monitoring visit is a critical component of organizational quality and confirmation of a CRAs performance.

CHAPTER 15

Adverse Events and Safety Monitoring

This chapter discusses adverse events and safety monitoring. It is critical that adverse events are monitored during clinical trials, for the protection of the subjects enrolled in the trial as well as future patients and proper use of the drug once it is marketed.

Monitoring safety during a clinical trial is one of the most important tasks a CRA performs. At the same time, safety reporting is one of the most difficult tasks for a study site. There are often misunderstandings about what is deemed necessary for reporting on safety issues in trials, stemming at least in part from the differences in clinical studies as compared to clinical practice, as well as inconsistent and changing reporting requirements on studies. Also, although the regulations charge the investigator with protecting the rights, safety and well-being of subjects in trials, they don't give much information about actual safety reporting. We will look at the regulations in detail.

Regulations and Definitions

21 CFR 312.64 (Investigator reports) requires investigators to report adverse events during clinical trials. It states:

> *Safety reports.* An investigator must immediately report to the sponsor any serious adverse event, whether or not considered drug related, including those listed in the protocol or investigator brochure and must include an assessment of whether there is a reasonable possibility that the drug caused the event. Study endpoints that are serious adverse events (e.g., all-cause mortality) must be reported in accordance with the protocol unless there is evidence suggesting a causal relationship between the drug and the event (e.g., death from anaphylaxis). In that case, the investigator must immediately report the event to the sponsor. The investigator must record

nonserious adverse events and report them to the sponsor according to the timetable for reporting specified in the protocol.

By signing form 1572, the investigator also commits to reporting to the sponsor adverse events that occur during the course of a trial, in accordance with 21 CFR 312.64.

ICH E6(R2) has somewhat more information. In the glossary, adverse events and adverse drug reactions are defined as follows:

Adverse Event (AE)
An AE is any untoward medical occurrence in a patient or clinical investigation subject administered a pharmaceutical product. It does not necessarily have a causal relationship with this treatment. An AE can therefore be any unfavorable and unintended sign (including an abnormal laboratory finding), symptom or disease temporally associated with the use of a medicinal (investigational) product whether or not related.

Adverse Drug Reaction (ADR)
In the pre-approval clinical experience with a new medicinal product or its new usages, particularly as the therapeutic dose(s) may not be established, all noxious and unintended responses to a medicinal product related to any dose should be considered adverse drug reactions. The phrase "responses to a medicinal product" means that a causal relationship between a medicinal product and an adverse event is at least a reasonable possibility, i.e., the relationship cannot be ruled out. Regarding marketed medicinal products: A response to a drug that is noxious and unintended and that occurs at doses normally used in man for prophylaxis, diagnosis or therapy of diseases or for modification of physiological function.

ICH E6(R2) also contains a section (4.11) on safety reporting. In this section, it states that all SAEs should be reported immediately to the sponsor except for those that the protocol or other document (e.g., investigator brochure) identifies as not needing immediate reporting. The immediate reports should be followed promptly by detailed written reports.

The FDA uses similar definitions on its web page on safety reporting for IND applications. These are regulatory definitions, not clinical definitions, which is an important distinction to understand when working with investigative sites:

IND application sponsors are required to notify FDA in a written safety report of:

- any adverse experience associated with the use of the drug that is both serious and unexpected, or
- any findings from tests in laboratory animals that suggest a significant risk for human subjects including reports of mutagenicity, teratogenicity, and carcinogenicity.

Adverse event means any untoward medical occurrence associated with the use of a drug in humans, whether or not considered drug related.

Suspected adverse reaction means any adverse event for which there is a reasonable possibility that the drug caused the adverse event. For the purposes of IND safety reporting, 'reasonable possibility' means there is evidence to suggest a causal relationship between the drug and the adverse event. A suspected adverse reaction implies a lesser degree of certainty about causality than an adverse reaction.

Adverse reaction means any adverse event caused by a drug. Adverse reactions are a subset of all suspected adverse reactions where there is reason to conclude that the drug caused the event.

Unexpected adverse event or suspected adverse reaction refers to an event or reaction that is not listed in the investigator's brochure or is not listed at the specificity or severity that has been observed; or, if an investigator's brochure is not required or available, is not consistent with the risk information described in the general investigational plan or elsewhere in the current IND application.

Serious adverse event or suspected adverse reaction refers to an event or reaction that, in the view of either the investigator or sponsor, results in any of the following outcomes:

- Death,
- A life-threatening adverse event,
- In-patient hospitalization or prolongation of existing hospitalization,
- A persistent or significant incapacity or substantial disruption of the ability to conduct normal life functions, or

- A congenital anomaly or birth defect.

Life-threatening adverse event or suspected adverse reaction is considered "life-threatening" if, in the view of the investigator or sponsor, its occurrence places the patient or subject at immediate risk of death. It does not include an adverse event or suspected adverse reaction that, had it occurred in a more severe form, might have caused death.

Important medical events that may not result in death, be life-threatening, or require hospitalization may be considered serious when, based upon appropriate medical judgment, they may jeopardize the patient or research subject and may require medical or surgical intervention to prevent one of the outcomes listed as serious.

Mandatory Safety Reporting

Initial reporting: IND application sponsor must report any suspected adverse reaction or adverse reaction to study treatment that is both serious and unexpected.

Unexpected serious suspected adverse reactions and observations from animal studies suggesting significant risk to human subjects must be reported to FDA as soon as possible but no later than within **15 calendar days** following the sponsor's initial receipt of the information.

Unexpected fatal or life-threatening suspected adverse reactions represent especially important safety information and must be reported to FDA as soon as possible but no later than **7 calendar days** following the sponsor's initial receipt of the information.

Follow-up reporting: Any relevant additional information obtained by the sponsor that pertains to a previously submitted IND safety report must be submitted as a Follow-up IND Safety Report. Such report should be submitted without delay, as soon as the information is available but no later than 15 calendar days after the sponsor receives the information.

All IND safety reports must be submitted on Form 3500A (if from clinical trials) or in a narrative format (if from animal or epidemiological studies) and be accompanied by Form 1571 (PDF - 830KB). The type of report (initial or follow-up) should be checked in the respective boxes on Forms 3500A and 1571. See Instructions for completing Form 3500A.

The submission must be identified as:

- "IND safety report" for 15-day reports, or
- "7-day IND safety report" for unexpected fatal or life-threatening suspected adverse reaction reports, or
- "Follow-up IND safety report" for follow-up information.

The report must be submitted to an appropriate Review division that has the responsibility to review the IND application under which the safety report is submitted. FDA recommends that sponsors submit safety reports electronically. Other means of rapid communication to the respective review division's Regulatory Project Manager (e.g., telephone, facsimile transmission, email) may also be used.

The reporting clock starts when the first person in the sponsor company hears of the event. If the sponsor is using a CRO, the CRO becomes, in effect, the sponsor company; in this case, the reporting clock starts even if a person in the CRO is the first to become aware of the event. Note that the first person may be a secretary or anyone else who happens to answer the telephone or receives the email or fax—it doesn't have to be someone involved with managing the study.

It is important to distinguish between the terms "serious" and "severe." The term "serious" is used with the definition above and categorizes events (i.e., they either meet the definition for serious or they don't). The term "severe" refers to the intensity of the event and can be used with any event, without regard to whether or not it meets the criteria for being classified as "serious." For example, a subject can have a severe headache, but it is not a serious event.

- **Related to or Associated with the Drug.** This means that there is a reasonable possibility that the event could have been caused by the investigational product (drug, biologic, device).
- **Expected/Unexpected.** An expected event is one in which the specificity and severity of the event are consistent with the information in the investigator brochure or labeling for the product. Unexpected events are all others.
- **Life-Threatening.** A life-threatening event is one in which the patient is in immediate danger of death unless there is intervention. It does not

mean that the patient may die at some time in the future from the event or may have died if the event had been more serious or specific.

- **Significant Disability.** A significant disability is one that causes substantial disruption to the person's normal life and activity.

Later in this chapter, we will discuss ways a CRA can work with sites to help investigators and their staff understand these definitions and how to apply them.

Adverse Events in Clinical Trials

CRAs will be most involved with AEs that occur during clinical trials of a drug still in the development process, before it's reached the market.

Most of the AEs seen during clinical trials will not be serious, as defined in the regulations. In general, these nonserious AEs will be recorded regularly on eCRFs/CRFs and will be reviewed and collected by the CRA during regular monitoring visits as well reviewed in between monitoring visits. Remember that nonserious events can be severe in intensity but still not meet the definition of serious.

Most sponsors would like all SAEs that occur during a trial to be reported to them by the investigator as soon as he or she becomes aware of them. This is for two reasons: first, to ensure the continued safety of subjects in the trial; and second, to meet the reporting requirements of the FDA.

Sponsors must still report (in writing) all AEs that are serious, related and unexpected to the FDA within 15 calendar days, and those that are also serious and alarming (death, immediately life-threatening) must be reported by telephone, electronic or facsimile transmission within seven days, with a written report within 15 days.

Safety Reporting Sections in Protocols

Every protocol for a clinical trial should contain a detailed plan for the collection and reporting of all AEs, both serious and nonserious. Several key items should be included.

Definitions. The protocol should include the regulatory definitions for an AE and a SAE, as well as the definitions for related/associated and for expected/unexpected events.

Sources of AEs. In general, the standard sources of all AEs will be the investigator reporting about:

- All directly observed events. [I see you have a rash on your arm...]
- Events elicited from the subject by means of a general nondirective question. [Have you had any problems with your health since you were here the last time?] The use of a specific question allows the sponsor to standardize procedures across all sites. A nondirective question does not prompt a subject to answer in a specific way. Asking subjects about specific events [Have you had any headaches?], although appropriate in some studies, will lead to a higher reporting rate for the specific event than a nondirective question.
- Events spontaneously volunteered by the study subject. [You know, Doc, ever since I started taking these pills, I have had an upset stomach.]
- Laboratory, EKG or other test results that meet protocol requirements for classification as AEs. [Such as laboratory values that are more than 10% outside the normal range.]

Event Collection Periods. The study periods during which AEs will be collected should be specified. Some protocols require them to be collected during a pre-treatment period as baseline data, while others require collection only during active treatment. It is also quite common to collect AEs during a post-treatment follow-up period. AEs are always collected during the entire period that a subject is on, or could be on (in the case of blinded trials), the investigational product or study drug.

Diaries and Other Data Collection Instruments. Whenever data collection instruments are used that may elicit information about AEs (e.g., quality-of-life questionnaires, patient diaries), the methods for handling these events should be specified in the protocol. Although they certainly have a place in data collection, instruments such as diaries can complicate the orderly collection of AEs. The problem is that subjects may write comments in diaries that refer to potential AEs, and there is often no orderly way to officially collect the pertinent information. There is an example of a patient diary with a written comment about a potential event in Table 1.

Table 1: Example: Patient diary

ACMEPHARMA STUDY 1234				Patient diary—Week 4
Name:	Betsy Smith			

Each day, please enter the time you took your study medication. Remember, you should always take one pill just before breakfast (about 8:00 am) and two pills before dinner (about 6:00 pm).

Sunday	Date:	2/2/18		
	Morning dose time		am	
	Evening dose time		pm	
Monday	Date:			
	Morning dose time		am	
	Evening dose time		pm	
Tuesday	Date:			
	Morning dose time	8	am	
	Evening dose time	6	pm	migraine—felt dizzy

Notice that this patient was filling in the times she took her investigational medication, but she also added some additional information—the migraine headache. Certainly, the study site personnel would want to know about the migraine, but this is not the place for it to be recorded. The study coordinator will need to ensure that this event is recorded on the appropriate AE CRFs, and not missed.

Unresolved Adverse Events. Sometimes AEs that occur during a study are unresolved at the time the subject's study participation ends. The protocol should state what is to be done in this case. Usually, serious AEs are followed to resolution, that is, until they resolve, disappear or become stable. There is often a time period during which any events that are ongoing at the end of the study are followed. Thirty days is a frequently used time period, but it varies depending on the compound, its half-life, the amount of time the subject was in the trial and the complexity of the diagnosis and protocol.

Exposure in Utero. If women of childbearing potential are allowed into the trial, then the protocol should include instructions for reporting exposure in utero and the subsequent outcome of the pregnancy. In general, the investigator will be required to follow up on any cases of pregnancy that occur during the study until the child is born or the pregnancy is terminated. There is usually no requirement for interim visits throughout the pregnancy, just an assurance that the subject will be contacted periodically to determine the outcome.

Timely Notification. The sponsor will want to be notified of serious events by the investigator in a timely manner, usually within 24 hours of the investigator's first knowledge of the event. It is extremely important that the investigator notify the sponsor of each SAE as soon as possible, even if all the details are not yet available. Additional details can be reported as they become available; the initial report should never be delayed while awaiting more information. An investigator may not know about an event for some time after it has occurred, especially if he or she is not the subject's primary physician. The study site may not know about the event until the subject comes in for his or her next appointment or fails to show up for the appointment because of the event. However, the investigator should inform the sponsor of the event as soon as he or she becomes aware of it. SAE reporting is accomplished by the investigational site via official SAE reporting forms or the EDC system SAE forms.

Nonserious AEs are also reported to the sponsor. This reporting is done by way of the eCRF/CRF and the regular data collection process. Final reporting is done within a reasonable time following completion of the study (usually within three months). There are no FDA requirements for expedited reporting of nonserious events.

Investigator Reporting Responsibilities

Investigators are required to collect, assess and report all AEs that occur during a trial. The following information is usually gathered for each event: onset (date/time), duration, severity (mild, moderate, severe), relationship to the study drug and whether or not it is serious. All events are to be recorded on the eCRF/CRF. In addition, if an event is serious, the investigator usually is expected to report it to the sponsor very quickly (e.g., within 24 hours).

Not only must the investigator report AEs to the sponsor, but he or she also is required to report these events to the IRB in the manner in which the IRB has requested. As with sponsors, some IRBs will want notification of all serious events, while others will want to hear only about events that are serious and related, or only those that are serious, related and unexpected. The IRB will tell the investigator what is expected, as well as the report timing and mechanisms. It is important that the investigator notify the IRB according to the rules the IRB has established.

It is a regulatory requirement that the investigator notify both the sponsor and the IRB of AEs. The investigator may receive IND Safety Reports (discussed in the next section) from the sponsor. Whenever one is received, the investigator must forward the information to the IRB.

Sponsor Responsibilities

Sponsors are required to review safety data throughout a trial, so appropriate adjustments can be made if there are any relevant safety issues. For example, the protocol might be amended; or, if there are serious safety concerns, the trial might be stopped. Remember that the sponsor is the only entity that has access to all the safety data for a drug; investigators and IRBs see safety data only from the site or sites with which they are involved. Therefore, the burden falls on the sponsor for prompt and thorough review of safety information as it is generated.

Sponsors have the responsibility of reporting AEs that are serious, related and unexpected to the FDA within the expedited reporting time frames, as discussed earlier.

Sponsors have an additional reporting requirement for SAEs in clinical trials; they must also inform all investigators who are currently working with the drug of any serious, related, unexpected AE. Investigators need to receive the same information that was sent to the FDA and within the same time period. These reports are called IND Safety Reports. Note that IND Safety Reports are sent to all investigators working with the compound, not just those doing the same protocol. The requirements for IND Safety Reports are found in 21 CFR 312.32.

Many sponsors use electronic portals to provide sites IND safety reports.

There may be rare instances in which an adverse finding or a series of AEs indicate that the drug has a safety issue that is so serious that its continued use in clinical trials is unacceptable. If this occurs, the sponsor must notify the FDA and all investigators who ever participated in a clinical trial with the drug of that decision immediately. This includes all investigators who ever studied the drug, not just those with currently active clinical trials. The investigators of open trials must then, in turn, immediately notify their IRBs of the trials' discontinuation for safety reasons.

In device trials, unanticipated adverse device effects (UADEs) are also collected. An UADE is defined as any SAE on health or safety or any death or life-threatening problem caused by or associated with a device if that effect was not previously identified in nature the investigational plan or application (21 CRF 812.3(s)). If an UADE occurs, the sponsor must immediately conduct an evaluation of the effect. If the sponsor determines that the effect presents an unreasonable risk to subjects, it must terminate all of its investigations, or at least the ones that present the risk, as soon as possible, but at least within five days after making the determination and within 15 days of receiving notice of the event (21 CFR 812.46 (b)(2)).

Differences Between Clinical Studies and Clinical Practice

One of the most important tasks of a CRA is training and working with investigative sites on AE reporting. One reason AE reporting is fraught with problems stems from the fact that clinical practice and clinical research are not the same thing, and it is easy to get the two confused when it comes to safety reporting. It is often difficult for investigators to understand that the definitions used for AE reporting in trials are regulatory definitions, not clinical definitions. A good CRA understands the definitions and reporting requirements and takes the time to thoroughly train each site on the requirements before subjects are enrolled. In this section, we will discuss some ways the CRA can help sites with the proper reporting of AEs.

First, the CRA should discuss with his or her sites the differences between clinical practice and clinical research. In studies, the investigator has a dual role as a physician and an investigator. It is a physician's duty to act in the best interest of the patient, while at the same time it is the duty of the investigator to perform good research. These duties are not necessarily in conflict, but there are differences between the roles that must be understood.

Some examples that a CRA may want to discuss with site personnel are:

- Concomitant medications that might normally be prescribed for a patient may not be allowed under the protocol.
- Treatment periods may be longer or shorter under the protocol than are usual in general practice.

- AEs that are "normal" for the disease usually must be reported under study rules.
- A worsening or progression of the disease may or may not be reported as an AE. For example, a worsening of anxiety in an anxiety trial would usually reported, while a progression of Alzheimer's disease in an Alzheimer's trial might not be reported, as it is a progressive disease.

Occasionally, investigators do not understand the importance of reporting AEs if the events do not seem to be connected with the trial or the study medication or if they are commonly seen with the disease under study. An investigator may say something to the effect of "we see that all the time in this disease" or "it's not connected to the trial" or "that isn't of any importance." These remarks signify a misunderstanding of the differences between clinical practice and research. As a CRA, you will want to be attuned to this type of misunderstanding and be aware of the need for additional explanations and training.

Sometimes it helps to remind the investigator and staff that the study is being conducted to find out about the investigational drug, including safety as well as efficacy. That is why studies are conducted—we never really know what we will learn about a drug or device when it is under investigation.

The investigator also may need to be reminded of his or her regulatory responsibilities with respect to conducting trials. He or she also is bound by the contract with the sponsor, and most contracts require the investigator to report AEs as mandated by the regulations.

Assessing the Relationship of an AE to the Study Drug

Investigators are usually asked to assess the relationship between an AE and the investigational product by picking the term that best characterizes the relationship of the AE to the investigational product: similar to not related, probably not related, possibly related, probably related, definitely related. Not much may be known about the product, so investigators could be uneasy about making a decision. The following are some aids a CRA might use when training investigators to make these decisions. It is always important to confirm that the PI and Sub-Investigators are assessing AE causality, not inappropriately delegated staff.

Temporal Relationship

Does the timing of ingesting the investigational drug strongly correlate to the timing of the event? For example, assume that the subject takes the drug, comes in two days later and is diagnosed with a cancer. The cancer is probably not related because it occurred too soon after taking the study drug. Or, assume that a subject has been taking the study drug without issue, but develops an AE just after the dose was titrated upward; in this case, the event might well be related to the drug.

Known Patterns of Reaction

Assume that the study drug causes a distinctive rash and a study subject develops that type of rash. Chances are good that the rash is related to the study drug.

Other Potential Cause

Is there something else that would explain the occurrence of the event? For example, assume that the subject is allergic to chocolate, but couldn't resist that piece of devil's food birthday cake last night. He ate some and ended up with hives. The hives are probably not related to the study drug, but to the chocolate.

Does it Make Sense?

Assume that a study subject suffers from regular migraines, takes the study drug and has a migraine. It's probably not related. Since starting the study drug, migraines have occurred every two-to-three days; whereas before taking the study drug, they occurred once or twice a month. They are probably related to the study drug. This might, in fact, be reported as an exacerbation of a previously existing medical condition (e.g., a change in severity).

Dechallenge/Rechallenge

In this scenario, the subject has an AE. The study drug is stopped (dechallenge) and the event stops. The study drug is restarted (rechallenge) and the event occurs again. It is probably related to the drug under study. This is a very definitive test, but it may not be done unless it is allowed in the protocol. Although an investigator may stop a study drug (dechallenge) at any time deemed appropriate, he or she may not restart it (rechallenge) unless it is allowed by the protocol or after discussion with and agreement by the sponsor.

It is important for CRAs to review all documentation related to AEs and causality during monitoring visits to ensure the appropriate individual (PI or Sub-Investigator) is completing the causality.

Common Reporting Problems

There are a number of common misunderstandings that result in incorrect AE reporting. Many of these errors can be avoided if the CRA takes the time to explain them to site personnel in advance. One of these misunderstandings involves symptoms vs. a syndrome. Usually sponsors would like a syndrome to be reported rather than individual symptoms, for example, flu versus cough, sniffles and sore throat all reported separately.

Another common error is the reporting of a procedure, as opposed to reporting the disease/condition that resulted in the procedure. An example of this is reporting a coronary bypass as the event, instead of reporting the heart condition that necessitated the bypass.

Changes in severity are frequently reported incorrectly, or not at all. The general convention is that if an event worsens in severity, it is reported as a new event, even if the event is in the pre-study history for the subject. Some protocols also require the reporting of changes in events when the change is for the better.

Although mentioned earlier in this chapter, it is critical for the CRA to ensure that his or her sites understand the distinction between the terms "serious" and "severe," where "severe" refers to the intensity of an event with no regard to whether or not it meets the criteria for being classified as "serious."

In case of exposure in utero, it is a good idea for a CRA to make a note to follow up with the investigator on any cases of pregnancy. It is easy to forget to do this when the subject is not being seen on a regular basis.

Dealing with Problems

If a CRA is having trouble with appropriate AE reporting at a site, the first step is to discuss the situation with the site personnel and conduct additional training, including a discussion of both the protocol and the regulations as they pertain to AEs. If training and retraining do not help the situation, the CRA should discuss the situation with his or her supervisor and the study project manager/study medical monitor.

At times, the sponsor will send people from the quality assurance/auditing group to assess the problem. This will usually get the attention of the investigator, as audits can tend to be somewhat frightening. If the problems are not resolved, the sponsor may need to take more drastic action and actually stop the trial at the problem site. (Note: In this case, you will not want to use the site again for another trial.) Stopping the trial for this reason is quite rare, as investigators usually become compliant earlier in the process. Most like to perform well when conducting a study and simply need the help of a knowledgeable CRA to keep things running smoothly.

Everyone involved in clinical trials must recognize that clinical trials differ from clinical practice and that subject safety is paramount. A CRA must have expert knowledge of the AE rules and regulations in order to help study sites remain compliant in this endeavor. Helping sites report AEs appropriately is one of the most difficult and important tasks.

Key Takeaways

- Subject safety is paramount in clinical trials.
- There are differences between clinical practice and clinical trials when it comes to reporting AEs.
- The definitions used in AE reporting are regulatory definitions, not clinical definitions.
- AEs that are serious, related and unexpected require expedited reporting to the FDA.
- All investigators working with an investigational drug must be informed of any event with the drug that is serious, related and unexpected. The sponsor sends an IND Safety Report to each investigator for any AE meeting these criteria.
- The investigator must inform his or her IRB of any IND Safety Report's received from a sponsor.

- Serious AEs must be reported to the sponsor of the study within a very short time period (usually 24 or 48 hours).
- Protocols should contain explicit directions for collecting, assessing and reporting AEs.
- CRAs must train their sites in proper reporting of AEs.

CHAPTER 16

Recruitment, Retention and Compliance

This chapter covers three of the most difficult aspects of conducting clinical trials: recruitment of subjects into the trial, retention of subjects after they have been entered and subject compliance with the protocol throughout the study.

Recruitment of Study Subjects

Finding, enrolling and retaining study subjects are some of the largest and costliest challenges facing clinical research professionals today. Given the enormous development costs, it is obvious that companies want to speed up the process as much as possible, allowing for more marketing time before their patent protection for the product expires. The timely enrollment of appropriate subjects into trials is critical to managing the timelines for a development program.

Estimating Enrollment Potential at Sites

Knowing the patient population and being able to accurately estimate the number of subjects that can be enrolled are critical to completing a trial within the given time period. Investigators frequently overestimate the number of potential subjects they have, often because they are looking only at the number of potential subjects who match the overall diagnosis, for example, depression. However, there are a number of other factors that must be weighed and taken into account, including the protocol inclusion criteria and the subjects themselves.

Protocol considerations include the inclusion and exclusion criteria, activities and logistics. The largest constraints on enrollment usually are the inclusion and exclusion criteria for study entry. These criteria delineate the specific characteristics of the population to be enrolled. They will include demographic parameters, such as age, sex, disease, diagnostic criteria and study-specific requirements. In a study of depression, for example, the following (simplified) inclusion/exclusion criteria might be found:

- Age 18 to 65 years.
- Men and women who are post-menopausal, surgically sterile or using acceptable birth control.
- Depression lasting at least six months, but no longer than one year.
- No previous depressive episodes before current episode.
- No previous treatment with anti-depressive medications.
- Not taking any other medications that might interfere with the study medication (list provided).
- Able to read and comprehend the informed consent document.
- Willing to sign the informed consent.
- Able to swallow pills.
- Able to make weekly visits to the clinic site for three months.

Let's look at how these criteria might affect the ability of a site to enroll subjects.

The upper age limit of 65 may restrict enrollment from sites that treat a large geriatric population. Depression is a disease that tends to recur in people over time, so the criterion that disallows previous depressive episodes would be a problem. The criterion disallowing previous treatment with antidepressants will be a big factor, because if these subjects are already in the care of the investigator many of them already will be on anti-depressive therapies. Willingness and ability to make weekly clinic visits are apt to interfere with a potential subject's life situation, especially when working. On top of these problems, many people just are not willing to participate in research, especially if the protocol requirements are burdensome and they do not see much potential value to themselves for participation.

How can these factors influence the ability to enroll? If a CRA takes the number of subjects a physician has in his or her practice who meet the diagnosis for the study (depression), then halves that number for each major inclusion/exclusion criteria, the number that remains is apt to be close to the number of subjects who will be enrolled. If we assume in our example that the site does not see many geriatric patients, then the four main criteria we need to be concerned with are: no previous episode, no previous treatment, no current medications for depression and willingness to sign a consent form. Let us also assume that the investigator says there are about 400 patients in the practice that suffer from depression. Take 400 and divide it in half for each of four major inclusion/exclusion criteria.

400 ▸ 200 ▸ 100 ▸ 50 ▸ 25

The CRA can assume the site probably will be able to enroll about 25 subjects into the study, in total. This number may be acceptable, but the rate of enrollment needs to be factored in as well. [Note that if a site regularly does research similar to the protocol in question, it may be able to estimate enrollment much more accurately based on its recent experience. In this case, there should be hard data about recent trials, including the inclusion and exclusion criteria, numbers of subjects enrolled and rates of enrollment to back up the estimate.]

The CRA must help the investigator analyze the requirements for the rate of enrollment. The sponsor may expect, for example, two patients to be enrolled every week, for the total of 25. Two patients a week does not seem too onerous, but remember that the study is three months in length and subjects are seen on a weekly basis.

Let's look at what happens as the site begins enrolling. (See Figure 1.) At week one, it enrolls two subjects. During the second week, it enrolls two more, for a total of four subjects on study. By week six, it is up to 12 subjects, and by week 10, it has 20 subjects on study. Since this is a three-month study, all of these subjects are still being seen on a weekly basis, and there are still five more to enroll. (It can be assumed that there are no dropouts for the purpose of this example.) The site must determine, with the CRA's help, if it is able to see and manage that many study subjects within a given week. The investigator's available staff and space must be assessed, along with the ancillary help needed for such things as scheduling visits and calling or emailing the subjects to remind them of their visits and other study responsibilities. Unfortunately, most sponsors and investigators do not look at the cumulative workload as the study progresses. This is an area in which a good CRA can make a significant difference in accurate assessments of enrollment and study load capacities.

Figure 1: Total subjects enrolled

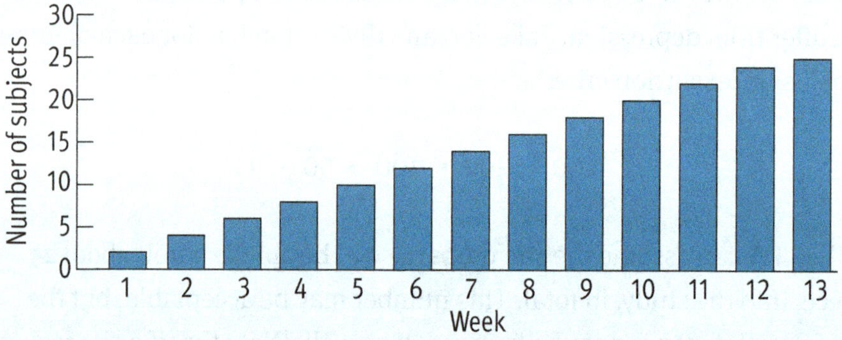

This information should be assessed during the prestudy visit and factors such as workload of study coordinators, number of study coordinators and personnel available to support the study efforts (patient visits, etc.) and availability of staff to recruit study patients should all be considered. During large vaccine trial site assessment visits, workload, average number of patients able to be screened daily/weekly, average number of visits the site conducts daily/weekly and how they triage, assign staff, etc. are all considered in the site evaluation process. A good site knows its capabilities and limits and can pivot staff, space and time to accommodate studies.

Before starting a study, the investigator should feel confident that his or her site could manage the enrollment rate and number of subjects appropriately.

It is especially important for a CRA to help new sites, those with very little or no study experience, to estimate the potential workload. Understanding what will be required in terms of time, staff and space throughout the trial will add to the overall chance of success.

Other Factors That Influence Enrollment

Another major factor influencing enrollment is competing studies. CRAs need to be aware of the enrollment problems that can result from having a competing study at an investigative site. Competing studies automatically reduce the resources available to your study, including the pool of available subjects. If an investigative site discloses during the feasibility or prestudy visit process that they have a competing study, the CRA must address this during the prestudy visit and obtain honest feedback from the investigator/site about how they will identify subjects for both studies. The type and transparency of the answer can impact site selection.

Even if the study is not competing for the same subject population, too many studies at a site can be a problem; they will compete for the other resources, including coordinator and investigator time and space.

There can also be a significant impact from other studies within the same community. These studies may be trying to enroll the same type of subjects and will draw from the same community pool of potential subjects. For example, in the early 1990s there were more than 150 different AIDS study sites in San Francisco. AIDS activists had a website and a toll-free number that listed all of the studies, plus the main inclusion/exclusion criteria for each as well as contact names and numbers. The people interested in these studies were very well informed and knew which had the most to offer in terms of potential benefit to subjects. Those studies with the newest and potentially best drug were meeting enrollment targets. Enrollment in the others languished. If a sponsor did not have an exciting compound, it was almost impossible to enroll sufficient numbers of subjects.

General interest in the trial, both on the part of the potential subjects and the investigator and staff, can have a major impact on enrollment. CRAs will want to remember that both investigators and subjects have a choice when it comes to participating in a clinical trial; the more exciting the trial and the compound, the more interest there will be in participating. It also helps if the CRA keeps the trial in the forefront of the investigator's and coordinator's minds; if they are thinking about the trial, they will be looking for potential subjects when they see patients in their regular practice. Consistent emails, phone calls and visits from a CRA can help encourage enrollment.

It is important for a CRA to consider the available staff and space at a site, even if there are no competing studies. If the coordinator and other involved personnel do not have sufficient time to conduct study activities or if there is no room to store study supplies and carry out study activities, they may be loath to enroll subjects. Sites sometimes underestimate the staff, space and time requirements for conducting a study; the CRA can help them realize what is involved and needs to be done to complete a successful study. The best way for a CRA to assess these things is to look around—check for organization, a relaxed attitude and happy employees. Think about what you see, and make an assessment of whether it appears that an additional study would create a workload problem.

Some sponsor companies require investigational sites to complete and sign a recruitment plan with their site CRA. This is usually done when study enrollment timelines are tight and the overall subject enrollment numbers are high. Or it is required of sites with poor or nonexistent patient enrollment. The purpose of the enrollment plan is to strategize effective enrollment tactics, to devise a plan to enroll a specific number of patients at specific timeframes (per week, per month) and obtain site assurance in writing that they will do their utmost to comply with the requirements of the recruitment plan.

Advertising for Study Subjects

Sometimes advertising for study subjects is planned right from the start of a study. In general, advertising planned from the start is used when it is expected that subjects will be difficult to find and enroll, when the timeline for enrollment is extremely ambitious or when a site routinely advertises for all its studies. In other cases, it becomes necessary to advertise for study subjects when enrollment targets are not being met as the study progresses (i.e., there is already an enrollment problem). However, the goal of advertising is the same no matter when it begins—to find and enroll suitable subjects into a trial.

The FDA has deemed that advertising for potential study subjects is not objectionable. In general, advertising is anything that is directed toward potential study subjects with the goal of recruiting them into the study. It may consist of radio or television spots, newspaper ads, posters on bulletin boards, flyers, internet postings, social media or any other methods to directly reach prospective subjects. For example, a large general practice that conducts studies has multiple copies of a notebook in its waiting room that contains a brief explanatory page for each study it is conducting with basic details about the study and whom to contact for further information. These notebooks are considered advertising.

The FDA considers direct advertising for study subjects to be "the start of the informed consent and subject selection process," according to an information sheet the agency released in January 1998, titled "Recruiting Study Subjects, Guidance for Institutional Review Boards and Clinical Investigators." Consequently, all advertising must be reviewed and approved by the IRB before use. Note that advertising may not be needed until later in the study, when it becomes apparent that enrollment goals are not being met. It does not matter that advertising materials were not submitted to the IRB when the study was first reviewed and approved; they simply must be approved before they are used.

But there are some items that the FDA does not count as advertising, according to the information sheet, including:

> (1) communications intended to be seen or heard by health professionals, such as "dear doctor" letters and doctor-to-doctor letters (even when soliciting for study subjects), (2) news stories and (3) publicity intended for other audiences, such as financial page advertisements directed toward prospective investors.

Investigators must keep in mind that ads written like news stories are still not news stories, but are more akin to "infomercials" or "advertorials"—ads with a newsy feel or element. They are still ads and all ads need to be approved by the IRB.

Somewhat confusing is the fact that there is a certain class of internet advertising that also does not need prior IRB review. Quoting from the same information sheet above:

> IRB review and approval of listings of clinical trials on the internet would provide no additional safeguard and is not required when the system format limits the information provided to basic trial information, such as: the title; purpose of the study; protocol summary; basic eligibility criteria; study site location(s); and how to contact the site for further information. Examples of clinical trial listing services that do not require prospective IRB approval include the National Cancer Institute's cancer clinical trial listing [in the Physician Data Query database] and the government-sponsored AIDS Clinical Trials Information Service (ACTIS). However, when the opportunity to add additional descriptive information is not precluded by the data base system, IRB review and approval may assure that the additional information does not promise or imply a certainty of cure or other benefit beyond what is contained in the protocol and the informed consent document.

Submitting all advertising to the IRB for review and approval is the best course of action. That eliminates all doubt and the need to make the determination of what is and is not appropriate material for the general public.

Advertising is reviewed by the IRB to ensure that it is not coercive and does not make promises about a cure or favorable outcome or promise things other than what appears in the protocol or the consent. This is especially important if the study involves subjects who are likely to be vulnerable to undue influence, such as children, prisoners and economically or educationally disadvantaged people.

For written advertisements, such as those designed for use in newspapers (print and online), the IRB will want to see finished copy to evaluate the whole ad, including type size and any visual effects. For audio and video advertising (radio, television, social media), the IRB will review both the written text and the audio version. Most IRBs will advise the investigator to submit the text first to be sure it is acceptable before the actual audio- or videotaping is done.

Advertising must not make any explicit or implicit claims that the investigational drug, biologic or device is safe and effective or that it is equivalent or superior to any other product. Remember that the reason for the trial is to determine these things; they are not yet known. The ads must explain that the test article is investigational or experimental. Using a term such as "new treatment" implies it is a proven and approved product and is not appropriate.

Advertisements may say subjects will be paid for participating in the study, but the payments should not be emphasized by big, bold type or other methods.

New Treatment for the Common Cold!!!

Cut your sniffle time in half!!!

Get paid $1,000 after only 7 days

Study subjects needed. Three shots a day for 4 days.

Call Success Clinical at 1-800-999-9999

Above is an example of an unacceptable advertisement. Note that it says "new treatment," promises to cut the time of the cold in half and emphasizes the overly high payment amount.

A more appropriate advertisement might be:

Research Study

Subjects needed for a study to investigate the effects of an experimental medicine on lessening the symptoms of the common cold.

Subjects must be seen by the second day of the cold and must be at least 18 years old. For details, contact Shirley Williams at Eastside Clinic. (222) 222-2000

What information should go into an advertisement? In general, the information should be limited to what prospective subjects need to know to determine if they might be interested in and eligible for the study. These may include the following items, according to the FDA information sheet:

> Generally, FDA believes that any advertisement to recruit subjects should be limited to the information the prospective subjects need to determine their eligibility and interest. When appropriately worded, the following items may be included in advertisements:
>
> 1. the name and address of the clinical investigator and/or research facility;
> 2. the condition under study and/or the purpose of the research;
> 3. in summary form, the criteria that will be used to determine eligibility for the study;
> 4. a brief list of participation benefits, if any (e.g., a no-cost health examination);
> 5. the time or other commitment required of the subjects; and
> 6. the location of the research and the person or office to contact for further information.

It should be noted that the FDA does not require inclusion of all of the listed items.

CRAs should be familiar with the information in the FDA information sheet, noted above, so they may better assist investigators in the proper development and use of advertising materials. The CRA should review all ads to make sure they are IRB-approved prior to use.

Established, Successful Recruitment Strategies

Google

It is very common for potential study subjects to conduct Google searches on their medical condition or even to look for possible clinical trials in which they might participate. If you want your web page to be available to potential trial subjects, there are two ways to make this happen on the Google search page. The first is in the unpaid section, called the "organic search" section. The other is in the paid section, "sponsored links." The sponsored links section is the list that shows up on the right-hand side of the page or in the top section.

The sponsored links are based on using Google Ads, which link your ad to a specific page on a website. This is based on a system that allows you to set one or more search terms. If the term is typed in by a Google user, the ad will show up; and if the user clicks on the ad, he or she will be directed to the specified web page.

Whether your ad actually shows up or not depends on how much you are willing to pay to direct a user to your website. This is called "cost per click" (CPC) and is paid only when the user clicks the ad and is directed to your web page. The CPC determines how often and how high your ad will appear in the sponsored links—the more you pay, the more often this will happen. The more specific your search term, the less competition there will be, so your term will cost less and show up more often. For example, a general term like "clinical trial" will require a higher CPC to outrank competition, while a term like "transcranial electronic stimulation" could show up high in the sponsored links with a relatively low CPC. In fact, if there were no other company using the search term, you could end up at the top of the sponsored links list at a small CPC. It's important that your web page is carefully and professionally designed for each trial with the appropriate keywords and information to both attract potential subjects and aid in achieving a higher level in the organic search section. Remember, all advertising, including internet advertising, must be approved by an IRB before use.

Note that many people may not trust ads, so a listing in the organic search section will usually result in a much higher click rate than a listing in the paid section. On the other hand, if a subject is searching for a new treatment for a disease, he or she might also click on an ad.

When you set up the Google Ads, you have the option of indicating a geographical region from which you want to attract searchers. This is called "geo-targeting" to indicate areas near your study site's locations. For example, if you had a study site in Chicago (or in Madrid), you could indicate that if a searcher in the Chicago area (or Madrid) is looking for information on transcranial electronic stimulation, you will pay the CPC amount to Google if your ad is shown and the searcher clicks on it. This could be especially useful for global trials.

The major benefits of using geo-targeting are that it allows directing a potential subject to your web page and if you have no presence in a certain region there is no need to pay to reach that region. This is an interesting technology for enhancing subject recruitment, especially in more difficult or esoteric trials for which enrollment is expected to be difficult.

Although Google is currently the largest search engine, others also might be worth using, such as MSN's BING. Note that different search engines may be more popular in countries other than the U.S. (e.g., Baidu in China).

Social Networks

Social media networks, such as Facebook, X (formerly Twitter) and Instagram, are increasingly being used for clinical trial recruitment. Used correctly, social networking can be an effective method for generating prequalified patient referrals.

Ads can run on social networks, as well as on Google. Since people have chosen to belong to these networks, they are more inclined to accept and act on messages received on these sites than from unsolicited advertising. Messages are also shared exponentially, without huge cost to the messenger.

Social networking sites have the ability to target ads to individual user pages based on information in the user profile, including location. Because these networks are global in scope, geo-targeting can be used to specify areas for desired recruitment of study subjects.

Social media-savvy sites can generate a large number of "likes" and visitors to their social media pages, which increases exposure and awareness of clinical trials they are conducting and services provided.

YouTube videos might also be used to disseminate information about a trial. A YouTube video can also have a link to a web page, so it can connect a viewer directly to your web page with additional information about a clinical trial.

Many trial sponsors have questions about the value and legality of reaching potential participants online. However, when it comes to using these networks for clinical trial recruitment, sponsors are not selling products or making any claims about treatment. They are only presenting clinical trials in IRB-approved advertising as an option to potential participants. This is really no different than any IRB-approved newspaper or radio ads that might be used. It is just the location of the ad that is different. Using social networks is simply another tool to reach a broader population and to help with the always difficult task of recruiting enough subjects for a clinical trial.

New Recruitment Strategies—AI and Clinical Research as a Care Option

The widespread use of social networks has created many new opportunities for the recruitment of subjects into clinical trials. In addition, artificial intelligence (AI) is now being used to troll through social media content to find potential trial participants. We are also seeing the growth of another new recruitment strategy—enrolling patients in clinical trials as part of their ongoing care.

AI can also be used to identify suitable patients for trials by analyzing medical records and to alert medical staff and patients about trial opportunities. This can help to reduce unnecessary screening. But AI has limitations. To be most effective, AI needs access to good quality data in a usable format, which is not always readily available.

Clinical Research as a Care Option (CRAACO) offers a way for research and clinical organizations to combine research with patient care by integrating their systems and data-sharing. An example includes research organizations partnering with health organizations to bring clinical trials to their existing patient population. The research organization brings research support staff and resources and integrates clinical trials into the health system infrastructure, physician practices and patient databases. CRAACO can use AI to identify patients most likely to benefit from the research. However, CRAACO faces obstacles because the healthcare system is not currently set up to enable widespread use. Once again, the available data will need to be easier to share in order to be most useful.

Other Recruitment Methods

Although advertising comes immediately to mind when discussing recruitment for study subjects, there are several other methods for finding subjects. The starting place for most sites is their own clinical/medical records. Many sites keep their patient information in an EMR, CTMS or e-source database that allows them to search based on diagnostic criteria. After they have found patients with an appropriate diagnosis, they are able to contact them to ascertain their interest and suitability for the trial. Contact made via telephone or email to database patients is an effective means of follow-up. In the case of studies in chronic diseases, such as diabetes or hypertension, most subjects will probably come from the investigator's own practice. In the case of acute diseases, such as pneumonia and other infectious diseases, searching the investigative site's records may not be particularly useful.

There are patient recruitment companies that have access to databases through partnerships or have the means to match patients and clinical trials.

In addition, there are clinical research advertising and marketing companies who use targeted digital advertising campaigns for their customers.

Many potential subjects hear about a trial by word-of-mouth, perhaps from a friend who is in the trial. Sites that conduct a number of trials often gain "free advertising" from current or past study subjects spreading the word. Subjects also find clinical trials by talking to people, searching the web and contacting organizations, including disease-related support groups and pharmaceutical companies.

There are many websites available to potential study subjects that list trials that are in progress or about to start. The website, clinicaltrials.gov, where clinical studies are listed by company, is often used by investigational sites. Potential subjects then find the studies and sign up. Additionally, there are specific websites for clinical trial advertisement purposes.

Advocacy groups for various diseases, such as AIDS, are sources of information about trials; sites may receive interested subjects from these groups or from people who have been in contact with them.

Frequently, other physicians or healthcare professionals will refer potential subjects to a trial. Investigators often contact other physicians in the community to inform them of the trial and ask that it be mentioned to suitable subjects. The investigator may make these contacts by phone or may send letters to other healthcare professionals in the community.

Usually, finding subjects for a trial is accomplished by a combination of methods. The more difficult it is to enroll, the more variety there will be in the methods used to attract potential subjects. It is important for a CRA to monitor enrollment and enrollment rates right from the start of each study and make suggestions for ways to enhance enrollment before it becomes a major problem. It is much easier to help when it begins to look like there may be trouble than to wait until there is a major problem. The way to fix enrollment problems is often by implementing several small ideas and suggestions. Not everything works in each case, and a single change is frequently not sufficient.

Author's Story

I once monitored a trial for a rare genetic mutation. Several investigators informed me that they were contacted by their patients about the trial, which is how the investigators became involved with the study and the sponsor. An example of patient centricity at its most admirable.

–Elizabeth

Payments to Research Subjects

It is quite common for subjects to be paid for participating in clinical trials, especially in the early phases of development. When subjects are paid, however, it is viewed by the FDA as a recruitment incentive, not as a study benefit. All payment schedules must be approved by the IRB in advance of the study, or in advance of being used. The IRB will look at both the payment amounts and the timing of the payments to be sure they are not coercive and would not present an undue influence on the subject's trial-related decisions. The payment amount must be included in the informed consent.

Subjects are usually paid on a regular basis throughout the trial, most commonly for each completed visit. It is rarely appropriate to pay subjects only if they complete the entire trial; this might encourage them to continue with the trial even if they otherwise would have discontinued due to side effects or other reasons. The FDA does allow a small payment as an incentive to finish the study, as long as it is not coercive. However, the IRB must determine that this bonus payment is reasonable and not so large that it would influence subjects to stay in the trial if they otherwise would withdraw.

The amount of the payments to subjects varies with respect to the complexity of the study and the involvement of the subjects. Payments are usually designed to cover any costs the subjects might incur by participating, such as transportation costs, parking, lunch and childcare. Payments must not be so large as to be coercive; that is, the subjects should not be entering a trial only because of the compensation. Before approving subject payments, the IRB will also take into account where the study is being conducted and the patient population. Payments of $25 per visit may be no enticement at all to people in some neighborhoods, but may constitute a great deal of money and enticement to subjects in other areas.

The exception for payments is in phase 1 trials in which healthy volunteers are the subjects. In this case, there are no real benefits for participating in the trial, so subjects are usually paid more. The amounts are not exorbitant, but are higher than in other trials and generally compensate the subjects for the greater amount of time required, such as overnight stays in the testing facility. Note that the FDA's January 2018 information sheet: Payment and Reimbursement to Research Subjects, Guidance for Institutional Review Boards and Clinical Investigators states:

> Paying research subjects in exchange for their participation is a common and, in general, acceptable practice. Payment to research subjects for participation in studies is not considered a benefit that would be part of the weighing of benefits or risks; it is a recruitment incentive. FDA recognizes that payment for participation may raise difficult questions that should be addressed by the IRB. For example, how much money should research subjects receive, and for what should subjects receive payment, such as their time, inconvenience, discomfort, or some other consideration. In contrast to payment for participation, FDA does not consider reimbursement for travel expenses to and from the clinical trial site and associated costs such as airfare, parking, and lodging to raise issues regarding undue influence. Other than reimbursement for reasonable travel and lodging expenses, IRBs should be sensitive to whether other aspects of proposed payment for participation could present an undue influence, thus interfering with the potential subjects' ability to give voluntary informed consent. Payment for participation in research should be just and fair. The amount and schedule of all payments should be presented to the IRB at the time of initial review. The IRB should review both the amount of payment and the proposed meth-

> od and timing of disbursement to assure that neither are coercive or present undue influence [21 CFR 50.20].

Some sites routinely pay subjects for participating in trials, while others never pay study subjects at all. Either is acceptable. What is important to remember about payments to study subjects is that they must not be coercive or present undue influence, and that they must be preapproved by the IRB.

Incentive Payments to Healthcare Professionals

There are two types of incentive payments: those paid by the investigator to other professionals to encourage them to find study subjects, and bonus payments by study sponsors to investigators and their respective staff to enhance enrollment.

Incentive payments to healthcare professionals by an investigator for the referral of study subjects are known as referral fees or finder's fees, examples of which are payments made to a coordinator or nurse, resident or intern physicians or other local physicians for each subject that is referred and entered into a study. These payments are usually not acceptable and may compromise the integrity of a trial. They may also be in violation of regulations or institutional policies.

Some states have laws that prohibit referral fees. For example, the California Health and Safety Code § 445 clearly prohibits referral fees. It states:

> No person, firm, partnership, association or corporation, or agent or employee thereof, shall for profit refer or recommend a person to a physician, hospital, health-related facility or dispensary for any form of medical care or treatment of any ailment or medical condition.

Also, the American Medical Association has stated in its Code of Medical Ethics that referral fees for research studies are unethical. Section 6.03 of the code, Fee Splitting: Referrals to Health Care Facilities, states:

> Offering or accepting payment for referring patients to research studies (finder's fees) is also unethical.

Many IRBs have taken a firm stand on the issue of finder's fees and will not permit them.

Incentive payments to healthcare professionals also include bonus payments by the study sponsor to investigators and coordinators for enhanced (faster or more) enrollment. True bonus payments are usually not acceptable because they may encourage the enrollment of "borderline" subjects, those that the investigator otherwise would not recruit. This creates a conflict of interest and should be avoided.

There is no problem, however, with a sponsor covering true extra costs for enrollment procedures. These payments might be for additional people to help with the screening of potential subjects, advertising costs or other direct costs borne by the investigative site. This is frequently decided upon before the study begins, even though not implemented unless necessary to increase enrollment or speed the rate of enrollment. For example, a sponsor may be willing to pay a per-screen amount for the prescreening of study candidates. In this case, there is usually a limit on the number of prescreens allowed in relation to the number of subjects actually entered into the trial. This ensures that the site is actually looking for and prescreening suitable candidates. The CRA will usually act as the liaison between the site and the sponsor on questions of appropriate support for enrollment.

If site personnel are not sure whether or not a payment plan is appropriate, they should contact their IRB for an opinion before implementation.

Summary

Timely and appropriate recruitment and enrollment of subjects into clinical trials are essential for a drug, biologic or device development program. CRAs must be aware of the regulations regarding recruitment and have an understanding of the potential problems and solutions for enrollment. It is important to remember that at each step, from potential patient identification through prescreening, screening and eligibility, the number of potential subjects decreases. The Venn diagram in Figure 2, patterned after one developed by Bert Spilker in his Guide to Clinical Studies and Developing Protocols, shows this in graphic form.

The CRA plays a significant role in subject enrollment by acting as an advisor to sites, by being aware of the rules and regulations regarding recruitment and by being the liaison between the sponsor and the site for managing enrollment concerns.

Retention of Study Subjects

Once subjects are enrolled in a trial, it is important that they stay in the trial until it is complete, if at all possible. CRAs should be familiar with both the reasons subjects drop out and how retention can be enhanced. The CRA should be the expert for helping sites with retention problems. In this section, we will explore the reasons that subjects leave trials and what can be done to increase retention.

Reasons Investigators or Sponsors Discontinue Subjects

Investigators and sponsors may discontinue a subject for a number of reasons. Some are medical, some are based on the patient's compliance and cooperation and some are trial-related. Some of the more common reasons for discontinuing a subject are listed below.

Medical Reasons for Discontinuation:

- Failure of the investigational drug to be effective.
- Intolerable adverse events.
- Patient's condition deteriorates.
- Patient's condition improves (eliminates need to continue).
- Patient develops an intercurrent illness (an illness other than the one under study but occurs during the course of the trial).
- Pregnancy.
- Abnormal laboratory values.
- Did not meet original entry criteria (discovered after study entry).

Patient Compliance and Cooperation Reasons:

- Unacceptable compliance with protocol activities.
- Unacceptable compliance in taking the study medication.
- Not keeping appointments.
- Not cooperating with study staff and/or study procedures.
- Use of nonapproved concomitant medications.
- Moved out of the area.

Trial-related Reasons:

- Trial was terminated by the sponsor due to safety concerns.
- Benefit so great trial is no longer ethical.
- Business reasons.
- Investigator no longer to continue the trial (retired, died, moved).
- Investigator did not meet enrollment targets in a timely fashion or did not comply with the protocol.
- Investigator had other problems or was put on the debarred list by the FDA. Since it was either the investigator or the sponsor who decided to discontinue patients or the trial for these reasons, there would be no further discussion.

The main concern for CRAs is helping sites retain subjects who would have decided to drop out of the study on their own.

Reasons Subjects Drop Out of Trials

It is important to differentiate between those subjects who choose to drop out on their own and those who are discontinued by the investigator or sponsor. There are many reasons study subjects decide to stop participating in a trial. Some of them are valid medical reasons, such as intolerable adverse reactions or a worsening of the disease. These cases are usually discussed with and agreed to by the investigator.

There are, however, other reasons that subjects drop out, that are not so compelling and could perhaps be avoided. This is when the CRA can help site personnel understand what causes some of the problems and how they might prevent them from occurring. The key for the CRA is catching problems, or patterns of problems, early so they can be fixed. The CRA wants to ensure that losses do not become the standard and that they do not exceed what normally would be expected during a study. Some reasons subjects drop out are:

- The subject does not understand the importance of remaining in the trial even when the disease condition has improved.
- The study requirements are too burdensome.
- The subject loses interest in the trial.
- The medication is unpleasant to take.

- The subject does not like some of the study staff or finds people at the investigative site unfriendly (which could be anyone, including the receptionist).
- The subject has to spend too much time at the clinic.
- Transportation, childcare or time off from work difficulties.
- The subject is upset about some aspect of the trial.
- Friends or family are unhappy about the subject's participation.
- The subject has a change in his or her personal life.

Maximizing Retention in Clinical Trials

The secret to subject retention in clinical trials is easy. It's not really a secret at all, but is just plain common sense. All site personnel have to do is be nice, treat subjects well, spend time with them, educate them, be transparent with them about trial responsibilities, listen carefully to what they are saying and communicate openly and often.

Investigators and study coordinators are very busy people. They get rushed and behind on things, have good and bad days and experience the same problems as the rest of us. Nevertheless, if a study is to go well, they must be able to set aside their concerns and problems when study subjects arrive for their visits. Study subjects want to feel that their contribution is important, and during their time with the investigator and/or coordinator they want to be the sole focus of attention.

When a study subject comes in for a clinic visit, he or she wants to be able to discuss what has happened since the last visit, to have any study concerns allayed, to be praised for doing well, to have questions answered and to be treated like an important partner in the study venture. In short, a study subject wants to be appreciated. After all, there are risks in becoming part of a study, there is no guaranteed outcome and it is voluntary. No one has to participate at all. People who volunteer for studies are special people, and they should be treated that way.

Given the premise of wanting to be treated well, there are many, frequently small, things that can make subjects decide that trial participation may not be worth the effort. Some of these things are:

- Having to wait when coming in for an appointment.

- Not being treated nicely and with respect.
- Not seeing the investigator or the coordinator, but being seen by a "substitute" they don't know.
- Not seeing the same person at each visit (developing a one-on-one relationship).
- Being rushed and hurried through the appointment.
- Feeling that the investigator/coordinator doesn't really want to see them.
- Not being asked about how they feel and how the study is going for them.
- Not having the opportunity to ask questions.
- Being afraid to ask study-related questions.
- Being made to feel dumb or silly when asking questions.
- Being berated for doing something wrong.
- Having the investigator or coordinator disparage the study.

There are also situations in which a subject does not return and is lost to follow-up, or in which a subject drops out but refuses to give a reason, other than personal choice, which is the subject's right—he or she doesn't have to give a reason. But that doesn't help site personnel understand if there is a more pervasive, underlying problem. These situations are difficult to prevent, so the investigative site cannot do much about them.

If there are many of these cases at a center, however, they should serve as a wake-up call. Chances are the real reasons are in the list above, but the subject doesn't want to say anything about them to site personnel.

These problems can all be fixed, but they first need to be recognized and acknowledged. It's critical to catch them early. Some problems are easy to fix. For example, if a subject has a logistics problem, such as transportation to the investigative site, a solution may be to pay for a taxi or other transportation vendor to transport the subject back and forth. If childcare is a problem, perhaps the visit time can be adjusted to an evening or weekend time so the subject can make appropriate arrangements. Questioning the subject about problems and being willing to help with arrangements or adjustments may allow the subject to continue participation. Subject payments in any form (cash, goods or services) should be reviewed by the IRB. It is fine to vary payments according to subjects' needs (taxi fare for one, but not another), but it would usually be stated as "payment for (actual) transportation costs," for example. Since these are actual costs to subjects, they would not be considered coercive. Coercion normally implies a sum of money above costs, with no purpose other than to entice people to enter the trial.

Some successful investigative sites have very clever ways of making their study subjects feel happy, important and wanted. Some of the ideas and little things that have added to retention success for sites are:

- Giving each volunteer a special study t-shirt.
- Giving them mugs, tote bags or gym bags for a study where there was exercise testing.
- Separate waiting room with coffee, tea and doughnuts—and current magazines and newspapers.
- Internet access while they wait for a study visit or during a study visit that requires timed testing with long waiting intervals.
- Reminder calls, texts or emails the day before each visit.
- Sending a cab to pick someone up if transportation is a problem.
- Thank you notes from the coordinator after a few weeks on a study.
- Thank you notes at the end of the subject's participation (leads to repeat volunteering).
- Balloons.
- Birthday cards.

For new investigative sites especially, though beneficial for most sites, it helps if the CRA meets with the investigator and coordinator at the beginning of the trial and plans out a strategy to help retain subjects. Many sponsors are willing to foot the bill for little extras (mugs, t-shirts) that might encourage subjects to feel good about their participation and remain in the trial until completion.

Any time there is a pattern of more-than-expected dropouts at an investigative site, the CRA should discuss the situation with the investigator and coordinator. Each case should be analyzed. Perhaps the reasons are clear-cut and recognizable, but perhaps they are not. It may be time to reflect on the atmosphere at the site and take a hard look at how subjects are being treated. The site personnel might even want to talk with subjects about their perceptions of how the study is going, how they feel when they come in for visits and if there are ways in which the investigative site could improve the study process.

Difficult as it is, site personnel must also take an honest look at their interactions with study subjects. Sometimes it helps to think about how you would feel if you were in the study, or how you would feel about having one of your loved ones participating.

Summary

Retention of subjects in clinical trials is critical to the completion of an informative, sound clinical trial. Site personnel should help subjects understand that a successful trial is a partnership between the subjects and the investigative staff. Respect, courtesy, honesty and open communication on the part of both subjects and investigators will increase the chances of successfully completing a study.

Subject Compliance

Clinical trials are conducted to assess the safety and efficacy of an investigational drug. To be able to accurately assess safety and efficacy, however, study subjects must take the medication as it is prescribed. Unfortunately, subjects do not always do this. In this section, we will look at compliance, what can go wrong and how to increase the probability of good compliance.

Undetected poor compliance can lead to invalid study results. Lack of compliance in one subject may affect only that particular subject; if several subjects are noncompliant, however, it can invalidate the entire study. Noncompliance can have the following results:

- An effective medication may look ineffective. This can mean that a medication that would be effective and that would be of benefit to patients never makes it to the marketplace. This is an unfortunate result for the sponsor that has made the investment in the investigational drug and even more unfortunate for those people who would have received benefit from it.

- An ineffective medication looks effective. This result is worse than the one above because, once marketed, the medication will be relied on to effect a cure and will not be effective in doing so.
- Failure to detect serious adverse events.
- Inappropriate dosage labeling. Depending on the noncompliance, the drug labeling could recommend either too high or too low a dose. This is not good in either direction—patients could be taking too little to be an effective treatment or more than they need, which could lead to an excess of adverse reactions.
- The effects of the investigational drug in noncompliant subjects cannot be extrapolated to compliant subjects. It is very important that all study subjects are as compliant as possible during their involvement in clinical trials.

Reasons for Noncompliance

Sometimes study subjects are noncompliant for disease-related reasons. One reason is a lack of symptoms, or what can be called the "antibiotic effect." As many of us know from personal experience, it is hard to remember to take medications when you feel better and have very few or no remaining disease symptoms. A prime example of this is the standard 10-day course of treatment with many antibiotics. After five or six days, when the patient appears to be better, it is very common to stop taking the pills. The subject has become noncompliant with the medication schedule; this happens in trials as well as in general practice.

There are also compliance problems with people suffering from terminal diseases. When a person knows he or she is going to die soon anyway, he does not have the same incentive to take a course of medications that he might otherwise have.

There are many other reasons subjects are not compliant when it comes to taking medication. Sometimes they just forget to take their pills. Sometimes there is a lack of belief in the treatment—"it isn't going to work anyway, I'm sure I'm on the placebo." If the medication is unpleasant to take, such as having a bad taste or pills being so big they are hard to swallow, compliance may be poor.

Noncompliance can result from the way the drug is packaged. Think about using safety containers (childproof lids) in an arthritis study, for example.

The subjects may not be able to open the containers without help, which will surely affect compliance. Sometimes a study drug is packaged in large blister packs containing several days' worth of the drug and with each day's drug clearly marked as to when it should be taken. At first glance, it appears this would help compliance, but think about it a bit more. What happens when a subject has to go to work? Most people do not want to carry a large blister pack to work with them and have other people asking about it. Consequently, subjects might take the day's drug out of the package and just carry it in a pocket, not knowing that the ordering of the pills for the day is important. They then become noncompliant.

Sometimes subjects just do not understand the dosing scheme, especially if it is complicated. "Oh, it's two white ones and one pink one? I thought it was two pink ones and one white one. That's why I ran out of pink ones last week." Sometimes it is the regimen that is confusing, with too many pills, too many different times per day to take them or confusion about the times and/or doses. It also can be the duration of the study, as subjects can lose interest over time.

Subjects may also become noncompliant because of adverse reactions. If a subject becomes nauseated after taking the medication or thinks it is causing headaches, he or she may not take it as often as required, if at all. A subject may not take medication appropriately because of mistrust, either in the medication or in the physician. A subject may be influenced by family or friends in ways that affect compliance; if people important to the subject do not want him or her to take the pills or be in the study, this may affect compliance.

Other ways in which subjects may be noncompliant related to the study medication are by prematurely discontinuing the drug or by sharing the drug with other people. Some of the other reasons subjects may become noncompliant include:

- Taking other medications at the same time, when the other medications are not allowed by the protocol.
- Using alcohol or other disallowed substances such as marijuana while in the study.
- Changes in a living situation that has an impact on when and how the study drug is taken.
- A mental condition that has an unfavorable effect on the ability to follow protocol instructions.

There are other compliance issues in studies that are not related directly to the medication. Subjects may also be noncompliant by missing visits or not coming in within the visit windows. They may not adhere to other study requirements, such as special tests (eye exams, for example), dietary requirements or keeping diaries. Subject compliance with diary entries is critical for some studies as it comprises part of the main safety endpoint. It is critical the patients are educated on the importance of diary entries early in a study and reminded at frequent intervals throughout the study. Fortunately, electronic diaries provide the means for site staff to track patient entries and results, and these systems send automated reminders for patients to complete entries and alert staff in the event of missed entries.

Sometimes compliance problems stem from investigator-related reasons. Subjects will be less compliant if it is difficult to schedule study visits, or if they are kept waiting when they arrive for a visit. If study staff do not keep appointments, subjects are apt to do the same. Worst of all is a poor physician-patient relationship. In general, subjects want to please the physician and do things correctly, but if the relationship is poor, the subject is not as likely to care about complying with study requirements.

Unfortunately, there are many ways to be noncompliant, both on purpose and by mistake. The key is discovering them and fixing the problem before it has a negative impact on the study.

Managing Compliance

Study protocols should be designed to enhance compliance as much as possible. They should also make it possible to monitor compliance.

CRAs should discuss compliance with site personnel and help them understand not only why it is important, but also how they can help to ensure compliance during the study. First of all, the CRA must help the investigator and coordinator understand that they need to work with their patients, both before and during the trial. There are certain things study patients must be aware of and do during the study. Just as clinical trials are different than clinical practice for investigators, they also are different for study subjects. The investigator and coordinator must ensure that potential study subjects are aware that if they are in the study, they must:

- Come in for all study visits on time and within the visit windows.

- Answer the questions truthfully, especially with respect to their medical histories and disease history.
- Cooperate fully with study procedures. This is one reason it is critical that the investigator fully explains the study to potential subjects.
- Allow tests to be done as appropriate, and on time.
- Take study medications as prescribed.
- Follow all study directions.
- Ask if something is not clear and inform the site of any problems.
- Report any new medications (OTC or Rx) before they take them or as soon as possible afterward.

The CRA should emphasize to the site that patients must be told how important it is to answer questions truthfully, especially about their compliance during the study. Patients need to know that it is better to let the investigator/coordinator know that they missed some doses than say nothing about it and that they will skew the results of the study if they are not forthcoming with this information. A CRA should remind the site personnel that they must thoroughly question each subject about compliance at each visit. They should be sure to let subjects know that they should call if they are having any problems complying with study activities or are confused about what needs to be done.

There are a variety of ways of testing for compliance in studies. Every study will have some way of asking about and maintaining drug accountability. Usually a record is kept for each subject of the amounts and dates study drug is dispensed and the amounts and dates of study drug returned. Subjects are told to bring back any unused medications at each visit. The returned study drug is counted and recorded by the coordinator. This is a reasonable way to assess compliance, but, unless the subject admits a problem, there is no way to know about the pill that fell down the drain or was swallowed by the vacuum. The person seeing the subject should also question him or her about whether or not all doses were taken.

Watching subjects take the pills in person would encourage good compliance, but studies are not usually set up in such a way that the subject is at the site each time a dose needs to be taken. This would work only if there is a single dose of medication being given, an IV drug is being administered or something similar.

Subjects are sometimes asked to keep diaries and record when each medication dose is taken. This is probably a good solution for very compliant subjects, but for others it is as easy to forget diary entry as it is to forget to take the medication.

The "gold standard" for testing for compliance is to check blood levels. This is done in some studies, but mostly only the very early (phase 1) studies. It is expensive and not feasible to do most of the time.

What can site personnel do to maximize compliance? First, it helps to know the subjects they enrolled. If an investigator and coordinator have worked with a subject before, they should have an idea of whether or not the person will be compliant. They should question subjects before entering the study on their willingness to comply with study activities, if they can swallow the pills, if they can come in for visits, etc.

The investigator and coordinator must pay attention to the signs of potential noncompliance. Does the patient show up for visits? Is the patient punctual? Did the subject complete all necessary prestudy activities? Is the person really interested in the study and aware of the requirements?

The coordinator should ask the subject about anything that may interfere with completing the study. Does the subject have a vacation planned during the time of the study? Does he or she understand what is involved in participating? Does the patient's lifestyle allow for complying with the study rules and activities? Does the distance the patient lives from the site preclude efficient and timely transportation to the study site for visits?

In short, if site personnel know or think a subject will not be a good, compliant patient, he or she should not be enrolled in the study.

When Noncompliance Happens

If the site is aware that a subject has been noncompliant, either in taking the medication or other study activities, the site should inform the sponsor of the noncompliance issue. Details of any noncompliance situations should be documented both in the CRF and in a note to the investigator's study file. The coordinator should discuss the situation with the subject and do some re-training in study procedures. If the subject continues to be noncompliant, he or she may need to be dropped from the trial. Keeping subjects who are not compliant in a trial is not good for the subject or for the trial. When subjects are dropped from a study for noncompliance, the relevant information must be recorded both in the CRF and in the subject's office chart or with a note in the investigator's study file.

By working closely with each potential subject before enrollment into a trial and by working closely with subjects throughout the trial, compliance can be maximized and study results will be more reliable than if there had been major compliance problems.

Good study designs and protocols will anticipate noncompliance and give instructions for minimizing it and for handling it, should it occur. If the CRA and the investigator do their jobs, both to minimize noncompliance and to detect and report it, the study should remain valid.

The Impact of Protocol Complexity on Subject Enrollment, Retention and Compliance

Not surprisingly, the complexity of the protocol has an effect on subject enrollment and retention in a trial, as well as on subject compliance. Tufts CSDD looked at the impact of protocol complexity on clinical trial performance, with some interesting results. (See Table 1.)

Table 1: Impact of protocol complexity on clinical trial enrollment

All therapeutic areas, phases 2-3

Subject	Less complex protocols	More complex protocols	Difference
Number of case report form pages per protocol (median)	55	180	+227%
Study volunteer enrollment rates	75%	59%	-16%
Study volunteer enrollment rates	69%	48%	-21%
Time from protocol ready to first patient first visit (median)	115 days	129 days	+12%
Time from protocol ready to last patient last visit (median)	413 days	714 days	+73%
Number of amendments	1.9	3.2	+68%

Source: Tufts CSDD

Notice that the enrollment rate goes down when protocol complexity goes up. This makes sense, of course; the more difficult a study will be for a potential subject, the less likely subjects are to volunteer and be involved. Complex studies require more time and effort from subjects.

Similarly, subject retention declines when complexity increases. This, too, is easy to understand; the more procedures subjects have to adhere to, the less likely they will want to remain in the trial. If the trial becomes too burdensome, in terms of time and/or activities, people will drop out rather than try to complete it.

Compliance is also an issue as trial complexity increases. More procedures mean more chances for something to go wrong. It's more difficult for subjects to remember and adhere to everything, as well as for site personnel to remember everything that needs to be done throughout the study.

This interrelatedness of all of the factors of a clinical trial should be addressed when the study is being planned. Thinking about the effect of complexity on study subjects in advance can lessen problems as the study progresses.

Key Takeaways

Recruitment

- Timely enrollment of subjects is critical to a drug, biologic or device development program.
- CRAs must help investigative sites accurately estimate the number of subjects they can expect to enroll in a study.
- Sites need to have the necessary personnel, time and space to handle the enrollment needed for each trial.
- Protocol requirements, especially the inclusion and exclusion criteria, are the primary limiting factors for enrollment.
- Assessment of the rate of enrollment is critical to managing a trial at the investigative site.

- Competing studies, both at the site and in the community, can have a significant impact on enrollment.
- Advertising for study subjects is allowed by the FDA, but must not be coercive or exert undue influence on potential subjects.
- All advertising must be approved by the IRB before use.
- Modern recruitment strategies include AI, clinical research as a care option, online search engines, such as Google and social networks including Facebook and YouTube.
- Most study subjects refer themselves to clinical trials.
- Payments to study subjects must be approved by the IRB and must not be coercive or exert undue influence.
- Finder's fees or referral fees are not acceptable and in some states are illegal.
- Sponsors will usually pay true extra costs for enrollment procedures.
- CRAs must be able to monitor enrollment and to suggest methods to increase enrollment if it lags behind expectations.
- The more complex the study, the harder it will be to enroll subjects.

Retention of Study Subjects

- Investigators may discontinue subjects from a trial for medical reasons, compliance or cooperation issues or because the sponsor is stopping the trial.
- Subjects have many reasons for dropping out of a trial, including medical reasons and logistics problems.
- Determining problems as early as possible is the first step to retaining subjects in trials.
- Respect and open communication are the biggest factors in subject retention.
- CRAs can help their sites achieve good retention.
- The complexity of the protocol has an impact on subject retention.

Subject Compliance

- Good compliance is critical for valid conclusions from clinical trials.
- Subjects need to be aware of the importance of compliance.
- Sites need to determine if potential study subjects are likely to be compliant and not enroll subjects who probably will not be compliant.
- There are many different ways in which subjects may be noncompliant with study procedures.
- Site personnel need to be alert to compliance problems throughout the study.
- If noncompliance occurs, the site should notify the sponsor.
- Compliance decreases as study complexity increases.

CHAPTER 17

Study Closeout

When a study has been completed at an investigative site, it must be officially closed. This is almost always the responsibility of the CRA. This chapter looks at the reasons studies are closed and what must be done officially to do so.

Reasons for Study Closeout

The primary reason to close a study is that the study has been completed: enrollment has stopped, all subjects have completed their study-related activities and the data are complete and correct. This is, of course, the best and most desired outcome. There are also reasons for closing a study before it is complete. Studies may be terminated early for both positive and negative reasons. Some of the reasons are listed below.

Positive Reasons for Early Study Termination

- The investigational treatment is so beneficial that it would not be ethical to conduct a trial during which subjects might not receive the active treatment.
- Overall enrollment is met in the trial, so all sites are being closed even if they did not complete the site enrollment goal.
- Statistical stopping criteria were set up in advance (in the protocol) and those criteria are met. This means that the endpoint is reached (either positive for the investigational treatment or not) and the trial will end. Whether or not the outcome is the one anticipated, there is no reason to expend additional resources on the trial.

Negative Reasons for Prematurely Ending a Trial

- The investigational treatment is found to be unsafe.
- The investigational treatment is not effective.
- It is not possible to find and enroll sufficient study subjects.
- The sponsor decides that the potential product was not viable for marketing.
- The sponsor terminates the program for another reason.
- The company runs out of funds. (This is being seen more frequently in small startup companies that rely heavily on venture capital.)
- The protocol is too difficult to execute.
- An investigator loses interest in the trial.
- An investigator dies, retires, moves, etc., and there is no replacement investigator.
- Problems arise in the manufacturing or stability of the compound.
- Compliance or other problems arise at the site.

As might be suspected from the length of the two lists, more studies are terminated early for negative reasons than for positive ones.

A trial may be discontinued at all sites at the same time or at individual sites at different times. Whatever the timing, the activity is essentially a single-site activity; that is, it must be done at each site without regard to activity at the other sites.

One cautionary note: If the study is stopped abruptly while subjects are still taking the study medications, there should be an orderly plan for discontinuing each subject. This plan will be formulated by the sponsor and communicated to each investigator. The CRA should be prepared to explain the plan to the site and ensure that it is followed correctly. The site also must be prepared to notify subjects promptly and assure them of appropriate therapy and follow-up outside of the trial.

The most common reason for closing a study is because it is finished and complete. It is also the easiest to handle. Site personnel are usually pleased that it was finished, hopeful of a favorable outcome and, frequently, hoping for additional studies from the sponsor in the future. In this case, the CRA is welcomed.

If a study was closed for a negative reason, it may affect all sites or just one. In this case, site personnel may not be happy about the closeout. Since the CRA is the sponsor's on-site representative, the CRA may be the recipient of the site's anger or unhappiness. This is the time for the CRA to use tact and interpersonal skills. If at all possible, you should want to leave the investigator and other site personnel on a friendly basis, even if they are unhappy friends.

No matter the reason for closing the study, the same procedures must be followed. In the rest of the chapter, we will discuss what must be done to close a study.

Closeout Procedures

A CRA will conduct in-person closeout visits at sites unless circumstances allow for remote site closeout. Possible scenarios for a remote site closeout visit could include a combination of these circumstances:

- The investigational site did not screen or enroll any study patients.
- The means to complete final review of the investigator site file and cross reconciliation with the sponsor/CRO eTMF could be accomplished virtually.
- The study site was able to destroy all study supplies or ship them back to the sponsor.
- The site never received the study drug.
- The investigator and staff are available virtually for final discussions.

A remote closeout visit would be feasible in these circumstances, with sponsor approval. There may be other circumstances under which a remote closeout visit is possible but those will not be covered in this chapter. The chapter will cover the requirements for on-site closeout visits and activities. The main items to be addressed during a closeout visit are: eCRFs/CRFs, drug accountability, the investigator's study file and administrative items.

Case Report Forms

If the eCRFs/CRFs have not already been completed, reviewed, corrected and verified, this must be done now. If the study has come to its natural end, this activity has probably been completed. If the study has been stopped abruptly or early, this may not be complete. It is always better to conduct a final closeout visit after the CRFs have been completed and reviewed, in the event final corrections need to be made before verification.

The CRA should make sure all CRFs are completed, verified and signed by the investigator and that any queries are resolved and closed.

SAE and Protocol Deviation Reporting

The CRA should take the opportunity during the site closeout visit to do a final reconciliation of SAEs and protocol deviations to ensure they have been reported to the sponsor and IRB according to study requirements. Though this should have been an ongoing process during study monitoring visits, especially if a CRA is conducting a closeout visit at a site he or she has not previously visited, the CRA should always conduct a final reconciliation of the SAE and protocol deviation listings with the source documents/eCRFs to ensure adequate completion.

Drug Accountability

If study drug supplies remain at the site, the CRA should complete a final inventory at the closeout visit. The study drug should then be packaged for return to the sponsor, in accordance with company policy, or destroyed by the site with the appropriate documentation and SOPs to support destruction activities and approval from the sponsor. A copy of the drug inventory form should be placed in the investigator's study file.

Drug reconciliation should have been done throughout the study, rather than left to the end. In this case, it should be relatively easy for the CRA and the coordinator to finish the reconciliation. Otherwise, drug accounting could be the most time-consuming study closeout activity.

Other Study Supplies and Equipment

The CRA will inventory and provide the site with return labels to ship back study equipment or supplies to the vendor, like blood pressure or ECG machines, thermometers, rulers, tablets or lab kits. Sometimes a site is permitted to destroy supplies, such as lab kits or rulers, if they have the sponsor's permission and an appropriate destruction documentation/process. On occasion the sponsor may allow the site to keep specific provided equipment.

Investigator's Study File

The CRA must thoroughly check the investigator's study document file at this visit. A reconciliation between the investigator study document file and site eTMF at the sponsor/CRO should have been completed prior to the closeout visit to ensure consistency, as well as during the closeout visit for the final reconciliation of documents, if needed.

It is wise to use a checklist (see Appendix C) during review of the investigator study document file, to ensure that nothing is overlooked. All documents must be present, including appropriate reapprovals and correspondence from the IRB, monitoring visit confirmation and follow up letters, IND safety reports, training logs, study manuals, etc. If there were protocol amendments during the study or amendments to the informed consent form, all versions should be in the file, including their dates of use.

Informed consent forms for each subject must be present. The CRA should double-check to be sure they were all signed and dated appropriately.

There should be documentation for any protocol variations, whether or not they were previously approved. The investigator brochure should be available with all revisions.

If any documents are missing from this file, the CRA should retrieve copies from the eTMF for the investigator study file. If the CRA keeps copies of missing documents on his/her computer, this is also a way to provide the site the needed copies for filing. When the file is complete and in order, it is ready for storage.

Investigator's Final Report to the Sponsor and the IRB

The investigator is required to make a final study report to the sponsor. This report should include an enrollment summary, including the numbers of subjects entered, those who completed, those who dropped out and their reasons for dropping out. It will also include information about AEs and any other information relative to the trial at that site.

The investigator will also make a final report to the IRB. It will contain the information above, in addition to any other information specifically requested by the IRB.

The investigator must also notify the institution that the study is complete, if appropriate.

The CRA should verify that these reports were completed, collect copies for the sponsor, if appropriate, and ensure that the reports are in the investigator's study file.

Administrative Issues

This may be the last visit the CRA will make to the investigative site for the trial, so any outstanding business or issues should be resolved before the study closeout is complete. Any loose ends should be resolved and taken care of before the site is completely closed.

The CRA should verify that all appropriate grant monies have been paid or requested. Be sure that the monetary amounts are in agreement between the investigator and the sponsor.

Any outstanding issues from previous visits or issues that arose during sponsor review should be resolved before the study is closed out at the site. If not documented elsewhere, a note detailing the resolution should be put in the investigator's study file.

The CRA should discuss record retention with the investigator. Not only do the records need to be stored and maintained, but there also must be a record of where they are stored. According to the regulations, records must be kept for two years after the NDA is approved for marketing. The same regulations apply if an NDA is not filed or is not approved after the investigation is discontinued and the FDA has been notified. However, most sponsors expect the investigator to retain all study records until notified by the sponsor that they may be disposed of; most often, this is stated in the contract the investigator signed before starting the study. The CRA must be sure that the investigator and site personnel are aware of and understand the retention period.

Investigative sites do not always keep study records as long as they should. Years go by and things happen—there may be a shortage of storage space, a move to a new facility or the erroneous thought that they don't need to "keep all that old stuff" around any longer. Unfortunately, these records may be needed years after the study is over. For example, the sponsor may decide to file a new application based, in part, on old studies; when the FDA visits investigative sites as part of the NDA review process, it will expect to see all the documents in place, even if the study was done many years earlier. It will be an embarrassment to the investigator if he or she has thrown them away, and it may have a negative impact on the sponsor's NDA.

CRAs need to impress upon their sites that record retention is important and not something to be taken lightly, along with the reasons to keep everything. Records must be kept until the sponsor has informed the site in writing that they may be destroyed. It is recommended that the boxes be labeled on the outside "DO NOT DESTROY" with the names of both the investigator and the sponsor as contacts for questions about them. If there is some reason a site can no longer maintain the records, the site should contact the sponsor. In most cases, the sponsor will arrange storage for these materials so that they are not destroyed. There are ways for sites to keep documents electronically, but this is specific to each site and their capabilities.

At this time, it may be best to remind the investigator of any publication terms for the study and to notify the sponsor of any impending FDA audit. When everything is complete and accounted for, the CRA should thank the site for its participation, being sure to include everyone who worked on the study. It is nice to follow up with a written letter of thanks.

Final Visit Report

The CRA must complete a visit report after this site visit, as for any other visit. Many companies have a special visit report for the closeout visit. This report documents that the study was officially closed.

In the final report, the CRA should verify that everything was checked, found complete and prepared for storage. If there were any outstanding issues from previous visits, the resolution of those issues should be documented in this visit report. The CRA should be sure that the report is clear and does not leave any unresolved loose ends.

Key Takeaways

- Studies can be stopped because they are complete or for a variety of other reasons—both positive and negative.
- The CRA is the person who will do a study closeout at an investigative site.

- All study documents, including CRFs, informed consent forms, drug accountability and study regulatory documents, must be completed, verified and filed (unless electronic) at the end of the study.
- All study drugs and other supplies must be returned to the sponsor or disposed of at the end of the study.
- The investigator must prepare a final study report for the sponsor and the IRB at the end of the study.
- The investigator must be aware of record retention requirements at the end of the study.
- In a final visit report, the CRA must verify that the study was properly closed.

CHAPTER 18

Quality Management

This chapter discusses some activities that can increase quality in clinical trials. Most of the data presented to regulatory agencies when seeking approval for a new drug is collected during clinical trials. If a regulatory agency has concerns or doubts about the integrity of the data, adherence to regulations and GCP or ethical concerns, this can lead to delays in the approval process. This is very costly for the sponsor. A quality management program that includes continuous monitoring and checking of quality-related measures can help ensure a smooth submission and review process.

There are three inter-related parameters that affect clinical trials and the data resulting from them: time, cost and quality. For example, if a sponsor cuts development time, it may be necessary to add more people or engage a CRO, which would increase cost. At the same time, data quality may decrease because there could be less time to properly collect and review it. There is the possibility that a decrease in available funds for a project might mean that there could be a delay to the start of some trials, or a lack of available resources to handle them expeditiously.

One way to manage quality is to be proactive about it from the beginning of the project. Designing good protocols and CRFs/eCRFs, obtaining expert advice and discussing the study protocol and CRFs/eCRFs with site personnel before they are finalized can eliminate problems once the study begins. Some sponsors have even field-tested the protocol and forms with a few subjects before finalizing them. This takes some time and costs money, especially for field testing, but these costs are often much lower than the cost involved in making fixes later on.

Continuous review of the data is another very effective quality management activity. One part of this is the timely review of the data from the first couple of subjects at each investigative site. If this review is done quickly, few potential subjects will be lost and an increase in quality should continue throughout the trial. Receiving feedback from the sponsor early allows misconceptions about processes and procedures to be corrected before they repeat over many subjects and multiple visits. This is also the time to work with any study coordinator (CRC) who is "error prone," whether due to misunderstanding or carelessness.

An additional quality measure with regards to screening/enrolling patients is the requirement for sites to submit eligibility documentation for a potential study subject to the study medical monitor or project manager for review and final study eligibility confirmation before enrollment. A number of studies require this; it is seen often with oncology studies as well as complicated therapeutic areas or study designs.

Continuous review depends not only on the CRA and monitoring visits but also on timely entry by site staff and timely review by data management. Whether the data are entered in the EDC system by the study coordinator or other site personnel, quality relies on timely and accurate information input as well as timely and accurate data review. Quality is facilitated by automated data checks in EDC systems and other electronic data collection measures used by sites, such as ePROs, eDiaries, etc. Study coordinators will learn from the queries they receive and will be less prone to making the same mistakes in the future. The CRA can also use the query information for specific training at sites.

With a good quality management plan in place, the overall rate of errors and problems at study sites should decrease as the study continues. The time spent upfront to put these activities in place will be more than compensated for by the time saved throughout the study. Stressing the importance of timely data entry to site staff, the importance of addressing and resolving queries at the beginning and continuing that throughout the study should allow the sponsor to have analysis-ready data very soon after the study is complete. This can result in earlier regulatory filings, which may then result in quicker approvals and additional marketing time for the product.

ICH E6(R2) details how a sponsor should institute quality management, using a risk-based approach as described below:

> 5.0.1 *Critical Process and Data Identification*
>
> During protocol development, the sponsor should identify those processes and data that are critical to ensure human subject protection and the reliability of trial results.

5.0.2 Risk Identification

The sponsor should identify risks to critical trial processes and data. Risks should be considered at both the system level (e.g., standard operating procedures, computerized systems, and personnel) and clinical trial level (e.g., trial design, data collection, and informed consent process).

5.0.3 Risk Evaluation

The sponsor should evaluate the identified risks against existing risk controls by considering:

(a) The likelihood of errors occurring.

(b) The extent to which such errors would be detectable.

(c) The impact of such errors on human subject protection and reliability of trial results.

5.0.4 Risk Control

The sponsor should decide which risks to reduce and/or which risks to accept. The approach used to reduce risk to an acceptable level should be proportionate to the significance of the risk. Risk reduction activities may be incorporated in protocol design and implementation, monitoring plans, agreements between parties defining roles and responsibilities, systematic safeguards to ensure adherence to standard operating procedures, and training in processes and procedures.

Predefined quality tolerance limits should be established, taking into consideration the medical and statistical characteristics of the variables as well as the statistical design of the trial, to identify systematic issues that can impact subject safety or reliability of trial results. Detection of deviations from the predefined quality tolerance limits should trigger an evaluation to determine if action is needed.

5.0.5 Risk Communication

The sponsor should document quality management activities. The sponsor should communicate quality management activities to those who are involved in or affected by such activities, to facilitate risk review and continual improvement during clinical trial execution.

5.0.6 Risk Review

The sponsor should periodically review risk control measures to ascertain whether the implemented quality management activities remain effective and relevant, taking into account emerging knowledge and experience.

5.0.7 Risk Reporting

The sponsor should describe the quality management approach implemented in the trial and summarize important deviations from the predefined quality tolerance limits and remedial actions taken in the clinical study report (ICH E3, section 9.6 Data Quality Assurance).

Site Metrics

A successful study site is one at which the enrollment goals are met in terms of both numbers of subjects and the time to complete enrollment and where the data generated are of high quality (accurate, valid and complete; see Chapter 14). Therefore, it is critical that a sponsor (or CRO) has systems in place to determine which sites will be good performers for clinical trials.

There are two facets to improve site quality: selecting good sites initially and helping ongoing sites. The probability of improving study success with both of these activities can be enhanced if sponsors keep some basic metrics on sites as part of their quality management program. To collect and maintain metrics, sponsors and CROs often develop their own in-house databases and analytical systems, or they may purchase available commercial programs/systems. Regardless, site performance data are collected and analyzed and used to categorize the site success level and this contributes to site identification. For new studies, looking at the metrics for sites used in the past can help when selecting good sites and avoiding sites that have not performed well. Some of the metrics that might be used for site identification are:

- Previous experience (number of studies and therapeutic areas).
- Time it takes for IRB review.
- Past enrollment data.
- Data quality measures from completed studies.

Some of these metrics may not be available for sites that the sponsor or CRO has not worked with in the past, but once a site has been used, this information can be collected. The use of these metrics will not guarantee good sites, but affords an opportunity to add another level of confidence to the selection process (more information on site selection can be found in Chapter 12).

For current studies, maintaining "real-time" site metrics can show the sponsor which sites are excelling, as well as which sites might need more training or closer monitoring. Not only is it easier to collect and maintain metrics throughout the study, as opposed to calculating them at the end, they can be put to good use throughout the study. Once the metrics are set up, they can be calculated based on ongoing data entry from eCRFs and other systems used to manage the study along with regular input from the CRAs and the sites (e.g., enrollment tracking). Since metrics are collected and reported primarily in electronic systems, this involves very little extra work and is potentially a big advantage.

These programs usually are not maintained by the CRA, but the CRA helps collect the information for them and has access to them. These metrics can be reviewed by the CRA and the CRA can use this tool to help improve quality at the study sites. A set of basic metrics might include the following:

- Number of subjects enrolled.
- Number of screen failures.
- Recruitment/enrollment time (from study start date to the date enrollment was completed).
- Number of subjects who discontinued the study early (dropouts), by category:
  - Ineffective study medication.
  - AEs.
  - Deaths.
  - Non-compliance.
  - Lost to follow-up.
  - Other categories, as appropriate.
- Number of protocol deviations.

- Number of AEs (or SAEs).

During the trial, the sponsor might want to compare sites based on these metrics. For example, an enrollment rate can be calculated by dividing the days of the enrollment time by the number of subjects enrolled during that time. This can be done before enrollment is complete and will show which sites are enrolling more rapidly. This allows the sponsor to investigate why some sites are seeing better, or worse, enrollment. Insights gained can be shared to help other sites. If sites are above or below average in any of these categories, the sponsor may want to find out why. Why are there more protocol violations at Site X? Why does Site Y have so many dropouts? Why is Site Z enrolling much more quickly than the average?

Table 1: Enrollment rates

Site number	Start date	Current date	Number of days	Subjects enrolled	Enrollment rate
1	12-5-2021	6-1-2022	178	21	0.118
2	12-16-2021	6-1-2022	167	3	0.018
3	1-4-2022	6-1-2022	148	14	0.095
4	1-23-2022	6-1-2022	129	25	0.194
5	2-3-2022	6-1-2022	118	6	0.051
6	2-3-2022	6-1-2022	118	19	0.161
7	2-25-2022	6-1-2022	96	34	0.354
8	3-21-2022	6-1-2022	72	9	0.125
9	3-24-2022	6-1-2022	69	13	0.188
10	3-28-2022	6-1-2022	65	17	0.262
Totals and overall rate			**1,160**	**161**	**0.139**

Let's look at an example of enrollment rates over a study with 10 sites. Table 1 shows that they did not all start enrollment at the same time, but a rate can be calculated by dividing the number of subjects enrolled to date by the number of days since each site started the study.

There are two sites in the chart that are enrolling much better than average—Site 7 and Site 10. This may be good, or it may not be. Are techniques being used for enrollment that other sites might not have thought to utilize? Or are sites enrolling too quickly and using inappropriate subjects? The CRA might want to visit both sites to see what is happening and why the enrollment is significantly higher than at the other eight sites.

Site 2 shows that enrollment looks very low. It would be a good idea to look into the reasons why enrollment is failing at this site, especially as it was the second site to begin. Site 5 isn't doing well, either.

Enrollment comparison is one tool that can help the sponsor manage the study.

Other site metrics that may be of interest can also be collected. Some to consider are:

- Time from commitment to IRB approval.
- Time to collect and submit study initiation paperwork.
- Number of coordinators.
- Number of sub-investigators.
- Time from subject visit to completion of CRFs.
- Turnaround time for queries.
- Error rate (e.g., queries per subject or queries per CRF page).
- Protocol-specific items.

Errors can be costly. The following example shows how this metric might be collected and compared over different investigative sites. Note that error rates could also be compared for different types of studies, or over different clinical programs.

In our example, let's assume we are looking at the same 10 sites we examined for enrollment rates. Although a bit unrealistic in a real situation, we will assume that each CRF page contains about 10 fields. Data management can tell us how many CRF pages have been entered to date for each site and how many queries have been made (each error means one query). Table 2 shows enrollment as well as the number of pages entered, queries sent and the error rate (queries divided by pages).

With enrollment rates, higher is better, but error rates should be as low as possible. Sites 4 and 7 look good here; not only have they enrolled well, but their error rates are low and they have enough pages entered to have confidence in what they are doing. Sites 3 and 9 look pretty good also, but note that there is not a great deal of data entered for them yet. Site 2 looks good, but with so few pages entered, you can't really get a good feel for how this rate will hold up.

Table 2: Query/error rates

Site number	Subjects enrolled	Pages entered	Queries sent	Error rate
1	21	314	51	0.172
2	3	24	2	0.083
3	14	140	13	0.093
4	25	450	35	0.078
5	6	62	15	0.242
6	19	250	76	0.304
7	34	342	29	0.085
8	9	60	24	0.400
9	13	150	12	0.080
10	17	235	46	0.196
Totals and overall rate	**161**	**2,027**	**306**	**0.151**

On the other hand, Sites 8, 6 and 5 have pretty high rates. It's probably too early to tell about Sites 8 and 5 since there are not many pages entered yet, but Site 6 could be a problem. It would be good for CRAs to check the sites with higher error rates quickly, so that any misunderstandings can be corrected before the errors are repeated.

The CRA is one of the primary resources for keeping the error rate low at study sites. It is the CRA who trains (and re-trains) study coordinators to complete the CRFs correctly. It is the CRA who is charged with reviewing the forms for accuracy and completion, alongside the data management team and internal system checks. It is primarily the CRA who reviews queries with the CRC to be sure they are understood and that errors don't repeat throughout the study. Because of this, CRAs must shoulder some of the responsibility for error rates at their sites. Therefore, an effective CRA will pay close attention to errors found at his or her sites and will work with the CRCs to ensure an understanding of how to complete the CRFs correctly, as well as the need for carefulness and accuracy. Pointing out the cost of errors and the amount of the cost borne by sites can help to reinforce the importance of doing things right the first time.

The collection of metrics has a huge payoff in terms of managing sites for current studies and selecting sites for future studies. Errors are expensive to fix, both in terms of resources and time. Poor sites can make a huge difference in overall data quality. Picking good sites can lessen the time to complete a study.

In summary, initiating a good quality management program can save time and money while increasing data quality and might, in fact, have a positive impact on the time to regulatory approval of a new product.

Key Takeaways

- The three interrelated parameters that affect clinical trials and the data resulting from them are time, cost and quality.
- Build in quality from the beginning of each project—be proactive.
- Continuous review of the data throughout a study can increase quality and ensure faster completion times.
- There are a number of site metrics that can be kept to help determine which sites might need additional help, as well as which sites might be best to use for future studies.
- CRAs should have regular access to site metrics so they can be used for training.
- The cost of errors is very high.
- Keep the quality up.

CHAPTER 19

Audits

During the clinical development process, the FDA may conduct audits (also called inspections) of investigative sites. Sponsors and IRBs may also conduct their own audits of investigative sites. The FDA also audits sponsors and IRBs. This chapter discusses these types of audits, as well as the CRA role in each. The chapter begins with audits conducted by sponsors and institutions or IRBs, but will concentrate primarily on those audits conducted by the FDA, as they are the most critical to the drug approval process and to the CRA.

Sponsor Audits of Investigative Sites

There are two main purposes for a sponsor to audit an investigative site. The first, and most common, reason is to ensure that a site is complying with regulations and protocol when conducting a study and that everything is in order in case of an FDA audit. These are referred to as routine audits. The second reason is that there is evidence the site is out of compliance and the sponsor wants to either verify the problem or be reassured that no problem exists. These are called for-cause audits.

A sponsor's right to audit a site is based on both the regulations and (usually) on the contract between the investigator and the sponsor. The contract will usually state that the investigator agrees that the sponsor may conduct audits of the site. The regulations under which sponsor audits are loosely covered are found in 21 CFR 312.56(a)(b), which states:

> (a) The sponsor shall monitor the progress of all clinical investigations being conducted under its IND, and (b) A sponsor who discovers that an investigator is not complying with the signed agreement (Form FDA1572), the general investigational plan, or the requirements of this part or other applicable parts shall promptly either secure compliance or discontinue shipments of

the investigational new drug to the investigator and end the investigator's participation in the investigation.

Sponsor audits are usually carried out by the sponsor's quality assurance (QA) department, if it has one. The CRA may or may not accompany the audit team but usually does not assist in the actual audit. If the sponsor company is too small to have a QA department or if the QA department does not have the resources to conduct an audit, the sponsor may contract with a CRO to do the work. In general, a sponsor may contract out routine audits but will usually do for-cause audits itself.

Routine Audits

If the sponsor knows or suspects that a site will be audited by the FDA, a routine audit may be conducted, either while the study is in progress or after it has been completed during the NDA review period. The sponsor knows the FDA will inspect some sites during its review of the NDA, so the sponsor will focus on the sites that are logical for the FDA to pick: those at which enrollment was the highest or at which multiple studies contributed to the NDA.

For a routine audit, the sponsor will send in an audit team, who will follow the same inspection plan used by the FDA. This inspection plan can be found in the FDA's Compliance Program Guidance Manual for Clinical Investigators (7348.811) on the agency's website.

A written report of sponsor audit results is usually not given to the investigator, because FDA inspectors do not have routine access to sponsor audit reports and sponsors do not want to have these reports freely circulating, either at the investigative site or internally. If a written report is sent to an investigator, the sponsor will usually ask that it be destroyed after corrective action is taken.

If any problems are found during the audit, the CRA most likely will be asked to work with the site to remedy them, with the goal being to ensure that the site is ready for an FDA audit. The CRA will report back on the final status at the site; this is sometimes done in a formal audit response, which is kept with the original audit report. Audit reports and responses are usually maintained in and by the QA department, and any other copies are to be destroyed.

For-Cause Audits

For-cause audits of investigative sites by a sponsor may be handled somewhat differently. These are audits conducted because of suspected noncompliance at a site, either with the regulations or with the protocol. They have the potential for being much more serious, both for the sponsor and ultimately for the investigator. The sponsor is unlikely to tell the investigator it is a for-cause audit; the CRA will probably know, since he or she most likely reported the information about the suspected problems to the sponsor. The audit team will look at most of the things it would inspect for any audit but will pay particular attention to the area of the suspected noncompliance.

Depending on the results of the audit, a number of things could happen:

- If everything appears to be in compliance, the results will be handled in the same way they would for any routine audit.
- If the problem was not found but is still suspected, another group may be sent to look. Or the sponsor might inform the FDA and ask it to inspect the site.
- If problems were found, they will either be rectified or enrollment may be put on hold pending further investigation or the study may be stopped at the site. In this case the FDA will be informed, if appropriate. If so, this will be done by the QA department, probably in conjunction with the medical monitor for the study and the sponsor's regulatory group.

The CRA is likely to be involved with for-cause audits in some way, especially if problems are found and enrollment is put on hold or the site is closed. These are not pleasant situations to be in, and the CRA will need a lot of tact and diplomacy in working through the problems.

Author's Story

Nightmare Audit

I had a nightmare FDA inspection several years ago that lasted more than two weeks. The one thing that kept me going was that I had personally done a good job from my end. I had no control over what was done to CRFs or source documents after the study was closed. I learned that, early on, I gave the site too many chances without documenting that there were prob-

lems; I had not wanted to "tell on them" without giving them a chance to correct them.

Document, document, document. Having to fax the FDA my visit reports (with my company's blessing) was quite a learning experience. I wished, of course, that there had been more on my reports about the problems I was aware of and had addressed with the site. I had communicated all the problems to the project manager on the phone, but not in writing, except too briefly on visit reports. This site had enrolled too quickly—60 patients when the average everywhere else was about eight.

–A CRA

IRB Audits of Investigative Sites

IRBs also visit or audit sites upon occasion. A central or independent IRB may visit sites simply because it is not located nearby and it wants to be assured the site is managing studies correctly. These are routine audits.

An IRB may also make for-cause visits if there is reason to think the site has ethics or compliance violations. IRBs are required to report to the FDA any instances of unanticipated problems involving risks to human subjects, serious or continuing noncompliance with the regulations or IRB requirements, or any suspension or termination of IRB approval.

CRAs will not be involved in IRB audits. Of course, the CRA would be involved in closing the study at a site if approval was withdrawn.

FDA Inspections

The FDA describes its Bioresearch Monitoring (BIMO) program as "a comprehensive program of on-site inspections, data audits, and remote regulatory assessments designed to monitor all aspects of the conduct and reporting of FDA regulated research. The BIMO program was established to assure the quality and integrity of data submitted to the agency in support of new product approvals and marketing applications, as well as to provide for protection of the rights and welfare of the thousands of human subjects and animals involved in FDA regulated research. It has become a cornerstone of the FDA preapproval process for new medicines, medical devices, food and color additives, veterinary products and tobacco products introduced to the U.S. consumer. The BIMO program also takes part in pharmacovigilance activities for postmarketing drug products. These activities serve to detect, understand, and prevent drug-related problems."

The BIMO program includes visits to investigators, sponsors, IRBs, CROs and animal labs. All FDA-regulated products are involved, including drugs, biologics, devices, radiological products, foods and veterinary products. Although the BIMO programs vary somewhat from product to product, they all have the same goals:

1. To ensure the quality and integrity of the information submitted to the FDA.
2. To protect human research subjects.

Copies of the FDA Compliance Program Guidance Manuals for clinical investigators are available on the FDA's website.

It would be useful for a CRA to read the FDA Compliance Program Guidance Manual documents for clinical investigators: program 7348.810 for sponsors and CROs; program 7348.811 for clinical investigators and sponsor-investigators; and program 7348.809 for IRBs. These documents delineate the particular items an FDA inspection team will concentrate on.

The FDA can make inspection visits to sponsors and IRBs at any time with the purpose of determining compliance to the regulations and the organizations' own SOPs. CRAs will not be involved in IRB inspections and only rarely would be involved in sponsor inspections, so there is no need to discuss these any further. However, we will discuss FDA audits of investigative sites in detail, as CRAs have a decided role and impact on this process.

FDA Audits of Investigative Sites

The FDA conducts three types of inspections at clinical investigative sites: study-related, bioequivalence study and investigator-related. Bioequivalence study inspections are conducted when one study is the sole basis for a drug's approval; we will not discuss these here. The two other types are important for a CRA to be aware of. For either study-related or investigator-related audits, the purpose is threefold:

1. To determine the validity and integrity of the data.
2. To assess adherence to regulations and guidelines.
3. To determine that the rights and safety of the human subjects were properly protected.

We will take a detailed look at both study and investigator audits.

Study-Related Audits

Study-related audits/inspections are almost always done on the studies that are important to an NDA or BLA that has been submitted to the FDA. These studies are the primary efficacy studies on which a sponsor relies for showing that the product works and should be approved for marketing.

The sites picked are usually those that contributed the most data to the application, either by high enrollment or by conducting multiple studies. Because of this, sponsors usually have a reasonable idea of which sites have a high probability of being audited. The sponsor also knows that studies will be inspected during the NDA review time

The primary efficacy studies are closed at this point, as the trials are complete and analyzed before being submitted in the NDA; in fact, they may have been closed for quite a while. Sometime early in the NDA review process, CRAs are often sent to the sites with high probability of being audited to ensure that all study materials are available and organized for FDA review. (Note that a site will usually inform the sponsor of an FDA-scheduled audit in which case the sponsor may send the CRA in to help the site prepare.) If the CRA finds missing documents or other problems, the site may be able to remedy the situation before an FDA audit occurs.

Investigator-Related Inspections

Investigator-related inspections are initiated for a variety of reasons, many of which are listed below:

- Investigators have done a large number of studies or have done work outside their specialty areas.
- An investigator has done a pivotal study that is critical to a new product application and it merits extra attention.

- The safety or efficacy findings of an investigator are inconsistent with the results from other investigators working with the same test product.
- The sponsor or IRB has notified the FDA about serious problems or concerns at the site.
- A subject has complained about the protocol or subject rights violations at the site.
- There was an unexpectedly high number of subjects with the diagnosis under study, given the location of the study.
- Enrollment at the site was much more rapid than expected.
- The study and investigator were highly publicized in the media.
- Any other reason that piques the curiosity of the agency.

Unless a sponsor alerted the FDA to problems at a site, the sponsor will probably not know in advance about an investigator-related inspection. (If the sponsor did alert the FDA, then it probably has already done its own QA audit.) Consequently, a CRA is rarely, if ever, involved in these audits.

Site Preparation

The best audit preparation is for the site to have done things correctly to begin with, in which case an audit will reveal no problems. However, once an audit is scheduled, the site should prepare by amassing all the study documents in one easily accessible place and reviewing them to be sure everything is accounted for, complete and well organized. The study documents that should be available for review include all informed consent forms, patient charts and other source documents, eCRFs/CRFs, and the study regulatory file. When an inspector asks to see a document, the site should be able to retrieve it easily and quickly. Sometimes, although this is seen most often when the FDA audits non-U.S. sites, the FDA may ask the site to send a letter of availability of records; this letter certifies that all study records will be available for FDA review upon its arrival.

The FDA's Office of Good Clinical Practice offered the following response to a question about FDA inspections and the agency's review of documents:

Question: A site on my study has an electronic medical record (EMR) system but staff print copies of the records for the shadow chart for monitoring/auditing as the EMR system is not [21 CFR] Part 11 compliant. The CRA has asked for the site to certify the copies and to look over the shoulder of the coordinator in order to confirm accuracy and completeness. However, the site will not allow the CRA to spot-check their EMR, stating that their SOP does not allow this.

Can you offer specific guidance on how the FDA views this site's policy?

Answer: Monitors will want to at least spot-check the completeness of records at the source—the electronic database. How they view them is at your discretion, however. Either looking over the shoulder of a study staff member or having limited access is common.

The reason at least a spot-check is necessary is that the records can be selectively copied. If certified copies are used, they may not be complete records. The monitor is checking to ensure that study inclusion/exclusion criteria are met and that there are no concomitant issues that would preclude the individual's participation in the study or confound the results.

In general, during an inspection, the FDA usually reviews original (source) records or certified copies of clinical trial records. For example, during an inspection of a clinical investigator (CI), the FDA investigator will evaluate the CI's practices and procedures to determine compliance with applicable regulations. Quite often, CIs maintain copies of certain records in their study files (e.g., records from a hospital or other institution that must maintain the originals).

The FDA refers to these as shadow files. While it is acceptable to keep shadow files in the study records, should the FDA conduct a bioresearch monitoring inspection of the study in question, the FDA investigator will expect to review at least a portion of the original source documents for such shadow files to verify their authenticity, even if the copies in the shadow files are certified as authentic copies.

I suggest you discuss with the site how you can bridge the gap between the research site and the monitor so that EMRs can be viewed by you as well as the FDA, when appropriate.

If there is time, and travel schedules allow, the CRA often goes to the site and assists in the audit preparation; if not, the CRA should be available at least by telephone to answer any questions the site may have or to send copies from the sponsor study file of any missing documentation. Sometimes a CRA can lend moral support by telling the site what to expect during the audit, how to interact with the inspector and what the process is. No one from the sponsor will be present during the audit; the audit is between the investigator and the FDA.

The Audit Process

The audit process begins with notification to the site. The inspector usually contacts the site by telephone to arrange a mutually acceptable time for the audit visit. Sites are generally given one weeks' notice. If the audit is investigator-related and if the FDA has concerns about subject safety or compliance, the time between the notification and the visit will probably be very short and delays will not be acceptable. If there are serious concerns, the FDA could just appear at the site without advance notice. Most sponsors ask and expect their investigators to let them know immediately about an impending audit.

The role of the investigator in the audit is to be present; to provide the inspector with a quiet, comfortable place to work; to assemble the necessary documents and to answer questions. The investigator should be polite, courteous, cooperative and reasonable when interacting with the FDA inspector; antagonism is inappropriate and will undoubtedly be regretted later. The investigator should provide all the materials/documents the inspector requests, but should never give the inspector unlimited access to the files. All questions should be answered, but extra information should not be volunteered. The inspector knows what he or she is asking for and will continue to question until the necessary information is obtained. The investigator should not offer the inspector anything beyond a cup of coffee; offering even a meal may be misconstrued. If the inspector is treated politely, the audit will be more pleasant for everyone. The CRA should go over these suggestions on conduct with the investigator and staff before an audit occurs.

When the inspector arrives at a site, he or she will present credentials (a photo ID) and a Notice of Inspections Form (482) to the clinical investigator.

If the inspector does not present these credentials, the investigator should ask for them. The investigator should check the date on the inspector's credentials to be sure they are still valid and note the inspector's badge number. During the inspection, the inspector will meet with study staff and review study documents. Two main aspects of the study will be looked at during the inspection: study conduct and study data.

According to the FDA's June 2010 information sheet on FDA inspections of clinical investigators:

> During an inspection at the site of a clinical investigator, the FDA investigator typically verifies compliance with the regulations governing the use of investigational products and human subject protections at 21 CFR parts 50, 56, 312, and/or 812, by inspecting records and talking to individuals involved in the conduct of the study to ascertain:
>
> - who performed various aspects of the protocol for the study (e.g., who verified inclusion and exclusion criteria, who obtained informed consent, who collected adverse event data);
> - whether the IRB approved the protocol, informed consent form, and any amendments to the protocol prior to implementation;
> - whether the clinical investigator and study staff adhered to the sponsor's protocol and investigational plan and whether protocol deviations were documented and reported appropriately;
> - whether informed consent documents were signed by the subject or the subject's legally authorized representative prior to entry in the study (i.e., performance of any study-related procedures);
> - whether authority to conduct aspects of the study was delegated, and if so, how the conduct of the study was supervised by the clinical investigator;
> - where specific aspects of the investigation were performed;
> - how the study data were obtained and where the study data were recorded;
> - accountability for the investigational product, including shipping records and disposition of unused investigational product;

- whether the clinical investigator disclosed information regarding his financial interests to the sponsor and/or interests of any subinvestigator(s), spouse(s) and dependent children;
- the monitor's communications with the clinical investigator;
- the monitor's evaluations of the progress of the investigation; and
- corrective actions in response to previous FDA inspections, if any, and regulatory
- correspondence or sponsor and/or monitor correspondence.

The FDA investigator also may audit the study data by comparing the data filed with the agency or the sponsor, if available, with records related to the clinical investigation. Such records may include the case report forms and supporting source documentation including signed and dated consent forms and medical records including, for example, progress notes of the physician, the subject's hospital chart(s), and the nurses' notes. These records may be in hard copy and/or an electronic format. For electronic records and/or electronic signatures, the FDA investigator may gather information to determine whether 21 CFR part 11 requirements have been met.

Notice that the monitor (CRA) is mentioned in two of these bullets. A CRA must communicate carefully with the investigator throughout the study and should make use of written communications to reiterate the points discussed during a monitoring visit. These communications should be kept in the investigator's study file, and copies should also be kept in the sponsor's file. The monitor should sign a study visit log at each monitoring visit to verify that the site was actually visited. This also underscores the need for complete and detailed monitoring visit reports, which were discussed in Chapter 14.

When the FDA inspects the study data, it will compare what was submitted to the FDA with the site records that support the data (i.e., investigator copies of the CRFs and all the available source documents, including patient charts, laboratory reports, other test reports and so forth). Sometimes the inspector will also have copies of the CRFs from the sponsor and will compare all three versions. The inspector will pay close attention to:

- The diagnosis.
- Whether the patients were properly diagnosed based on their past history.

- Whether or not the subjects met the protocol inclusion/exclusion criteria.
- Concomitant medications, especially those that were not allowed.
- Appropriate follow-up of AEs.

The inspector may look at data for only a sampling of subjects; or if there appears to be problems, he or she may look at the data from all of the subjects. All informed consents are usually reviewed.

An FDA audit usually takes one to two weeks, although it depends on the amount of data to review, the findings and the amount of time the inspector has available for the audit. The days may not be consecutive for the entire period, but rather a day or two at a time at the site until the review is complete.

The inspector should meet with the investigator throughout the process to review the audit findings. During these meetings the investigator may ask questions about anything that is not understood and may clarify anything the inspector has interpreted incorrectly. Sometimes a misunderstanding or negative finding by the inspector can be explained satisfactorily at this point. The inspector can also use this as an opportunity to investigate further. If there are significant findings, the inspector may issue a Form FDA-483 (Notice of Observations) to the investigator. This form will detail the findings from the audit that may constitute compliance violations.

Most sponsors ask that an investigator call them after the inspector leaves and let them know the results of the audit. If the investigator has received a 483 form, the sponsor will help the investigator formulate his or her reply (a written reply is not required but highly recommended).

After the Audit

After the audit has been completed, the FDA inspector prepares an Establishment Inspection Report (EIR). This report goes through FDA compliance channels, and a classification is assigned to it. The timeframe for when the investigator will receive a copy of the report varies, but it will typically take several months. The report is also available through the Freedom of Information Act, and most sponsors will request copies for their files.

There are three classes of EIRs that result from an FDA inspection:

- No Action Indicated (NAI). This is the best outcome and means that no significant deviations from the regulations were found. The clinical investigator is not required to respond to this report.
- Voluntary Action Indicated (VAI). This report provides information about findings of deviations from the regulations and GCP. The letter may or may not require a response from the investigator. If a response is required, the letter will specify what is necessary. A contact person also will be listed for any questions.
- Official Action Indicated (OAI). This is the worst result to receive. It identifies serious deviations from the regulations that require prompt action from the investigator. In most cases, the FDA will issue a warning letter that outlines problems the agency expects to be corrected. The FDA may also inform the sponsor if the agency feels that monitoring of the study was deficient (beware, CRAs). In addition to issuing the warning letter, the FDA may take other action such as regulatory and/or administrative sanctions against the investigator. All in all, this is a very unpleasant process and should be avoided at all cost.

Figure 1: BIMO program inspection classifications (2019 to March 2023)

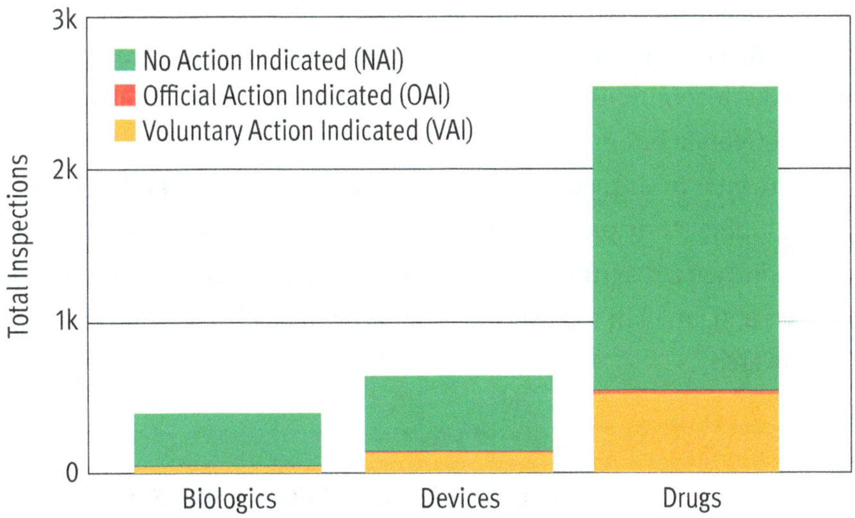

Source: FDA

Consequences

The consequences of problems found during audits can be significant, especially when they have an impact on a large amount of the data for a pivotal trial. The study at a particular site may be invalidated, especially if sufficient source documents were not available, if there were significant unreported concomitant therapies or if there was a failure to follow the protocol. If the site was a high enroller and generated a significant amount of data in support of the sponsor's NDA, these problems could delay the NDA or result in a disapproved application. A sponsor may even have to repeat a study, which could add years to the drug development cycle.

There are also significant consequences for the investigator in these cases. An investigator may be disqualified or restricted from conducting clinical trials. This puts him or her on the infamous "black list," known more formally as the List of Disqualified and Restricted Investigators. An investigator can be added to the list through a court hearing or through a consent agreement; he or she can be disqualified from ever conducting clinical studies or may have other restrictions placed on him or her, such as conducting studies only as a sub-investigator or conducting not more than one study every two years, etc. Once on the list, the investigator stays on the list forever, even if corrective actions are taken.

It does not happen often, but in the worst cases an investigator can be fined and/or sentenced to prison. For example, look at the case of Dr. Richard Borison, a psychiatrist, and Dr. Bruce Diamond, a pharmacologist. They conducted schizophrenia trials for eight years using resources at the Medical College of Georgia but pocketed the proceeds. They also encouraged psychotic patients to enter trials by giving them money and cigarettes and had untrained staff performing study procedures, including blood draws. These abuses were discovered when a disgruntled employee informed the university. The doctors were fined and jailed in 1997 and were ordered to pay back millions of dollars to the university.

Remote Regulatory Assessments by the FDA

The FDA issued a draft guidance in July 2022 on Conducting Remote Regulatory Assessments, describing remote inspection practices implemented during the COVID-19 pandemic. Based on the experiences during the pandemic, the agency concluded that remote regulatory assessments (RRA) should be used for certain scenarios beyond the pandemic and for all types of FDA-regulated products. The 16-page guidance describes the agency's current thinking on the use of RRAs and includes answers to frequently asked questions:

> FDA uses a variety of tools for oversight of FDA-regulated products and establishments. In this guidance, the term "establishment" includes any facility, entity, person, importer, or site, whether foreign or domestic, subject to the laws administered by FDA. During the COVID-19 pandemic, FDA has used RRAs to help the Agency conduct oversight, mitigate risk, and meet critical public health needs with respect to certain FDA-regulated products. To date, RRAs have included review of records or other information submitted upon request from FDA under sections 704(a)(4)6 and 8057 (the latter hereinafter referred to as "requests for Foreign Supplier Verification Program (FSVP) records under 21 CFR 1.510(b)(3) or 1.512(b)(5)(ii)(C)" or similar) of the Federal Food, Drug, and Cosmetic Act (FD&C Act) (mandatory RRAs); and records assessments and/or interactive evaluations (such as remote livestreaming video of operations, teleconferences, and screen sharing) conducted pursuant to voluntary participation by industry (voluntary RRAs).
>
> FDA's experiences so far have identified significant benefits in using RRAs. For instance, RRAs have assisted FDA in verifying corrective actions taken in response to inspections of previously compliant manufacturers and in gaining compliance insight when it was not practicable to inspect. RRAs have also provided information about deficient practices, which led FDA to take regulatory actions, conduct inspections, and have informed future inspection planning. RRAs have been used to help support, and reduce delays of, approval or authorization of marketing submissions for FDA-regulated products during the COVID-19 pandemic. In the food program, they have assisted in determining compliance with veterinary feed directive regulations, assessing foreign manufacturing process records, adding foreign firms to import alerts, and with issuance of warning letters.
>
> Based on these experiences, FDA has determined that RRAs are valuable and, under certain circumstances, will continue to assist FDA during and beyond the COVID-19 pandemic in its mission to protect public health, oversee regulated industry, and ensure all types of regulated products comply with FDA requirements.

FDA had previously issued guidance regarding the use of voluntary remote interactive evaluations of certain establishments during the COVID-19 public health emergency; a remote interactive evaluation is a type of RRA. The Agency believes that FDA's use of both voluntary and mandatory RRAs, as applicable, for all types of FDA-regulated products is in the interest of the public health, and the Agency is issuing this guidance to provide further transparency to stakeholders about the circumstances in which RRAs may be used both during and beyond the COVID-19 pandemic and promote greater consistency in the way RRAs are conducted. "

Section III. Questions and Answers

This section is intended to provide FDA's current thinking regarding the requesting, conducting, and use of RRAs by FDA.

1. *What is an RRA?*

   An RRA is an examination of an FDA-regulated establishment and/or its records, conducted entirely remotely, to evaluate compliance with applicable FDA requirements. RRAs assist in protecting human and animal health, informing regulatory decisions, and verifying certain information submitted to the Agency. RRAs are a tool FDA may use to support regulatory decisions and oversight activities. Currently, requests for records or other information from drug establishments under section 704(a)(4) of the FD&C Act, and requests for FSVP records under 21 CFR 1.510(b)(3) and 1.512(b)(5)(ii)(C), are RRAs that FDA conducts for which participation is mandatory (i.e., are not voluntary). RRAs that are not conducted under statutory or regulatory authority are voluntary in that an establishment can decline to participate or withdraw participation during the RRA, in which case the Agency would consider other tools for evaluating compliance with FDA requirements. RRAs complement FDA's authority to conduct inspections under section 704(a)(1) of the FD&C Act and other applicable FDA authorities. RRAs do not limit the authority of FDA to conduct inspections under section 704(a)(1) of the FD&C Act and other applicable FDA authorities.

2. *Who may be subject to an RRA?*

   - *Voluntary RRAs*

   If an RRA is not mandatory (or FDA opts against exercising its mandatory RRA authority in a certain instance), FDA may request that any establishment (e.g., food producers, tobacco product manufacturers, drug or medical device manufacturers, clinical investigators, or others) participate in a voluntary RRA.

- *Mandatory* RRAs

Mandatory RRAs include the following: Establishments that engage in the manufacture, preparation, propagation, compounding, or processing of a drug are subject to section 704(a)(4) of the FD&C Act. Under FSVP, importers, as defined at 21 CFR 1.500, are subject to section 805(d) of the FD&C Act and implementing regulations in 21 CFR 1.510(b)(3) or 1.512(b)(5)(ii)(C), as applicable. Drug manufacturers include establishments that engage in the manufacture, preparation, propagation, compounding, or processing of a drug. A drug includes human and animal drugs (including drug products produced by facilities registered as human drug compounding outsourcing facilities under section 503B of the FD&C Act), and biological drug products for humans. Regarding application of this guidance to combination products (defined under 21 CFR Part 3), the opportunity to participate voluntarily in an RRA applies to all combination products that are not subject to the authorities under section 704(a)(4) of the FD&C Act. Elements of the guidance specific to drugs (i.e., a 704(a)(4) request) also apply to drug-led combination products (see section 503(g)(1)(C) of the FD&C Act), including the drug constituent part(s) (defined under 21 CFR Part 4) of such combination products.

3. *Are RRAs replacing other established means of obtaining information outside of inspections?*

   No, RRAs are not intended to limit or replace other established means of obtaining information necessary for FDA to accomplish its public health mission outside of inspections, including, among other things, applicant information request letters, registration confirmations, meetings, product submission or application assessments, or follow-up communications during outbreaks or other emergencies. Similarly, if, for example, FDA calls an establishment to inform them that a submission or application is missing certain information, this is not an RRA. Although these activities may be conducted remotely, the Agency does not consider these RRAs.

4. *Is an RRA an inspection?*

Generally, an inspection, such as described in section 704(a)(1) of the FD&C Act, involves duly designated officers or employees of the FDA physically entering (at reasonable times and in a reasonable manner), establishments subject to regulation under the FD&C Act to determine compliance with applicable FDA requirements. For this reason, we do not consider an RRA to satisfy statutory requirements that specify inspection under section 704 of the FD&C Act (e.g., section 510(h) or 503B(b) of the FD&C Act). However, remote requests for FSVP records are under the authority of section 805(d) of the FD&C Act and FDA's implementing regulation. These record requests function as inspections in that FDA uses these records requests to evaluate a food importer's compliance with FSVP.

5. *When may FDA initiate or request to conduct an RRA?*

FDA may initiate or, in the case of a voluntary RRA, request to conduct an RRA, whenever we determine an RRA is appropriate to help fulfill the Agency's regulatory responsibilities and protect human and animal health. For example:

- When FDA cannot conduct an inspection due to travel limitations brought on by pandemics, natural disasters, or other unstable situations making travel infeasible.
- When FDA determines that an RRA will assist FDA in conducting elements of establishment oversight or support regulatory decisions. Examples include preparing for an already planned inspection, following up on a consumer complaint, assisting in verifying that an establishment completed certain corrective actions (e.g., in response to a previous inspection, or previous RRA), or supporting the review of a marketing submission.

FDA will use a risk-based approach to determine whether to initiate or request an RRA. Factors that may be considered include, but are not limited to, firm location, inspection history, complexity of product and process, and travel restrictions. Programs and centers within FDA may assess risk differently based on the product. The above examples are illustrative, and the ultimate decision to initiate or request an RRA rests with FDA as FDA retains discretion to deploy RRAs as appropriate. At this time, we do not accept requests for FDA to perform an RRA.

6. *Will FDA use RRAs during or as part of an FDA inspection of an establishment?*

   No, at this time, FDA does not plan to conduct RRAs and inspections of an establishment simultaneously. An RRA is conducted remotely by FDA staff without FDA staff present at an establishment conducting an inspection. However, an RRA could precede, prompt, or be a follow-up to, an inspection. When an RRA precedes an inspection, FDA will generally conclude the RRA prior to initiating the inspection. FDA may combine any information gained from the RRA with any resulting observations from the subsequent inspection. In such circumstance, FDA would confirm any observations from the RRA during the inspection before including them on the Form FDA 483 Inspectional Observations. Additionally, FDA may conduct an RRA following an inspection in order to conduct follow-up activities with the establishment or to assist in verifying corrective actions, if appropriate. When oversight activities are conducted by a party other than FDA (e.g., state and foreign regulatory partners), FDA may conduct RRAs (e.g., livestreaming) during these oversight activities.

7. *What are the benefits of an RRA?*

   FDA, industry, and the general public can all benefit from RRAs as RRAs help the Agency to meet critical public health needs. These potential benefits can include, but are not limited to:

   - Allowing FDA to remotely evaluate compliance of FDA-regulated products, clinical studies, and establishments, as appropriate. This may identify issues that lead establishments to promptly make corrective actions, which may enhance the establishment's preparedness for their next FDA inspection.
   - Having an RRA precede an inspection under section 704(a)(1) of the FD&C Act could reduce resource expenditure by (1) potentially reducing the time FDA is present at the establishment, and (2) helping optimize FDA's time on-site, by reducing the extent of records to be reviewed during the inspection.

- FDA can make regulatory decisions, including the approval of an application or authorization for emergency use, without an inspection, when appropriate conditions are fulfilled, such as, the ability to verify information in the marketing submission. In such cases, the application approval, or the authorization, must still meet applicable standards.
- Providing FDA additional information to incorporate into a risk-based inspection schedule, thereby helping FDA use inspectional resources more efficiently and effectively.
- Assisting FDA in verifying corrective actions taken in response to inspections of previously compliant manufacturers.
- Helping to support, and reduce delays of, approval or authorization of marketing submissions for FDA-regulated products.

Key Takeaways

- Sponsors audit investigative sites for studies that contribute highly to their development programs. They also audit sites at which it appears there may be compliance problems.
- IRBs can also audit sites, especially if they suspect ethics violations.
- The FDA performs both study-related and investigator-related audits.
- The best preparation for an audit is to perform the study correctly.
- CRAs should help their sites understand the audit process and prepare for them.
- There are three classes of EIRs that result from an FDA inspection: NAI, VAI and OAI.
- The consequences of noncompliance are great and can result in delays in an NDA, and/or in disqualification and other penalties for investigators.
- There has been an increase in compliance problems during the past few years.

- CRAs must be educated about the correct procedures for clinical trials and must watch their sites closely to ensure compliance.
- The FDA conducted RRAs in response to the pandemic.

CHAPTER 20

Errors, Misconduct and Fraud

This chapter discusses some serious situations that CRAs face: errors, misconduct and fraud. The discussion will be limited to the occurrence of these unfortunate events at investigative sites and will focus primarily on the CRA's role in detecting and coping with these problems. The chapter will start by defining each term and then looking at the impact of each on a clinical trial and on the CRA.

Definitions

If you consult a dictionary, you will find the following definitions for error, misconduct and fraud:

- **Error:** an act involving an unintentional deviation from truth or accuracy.
- **Misconduct:** intentional wrongdoing.
- **Fraud:** intentional perversion of truth in order to induce another to part with something of value or to surrender a legal right.

As you can see, these are listed in increasing severity, and the same is true of their impact on a clinical trial and on the CRA. We'll consider each category in detail.

Errors

If you think about the definition of an error, it contains two key ideas. The first is that an error is a deviation from truth or accuracy, and the second is that it is unintentional. There is no doubt that a CRA will see errors when monitoring studies; in fact, the CRA can expect to see some errors at every study site he or she monitors, assuming the sites enroll any subjects at all. Most commonly, the errors CRAs will see are those in eCRFs/CRFs, although these are not the only errors that can occur during a study. Errors may also occur in drug dispensing, study documents, protocol conduct or any other aspect of study performance.

Some of the errors may occur during a study, starting with eCRFs/CRFs. Errors commonly seen on CRFs result from omissions (missing values), inconsistencies, incorrect entries, out-of-range entries, illogical entries and undecipherable entries.

This example uses one of the standard questions that is asked in almost every study. See how it can be answered (on a CRF) to meet one of the error types listed above. The question is:

Sex: Male ☐ Female ☐

It looks very straightforward and should be easy to answer without making an error. Here is the error of omission:

Sex: Male ☐ Female ☐

Notice that neither box is checked—the question was not answered.

An error of inconsistency would be, in this case, that the subject was listed as a male in one place and as a female in another. Most CRFs will not ask this question directly more than once, but there may be other questions where the sex is implied by the answer. One common question in the inclusion/exclusion criteria asks if the female subject has had a pregnancy test. The answer can be assumed to be "Yes," but then the entry for the gender example is:

Sex: Male ☒ Female ☐

There is an inconsistency between the two entries. An incorrect entry is easy—the wrong box was checked.

For this question, out-of-range entries would probably not be seen. An out-of-range entry occurs when an answer is supposed to fall between two values and doesn't. For example, when the answer to "Rate the subject's pain on a scale of 1 to 10" is recorded as "12." An illogical entry for this same question would be "Better" or "D." Neither entry makes sense, given the question and the way it is worded.

Undecipherable entries are sometimes illegible answers, those that cannot be read because of poor handwriting. They also may be entries like:

Sex: Male ☒ Female ☒

Overall, errors run the gamut from small discrepancies to glaring inconsistencies.

Electronic CRF systems have built-in edit checks to address some types of errors, with the exception of missing answers, inconsistent answers or answers out of range. When the eCRF system notes an error, the system queries the user for clarification/correction.

Because errors are unintentional, there is hope of eliminating, or at least reducing, their occurrence over the course of a study. Chapter 11 discussed different ways in which the CRA can help lessen or eliminate errors at sites. It also discussed the impact of errors and the cost of errors. It is important to realize that the CRA can make a significant contribution to studies by working with his or her sites to eliminate errors made on eCRFs/CRFs.

In general, errors are relatively easy to find and easy to fix. Although it depends on the parameter, the impact of errors on the study is usually quite low, since they are fixable. If the CRA is doing a good job, the error rate should decrease as the study progresses. The following are some things the CRA can do to help decrease or eliminate errors:

- Review the first patient or two very soon after enrollment. Conduct a very thorough review. Quick feedback to the site can do more than anything else to eliminate future errors. Many errors, especially at the beginning of a study, are due to misunderstandings on the part of the study coordinator and other site personnel. If these problems are found and corrected early, they usually will not occur in the future.
- Look for systematic errors and instruct the site on the correct way to record the data. Systematic errors also usually are due to misunderstandings and can be eliminated by quick feedback. For example, the CRF may have a question that reads: Have there been any changes in concomitant medications since the last visit? The site may be record-

ing only new or stopped medications, rather than including changes in dosage for medication during the study. Once this is clarified, these systematic errors should not continue.

- Train your sites well in the beginning, and re-train them if:
  - There are misunderstandings.
  - New personnel are added.
  - The study or procedures change in any way.
- Demand good work, nicely. This is especially important when there are errors due to carelessness. One of the techniques a CRA may find helpful is to remind the site of the high cost, both in time and money, of correcting errors. An estimate of the cost of each error for a site is about $20 and 15 minutes of time.

The CRA also has great influence when it comes to eliminating other errors in studies, such as those that occur in drug dispensing, study documents, protocol conduct and other aspects of study performance. Remember that the CRA is the sponsor representative who visits the site most often and may, in fact, be the only sponsor representative who ever visits an investigative site. No one else has a better opportunity to eliminate errors in a study than the CRA who monitors it. It is the responsibility of the CRA to:

- Be aware of problems that might occur.
- Be aware and vigilant when looking for problems.
- Instruct site personnel how to handle problems if they occur.
- Train site personnel to decrease and/or eliminate problems in the future.

To summarize, most errors are caused by misunderstanding or inattention. The impact of errors on study results is generally low, because they are usually correctable once they are caught. They can be eliminated, or at least reduced in number by training, which includes feedback. The dual role of the CRA is checker and trainer; actual error correction must be done by site personnel.

Misconduct

Misconduct is a degree more serious than error. Misconduct implies that someone knowingly did something that was wrong. In studies, some of the more commonly seen types of misconduct are enrolling without permission subjects who "almost qualify", guessing at vital signs and easing things into compliance, examples of which can be found later in this section.

Investigators are under enormous pressure to enroll subjects quickly into clinical trials. The pressure has increased even more over the past few years with the widespread use of "competitive enrollment." Sponsors sign more investigators than they expect to need for a trial and allow enrollment of subjects to continue only until the necessary number of subjects is reached. If investigators enroll quickly, they will remain investigators for the trial; if they enroll slowly, they may have very few subjects entered when enrollment is halted, perhaps none, which would result in being dropped from the trial. Some study-related activities must take place at a site before subjects can be enrolled. It is possible that an investigator can even lose money on a study if he or she has no, or low, enrollment when the enrollment period is closed.

Given this enrollment scenario, an investigator may use all means available to find suitable subjects. Due to the fact that some of the inclusion and exclusion criteria for studies have measurements that are somewhat imprecise or could lend themselves to differing interpretations, such as blood pressure readings or rating scales such as the Hamilton Rating Scale for Depression (HAM-D), it could be tempting, and fairly easy, to ease these readings or ratings into compliance. For example, if a subject in a hypertension study was supposed to have an initial diastolic blood pressure between 90 and 100 mmHg, and the person being evaluated for the study is perfect in every way except that his initial diastolic blood pressure is 88 mmHg, who would know if the investigator recorded it as 90 or 91? No one would, as long as the office chart and the CRF match. But if it is incorrect and was done on purpose, it is an example of misconduct.

Another example is a case in which subjects were to read an eye chart from a distance of 15 feet. Each subject did this at every visit. It wasn't until a new and astute CRA measured the distance that it was found to be only 13 feet, rendering the data unusable. The investigator knew he didn't have a 15-foot span to use, but figured it was "close enough" and that no one would measure.

The investigator was aware of the discrepancy, but didn't really think it made any difference, so he never mentioned it and continued to use the shorter span. This is misconduct.

Misconduct can have a more pronounced effect on studies than errors, simply because it may not be discovered or it may be unfixable if it is found. In the eye exam example, the misconduct was discovered but the data for about 25 subjects was unusable. It was in a very difficult study in which every subject enrolled was critical. When misconduct is not discovered it can, depending on the magnitude of the problem, affect the results of a study. It could make an investigational drug look effective or safe when it is not, or vice versa; neither is a good outcome for consumers.

It is much more difficult for a CRA to root out misconduct than errors. A CRA must be vigilant when performing source document review, particularly when it comes to verifying the inclusion and exclusion criteria for a subject. Sometimes site personnel may change things slightly in the CRF to make the subject fit the study, without thinking about past entries in an office chart. The CRA must also be aware of the pressures to enroll and be cognizant of enrollment that seem a little too good to be true. Things that seem too good to be true often are.

CRAs also need to think about what is needed in a study and should not be afraid to verify that they are correct. What a difference it could have made if the original CRA on the eye study had measured the 15-foot distance before subjects were enrolled.

Fraud

Fraud is the most serious offense of the three and the most difficult to discover. Fraud is willful deception. The impact of fraud on a study is apt to be very large, but can be measured only if it is discovered. It is a nightmare for the sponsor(s) involved and for the CRA. A CRA will not see cases of fraud often. We will discuss some publicized cases of fraud later in this chapter.

Fraud can manifest itself in various ways. Some of the more common ways are the use of fictitious trial subjects and/or data, faked test results and fraudulent study documents. Fraud is usually committed in order to increase revenue from the trial—either by enrolling more subjects, enrolling more quickly or cutting actual costs. After discussing some examples of fraud, we will talk about what a CRA can do to lessen the chances of fraud, how to look for fraud and what can be done when it is discovered.

Fraud is difficult to discover. The perpetrator of fraud is usually careful to do as much as possible to keep the deception hidden. However, there are some techniques a CRA may find useful when reviewing data that may point to situations that should be investigated further. It is important to keep in mind that the incidence of fraud in clinical trials is very low, and most CRAs will never encounter fraud. Still, it is important for CRAs to remain vigilant and aware of its potential.

Real-life Examples of Fraud

In a study at one investigative site, everything looked fine. The study went well, enrolled well and no one suspected that it was not handled correctly. It was only during a routine FDA inspection during the NDA review that a problem was found. The FDA inspector took all of the informed consents, stacked them up and fanned through them looking at the signatures. What he saw looked something like this:

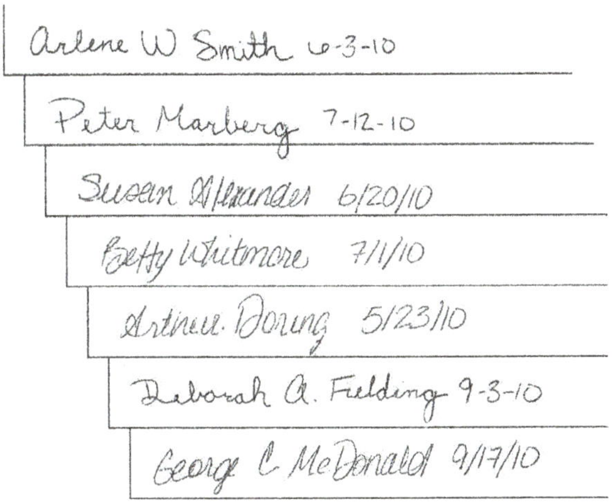

It became apparent to the inspector as he rifled through them that all of the consent forms were signed by only three different people. The names on the form were different, but the handwriting was the same. As it turned out, in this case, they had been signed by the investigator and two research nurses. Study subjects did not exist at all, but were part of a carefully laid plan to collect the grant without actually enrolling subjects. The subjects were fictitious, as were the data. It was cleverly done and might not have been discovered at all, except for the savvy inspector who looked at all of the consents together.

Why didn't the CRA find the consent problem? Because the consents were checked individually, as each subject was enrolled. Each one was signed and dated before the subject was entered into the study. The consents were each kept with the individual study chart and CRF, not together in one place. It never occurred to the CRA to pull them out and fan through them. It is a good practice for CRAs to look at all the consents together occasionally, rather than individually as each subject is enrolled.

This investigator had contributed heavily to the data submitted for approval of this drug, so the sponsor company was required to re-analyze all of the data without including this investigator. It was an enormous job and cost the company dearly in terms of time and resources.

In another case, the investigator had subjects but didn't want to take the time to have their blood drawn. Instead, he drew blood from his own staff in greater quantities, divided it up and labeled it with the initials of each subject.

This way it could be done all at one time and stored ready to ship.

In this study, all of the blood samples were shipped to the sponsor. They were batched and sent every two-to-three months. The problem at this site was discovered when the samples for August and September came in and the vials were marked for October—someone had grabbed them by mistake. The CRA investigated, checked the freezer and there they were, neatly labeled and stored for months in advance. Needless to say, the data were not usable. Would this have been caught during routine monitoring? Probably not, unless the CRA happened to look in the freezer and see them. Had the site known the freezer would be checked, the samples probably would have been moved or disguised. One hint that might have caught the notice of that CRA beforehand was the site's lack of "busyness." If you don't see many subjects during your monitoring visits, it may be time to suspect fraudulent practices.

In 2010, a prominent anesthesiologist researcher on the East Coast was found guilty and sentenced to six months in prison for falsifying data in some clinical trials and inventing other trials entirely. He admitted to faking dozens of studies, and 21 published papers written in support of pain-killing medications had to be retracted. He had never applied for IRB approval at the medical facility where these trials supposedly had been conducted.

When questioned about the incidence of investigator fraud, according to an article in Scrip Clinical Research, an FDA spokesperson stated, "despite concerns that falsification may be difficult to identify, investigator fraud in clinical trials is generally believed to be rare. Published estimates of the proportion of clinical trials affected by fraud range from 1% to 5% of clinical trials, with less than 1% of all investigators involved in engaging in data falsifications."

Do Subjects Really Exist?

People who revert to fraud are usually quite clever at disguising their fraudulent practices, which makes them difficult to discover. However, there are some things a CRA can do when monitoring an investigative site to help uncover signs of potential fraud. First, think about whether or not subjects actually exist. When you are at an investigative site, look for signs that point to the existence of actual subjects/patients being seen. Do you see patients in the waiting room? Is the practice bustling? Are the phones ringing? Do you hear appointments being scheduled?

When the CRA is reviewing source documents, particularly office charts, or the EMR system, there are things you would expect to see. Office charts usually contain the patient's name, address, phone number, social security number, date of birth and insurance information. If it is not there, where is it? Does the chart look like most office charts, with entries done over time, in different handwriting, with different pens? Are lab reports available in the chart? The CRA should think about whether or not the patient charts look like standard office charts in most medical practices.

Look at the dates of study visits and compare them on a calendar. Are people coming in on appropriate days of the week, or are there a lot of weekend and/or holiday visits? Look for things that you would not expect to see. A site may see study patients on a Saturday, or even in the evenings, but you would not expect to see Sunday visits or visits on holidays (Thanksgiving, Easter Sunday, July 4th, etc.).

Think about the accrual rate of subjects into the trial. Is the rate faster than expected? Faster than other sites? How can this site enroll well if others can't? If there is no explanation, a wise CRA will thoroughly check the source documents and look closely at the data and the screen failure rate. Is it similar to other sites' or lower than expected?

Numeric Data

There are also things to consider when reviewing numerical data, such as blood pressure readings. Look at the blood pressure readings listed below:

120/80	120/85	115/80	120/75	110/70
120/80	110/70	115/80	120/90	110/70
120/85	110/80	120/80	120/80	110/65
120/80	110/80	120/80	120/85	115/80

The first thing you should notice about these numbers is that they all end in either 0 or 5. You would not expect all blood pressure readings to end in 0 or 5, when presumably they could end in any digit. Unless the instrument used is calibrated only in increments of five, this will not happen.

With numerical data, look for other digit preferences, as well as 0 and 5. You should expect to see a pretty random distribution of the last digits; you would not expect to see mostly 7 or 3, for example. Look also for other invented patterns of numbers (lots of 77s or 123s, for example) and for more duplicate numbers than you would expect.

Look also for too few or too many outliers (outliers are the data values that lie outside the range you would normally expect to see). If you are dealing with a population of subjects whose blood pressures are "normal," as opposed to a hypertension study, for example, you will expect to see some people with higher-than-normal pressures and a few with lower-than-normal pressures. If you are seeing too many that are outside the normal range, you may want to investigate further. The same is true if you see no one outside the normal range. The data may be valid, but it is worth checking the source documents for verification or asking about it.

Commonly Chosen Data for Fabrication

According to Iber, Riley and Murray in their book "Conducting Clinical Trials," the data points commonly chosen for fabrication, with comments in italics added, are:

Entry Criteria:

- Known disqualifying factors are suppressed, such as taking a non-allowed medication prior to entry.

- Birth date altered to meet eligible age range; weight or height altered. It's more difficult to alter the birth date in source documents, since it appears in many places. Weight is variable and may fluctuate, making it more likely to be changed.
- Dates of prohibited medication use altered or suppressed. Example: no previous treatment with an antibiotic was allowed in an infectious disease trial. The subject was treated, but it was not put in his chart or on the CRF.
- History of drug or alcohol abuse or mental illness suppressed. If this information already appears in the chart, it is difficult to suppress. If it is a new patient; however, this information can just be omitted from the chart when the history is taken.

Safety Checks:

- Reports of procedures from previous visits or from other patients are used for the current visit. Laboratory reports, ECGs, etc. are either from a previous subject visit or might be from a completely different person as with the blood sample example.
- Blood and urine samples substituted from other patients. This can happen when the subject doesn't qualify. A sample from someone who does qualify might be split and relabeled with the ineligible subject's identifiers.

Visit Data:

- Visit dates altered to fit permitted windows. This keeps the patient in compliance and the visit from being missed.
- Visits fabricated. This can be easy to do, especially with phone visits or visits when laboratory tests, ECGs, etc. are not completed.
- Medication counts falsified, with tablets discarded so inventories match false reports. This makes it look like they are in compliance when they are not. It can also cover up incorrect dispensing on the part of site personnel.

- Diaries fabricated. Note that the handwriting in diaries can be checked in the same manner as the writing on consents—look at them all together, both for a single subject and for all subjects.

Suspicion of Misconduct or Fraud

When a CRA suspects that things may not be quite right at a site, there are a number of things that can be done. The first is to thoroughly monitor everything, doing more than you might do under normal circumstances. Be thorough when reviewing source documents, taking the time to check all variables. Check carefully across visits, thinking about whether the new data seems consistent with older data in light of what you know about each subject. Do you see differences in the data that appear odd or unusual?

The CRA can also check the laboratory reports and other test results. Be sure the patient identifiers are consistent (name, age, date of birth, etc.). If someone is falsifying information, he or she is apt to make mistakes on the small, non-essential information rather than on the primary information. If you notice discrepancies, ask the study coordinator or the investigator about them and listen carefully to the explanations they give you.

If you have checked carefully and your suspicions remain, call someone to help. Ask your supervisor or another (senior) CRA to monitor with you and see what they think. If there still appears to be a cause for concern, ask your Quality Assurance (QA) group to send someone to perform an audit. At this point, the investigative site may not need to know about any concerns involving misconduct or fraud. It may be best not to alert the site, as some may be tempted to cover up the issues. Also, if there was no misconduct or fraud, the relationship may be damaged by the accusation. Remember, you need to continue working with them. If your company has determined that there is probably fraud, it must be reported to the FDA. In this case, the FDA most likely will do a for-cause audit of the investigative site, which was discussed in the previous chapter.

Consequences of Fraud

The consequences of fraud can be disastrous for a sponsor. The data from the fraudulent site may not be usable, which may result in losing a complete study. This can delay the NDA or cause the FDA to declare it as "unfileable." This can set a development program back by several years or may cause the program to be completely halted. At the very least, a sponsor will probably need to re-analyze the data, which will eliminate all data from the questionable site.

The consequences for investigators who have participated in fraud are also severe. They may be placed on the FDA List of Disqualified and Restricted Investigators or they may be barred from participating in clinical research. In the worst cases, they also may be fined and/or sent to prison.

There can be consequences for a CRA if fraud has been found at his or her site. If the CRA found the problem through diligence and good monitoring and found it early, he or she will probably be credited with a job well done. Given that fraud can be very difficult to detect, a CRA might not have found it even while doing a superb job of monitoring; in this case, there are not likely to be any tangible repercussions for the CRA. There may be intangible repercussions, however; memories are long when it comes to cases of fraud. Even if the fraud was cleverly perpetrated and disguised and even if there was no blame placed on the CRA, it's not pleasant to have to explain (for years) what happened at "your" site. Of course, if the CRA did not find problems because of improper monitoring, the outcome won't be as rosy. CRAs can be severely reprimanded, or even lose their jobs, in this situation.

The best steps a CRA can take to minimize the potential for fraud at a site, or to detect it if it is present, are:

- Monitor carefully and thoroughly. Don't cut corners. Ask questions if you are seeing discrepancies.
- Think about what you are seeing and doing. Does it make sense?
- Pay attention to small signs and problems. Be aware of what is going on around you. Pay attention to your "gut feelings."
- Listen. Be approachable. Many times fraud is uncovered because an employee tells someone else about it.

- Bring in another set of eyes. The site does not have to know why you have someone else with you—it can just be a joint monitoring visit or a training session.
- If you see potential problems, share them with your supervisor. The problems will not take care of themselves.

Key Takeaways

- Errors are unintentional, usually due to misunderstanding or carelessness, and can be fixed. They usually have a low impact on a trial.
- Early detection of errors and close cooperation with site personnel will generally reduce errors in a study.
- Misconduct and fraud are classified as intentional wrongdoing, are difficult to detect and can have a major impact on a trial.
- Fraud is usually committed for personal gain, while misconduct is often committed for expediency.
- The CRA is the first line of defense against errors, misconduct and fraud.
- Good monitoring and awareness can help prevent and detect misconduct and fraud.
- The FDA is relying on help from CRAs to discover noncompliance at investigative sites.

CHAPTER 21

The Future for CRAs

CRAs, who have long had an essential role in ensuring the quality and integrity of clinical trial data, continue to find their responsibilities changing and expanding beyond traditional monitoring duties. Based on today's trends, it is likely that the CRA job will evolve further.

Impact of Technology

Since the mid-1990s, industry thought leaders have predicted that technology would ultimately replace the role of the study monitor. But technology has actually helped expand and change the CRA's role in clinical research.

While EDC can improve a monitor's efficiency, it won't eliminate the need for source document verification and general study oversight. A CRA does much more at site visits than review CRFs and source documents; EDC doesn't affect these other activities.

EDC has changed how CRAs complete monitoring activities but not the basic premise of the site visit or monitoring activities. EDC allows field monitors to examine patient enrollment, look at actual data, review queries that have been generated, run reports and make sure the data entry is up-to-date before visiting a site. The technology also gives CRAs the ability to analyze information and to query data directly with the sites, making source verification activities more efficient while on site. IRT (IVRS/IWRS) platforms allow CRAs to track study drug shipment, receipt and drug assignment, as well as inventory and new study patient enrollment, both before a site visit and in real time while on site.

These are all elements of drug accountability and review.

Central vendor portals (imaging, lab, ECG) allow CRAs to track site compliance with image uploading, review lab and ECG results, and track site compliance with sample shipments.

CRAs can use ePRO/ediary website portals to review diary entry and compliance by sites, as well as monitor for possible adverse events. And eTMF systems allow CRAs to upload study documents directly from sites and retrieve documents for site study files during monitoring visits, while eConsent allows CRAs to sometimes review consents before the site visit.

These systems allow CRAs to conduct some monitoring activities and preparation before the site visit so they have an understanding of the site status and what needs to be done while on site, for greater productivity. This makes for a more efficient and holistic site management process and emphasizes the importance of monitoring activities, before, during and after an on-site visit. CRAs are no longer limited to completing most monitoring activities while on site. These platforms have revolutionized how monitoring activities are executed.

Data analytics, collection and review will become more and more critical in overall site management and site risk analysis. Regulatory portals and shared databases are expediting study startup and IRB submission activities, which require CRAs to become adept at using a variety of databases to conduct their jobs. CRAs must have experience with computer- and cloud-based systems in the conduct of job responsibilities; gone are the days when a mere "comfort level" with the technology was good enough for performing monitoring tasks.

As noted in Chapter 14, risk-based monitoring and remote/central monitoring have led to a decrease in some on-site monitoring activities and to a more efficient means of reviewing and transmitting study data. It has also further contributed to the separate, emerging role of the remote monitor and the partnership of the CRA and remote monitor in site management.

AI and Machine Learning Impact the CRA's Role

AI and machine learning concepts are integrating into the clinical trials landscape in remarkable ways, including boosting patient identification efforts as described in Chapter 16 (recruitment, retention and compliance).

Machine learning is a branch of AI that uses data and algorithms to imitate how humans learn, which means a computer can keep getting better at its task as it absorbs more data and recognizes the patterns.

AI also has great potential for digitizing clinical trial processes and automating reports, enabling faster completion of trials. A survey in 2021 by Deloitte Consulting found that 76 percent of life sciences companies are investing in AI for clinical development and that, so far, they have only "scratched the surface of AI's potential." For example, AI can make use of databases developed for previous trials, but most trials currently create databases from the ground up, which means there is a lot of duplication of effort.

Increased Responsibility

Although specific approaches differ widely by company, drug sponsors are beginning to rely on CRAs to help build stronger relationships with investigative sites. Increasingly, sponsors give study monitors additional responsibility for site management activities, such as evaluating patient enrollment plans, helping to solve patient recruitment problems and participating in site selection. This often means not only monitoring data and ensuring investigator compliance, but also solving day-to-day problems at sites and acting as the liaison between the drug sponsor and the investigator.

More companies are empowering their CRAs to be influential in site selection. The majority of sponsors/CROs already have their monitors conduct pre-study site visits to evaluate the investigator, staff, facility and lab and then make recommendations about whether the site should participate in a study. This can result in more successful studies because the monitors, who work with investigative sites on a regular basis, know the quality—or lack thereof—of individual sites.

If a CRA has developed a good relationship with an investigator and site personnel and helps select that site for a study, the investigator is apt to work harder to make the study successful. Working with the same monitor on repeat studies can also help improve communication and expectations between investigators and field monitors. Both sides benefit from these monitor-investigator relationships. Monitors may be able to alert investigators about potential studies in the pipeline, while investigators develop a sense of loyalty that extends to giving that drug sponsor preference when competing studies arise. At the same time, this type of relationship can go a long way toward helping to solve problems that occur during a study.

Impact of Diversity on the Clinical Trial Landscape

The lack of diversity in study patient recruitment has drawn increased attention from the FDA and other regulatory authorities in recent years and more steps are being taken to improve the situation.

In April 2022, the FDA issued a draft guidance entitled Diversity Plans to Improve Enrollment of Participants from Underrepresented Racial and Ethnic Populations in Clinical Trials, advising sponsors of medical products to develop a Race and Ethnicity Diversity Plan to enroll "representative numbers of participants from underrepresented racial and ethnic populations in the United States, such as Black or African American, Hispanic/Latino, Indigenous and Native American, Asian, Native Hawaiian and Other Pacific Islanders, and other persons of color in clinical trials."

The FDA noted that individuals from these populations are frequently underrepresented in biomedical research despite having a disproportionate disease burden for certain diseases. The agency went on to state that:

> Adequate representation of these populations in clinical trials and studies supporting regulatory submissions helps ensure that the data generated in the development program reflect the racial and ethnic diversity of the population expected to use the medical product, if approved, and may potentially identify effects on safety or efficacy outcomes that may be associated with, or occur more frequently within, these populations.

The FDA also advised sponsors to seek diversity in clinical trial enrollment from underrepresented populations defined by demographics, such as sex, gender identity, age, socioeconomic status, disability, pregnancy status, lactation status and comorbidity, adding that:

> The agency recommends that a plan to enroll representative numbers of participants from historically underrepresented racial and ethnic populations be submitted to the investigational new drug (IND) application, for a drug, including biological products regulated as drugs, or the investigational device exemption (IDE) application, for a device. This plan should be discussed with the FDA as soon as practicable during medical product development. For drugs, this should occur no later than when a sponsor is seeking

feedback regarding the applicable pivotal trial(s) for the drug (often during the End of Phase 2 (EOP2) meeting).

Impact of Diversity on the CRA Role

Increased diversity is not just a goal for clinical trial participation, it is also reflected in greater job opportunities for CRAs from different cultures, countries and orientations. For example, groups such as Latinos in Clinical Research and Black Women in Clinical Research provide educational opportunities for their members with webinars and educational events, as well as networking events, to promote awareness and job opportunities for their members. These groups and other organizations seek to promote diversity within pharma by encouraging organizations to consider everyone equally for positions, as well as help offer resources to people of all backgrounds to help them move into positions in clinical research.

Regional Monitoring

CRAs have seen their roles shift, in part, due to wide-spread adoption of the regional field monitor structure by major pharmaceutical companies/CROs. Many of the top drug companies use this approach as opposed to sending CRAs from a centralized office to far-flung investigative sites. This regional structure has allowed drug companies to cut travel costs and has also led to improved job satisfaction and decreased turnover rates of CRAs.

At the same time, sponsors have realized another benefit of a regional study monitor structure: regional monitors, who repeatedly visit the same sites and spend many hours with investigators and coordinators, have become an invaluable source of information about site operational issues, such as the professionalism of a site, the efficiency of the coordinator and how staff handle data. Study monitors might notice other factors that could affect the success of a study, such as signs that the coordinator and ancillary staff are overworked or frustrated. They are the eyes and ears of the sponsor.

The demands placed on regional monitors, who work out of their home offices with minimal supervision, require a higher level of skill, experience and training. Many CRAs not only have degrees in nursing or life sciences but are trained physicians from different countries. Many CRAs have years of clinical experience as medical technologists, medical assistants, pharmacy technicians, etc. but also have studied business, accounting, sociology or psychology.

Conclusion

Pharmaceutical companies/CROs rely on the skills of experienced CRAs. Pay and benefits have increased to reflect this. Because travel requirements have often been reduced and duties have expanded beyond ensuring the quality of data, job satisfaction has improved. The CRA position has become more of a career choice and less of a stepping stone to another position in clinical research.

As their roles and responsibilities continue to grow, CRAs are becoming even more critical to the success of clinical trials. Investigative sites consistently have rated the quality of CRAs as one of the top five most essential factors contributing to study success. For the sponsor or CRO, the study monitor is the person who can make or break a study.

Key Takeaways

- EDC and electronic systems/portals used to manage and complete study activities have changed the way monitoring activities are completed.
- Technology enables CRAs to analyze and review site data and metrics before a site visit as well as in real time during site visits.
- AI and machine learning are being integrated into the clinical trials/study structure.
- Risk-based and remote monitoring practices have reduced the need for completion of some on-site monitoring tasks.
- Diversity of underrepresented populations enrollment into clinical trials is critical.
- Monitors are expanding their duties beyond checking to see that sites comply with regulations and verifying source documents.

- Companies are empowering regional monitors to be influential in site selection and in communication with investigators.

APPENDIX A

Resources

Books and Videotapes

Acres of Skin: Human Experiments at Holmesburg Prison—A True Story of Abuse and Exploitation in the Name of Medical Science
Allen M. Hornblum, 1998

Bad Blood—The Tuskegee Syphilis Experiment
James H. Jones, 1981

Code of Medical Ethics
American Medical Association, 150th Anniversary Edition, 1997

Factories of Death—Japanese Biological Warfare, 1932-45, and the American Cover-up
Sheldon H. Harris, 1994

Guide to Clinical Trials
Bert Spilker, Lippincott-Raven, 1996

Human Radiation Experiments—(The) Final Report of the President's Advisory Committee
Advisory Committee, 1996

Nazi Doctors—(The) Medical Killing and the Psychology of Genocide
Robert Jay Lifton, 2000 (reprint)

(The) Placebo Effect
Edited by Anne Harrington, 1997

(The) Plutonium Files—America's Secret Medical Experiments in the Cold War
Eileen Welcome, 1999

Protecting Human Subjects—A Series of Instructional Videotapes—Evolving Concern; Protection for Human Subjects (3 videotapes)
OPRR/OHRP

Protecting Study Volunteers in Research—A Manual for Investigative Sites
Cynthia Dunn,M.D.; Gary Chadwick, Pharm.D. MPH, CIP, 2002

Tuskegee's Truths; Rethinking the Tuskegee Syphilis Study
Susan M. Reverby (Editor), 2000

Agencies

Center for Drug Evaluation and Research (CDER)
Clinical Investigator Information
www.fda.gov/AboutFDA/CentersOffices/CDER/default.htm

FDA
www.fda.gov

International Council for Harmonization
www.ich.org

OHRP Site
www.hhs.gov/ohrp

World Medical Association
www.wma.net
The World Medical Association (WMA) is the organization that issued the Declaration of Helsinki and is responsible for its updates.

Bioethics Resources on the Web
http://bioethics.od.nih.gov
This site is maintained by the National Institutes of Health and provides links to a wide variety of bioethics resources on the web.

Human Subjects Research and IRBs
http://bioethics.od.nih.gov/irb.html

ClinicalTrials.gov
www.clinicaltrials.gov
The U.S. National Institutes of Health, through its National Library of Medicine, has developed ClinicalTrials.gov to provide subjects, family members and members of the public current information about clinical research studies.

HIPAA References

Background/Overview

HHS HIPAA implementation process
http://aspe.hhs.gov/admnsimp/kkimpl.htm

Privacy

Summary of the HIPAA Privacy Rule
www.hhs.gov/ocr/privacy/hipaa/understanding/summary/index.html

Other Information

Department of Health and Human Services (HHS) Protection of Human Subjects Regulations
www.hhs.gov/ohrp/humansubjects/index.html

Belmont Report
http://ohsr.od.nih.gov/guidelines/belmont.html

FDA Forms
www.fda.gov/opacom/morechoices/fdaforms/cder.html

FDA Information Sheets
www.fda.gov/oc/ohrt/irbs/default.htm

Declaration of Helsinki
www.wma.net/en/30publications/10policies/b3/

Nuremberg Code
http://ohsr.od.nih.gov/guidelines/nuremberg.html

NIH Required Education in the Protection of Human Research Participants

http://grants.nih.gov/grants/guide/index.html

Sources of Potential Investigators

www.centerwatch.com

www.clinicalinvestigators.com

APPENDIX B

Hints and Tips

Hints for Independent CRAs

As was mentioned in Chapter 1, many CRAs are currently self-employed as independent contractors. There are advantages and disadvantages to working as an independent contractor. The advantages are that you are essentially your own boss. There will be someone at the sponsor company or CRO to whom you "report" for a specific job, but you are usually on your own as far as planning your schedule and hours. You are also able to work from your home, away from the hustle, noise and politics of a corporate office.

Probably the biggest hurdle for independents is finding work. You have to "market yourself," and this can be difficult and time-consuming to do. Working as an independent also requires a significant amount of personal discipline. Many people prefer to work in an office environment with other people around to have coffee and lunch with, and with whom to discuss problems and job situations.

Because there are special considerations when working as an independent CRA, here are some helpful hints that may be of value:

- The IRS considers an independent CRA as a small business. Consequently, you must maintain your records and tax documents appropriately.
- Find yourself a good tax accountant/CPA. You will probably gain more than you spend to pay for this service.
- Always have a contract for the services you provide.
- You may want to discuss your company organization with an attorney.

- There are many kinds of small business organizations, and the appropriateness of each type varies according to personal situations and desires.
- You may also want the services of an attorney if you are not comfortable dealing with contracts.
- Build some structure into your workday, including break times for coffee and lunch.
- Save your household chores for the non-working times of the day.
- Keep yourself organized.
- Set up a good filing system and keep current on your filing.
- Have a separate credit card that you use only for business.
- Keep a separate checking account only for business.
- Invest in a good computer program for tracking your financial information. There are several on the market. (Ask your accountant or CPA for advice.)
- Have business cards made. Since you may work for multiple companies, you might want to have a "generic" card that lists only your name and contact information.
- Develop a system for keeping track of your expenses. Be sure to write them down as they occur. This is important if you are being reimbursed, or for tax purposes if you are not reimbursed.
- Keep your receipts. File them in such a way that you can retrieve them when needed.
- Pay for most things using your credit card. This helps to track expenses.
- If you take someone out for a business meal, jot on the back or bottom of your receipt who was present and the reason.
- Maintain confidentiality. Never discuss one sponsor's program with another sponsor.
- If you are able to combine travel for multiple sponsors, let each sponsor know, and split the expenses appropriately.

- Many independent CRAs work on an hourly basis. Record your time honestly.
- Repeat business is critical. Do not do anything to jeopardize your reputation with a company.

Maintaining Ties With Sites Between Studies

- Telephone them every couple of months to say hello.
- Know the coordinator's birthday and send him or her a card.
- If you see something written about the site (or any of the staff) in the paper, etc., drop them a note.
- If you happen to be in the vicinity and have time, drop by for just a minute to say hello. Keep the visit short so that it's not disruptive.
- When the drug they worked on is approved, drop them a note to tell them.
- Send a card (with a personal note) at the holidays.

Hints for Monitoring

- If you aren't sure where the site is, scope it out the night before.
- Some computer sites that help you locate addresses are google maps, mapquest.com and expedia.com. Most smart phones have a maps option, or you can download a map application.
- Don't be late.
- If you are going to be late, call the site to let them know.
- Do not expect site personnel to stay late for you because you were late in arriving. They have other commitments also.
- Don't spend your time at the site on the phone to other sites.
- Be polite. Good manners are important.

- Know the study you are monitoring. Be very familiar with the protocol. Never visit a site without reading the protocol first. Be sure you understand it—don't embarrass yourself by not being able to discuss it intelligently.
- Always use checklists.
- Carry a "Pocket Pharmacopoeia" by Tarascon with you.
- Remember that your smart phone has the ability provide internet access via the hot spot, but be aware of your company data plan and any additional charges
- Use your own supplies. Don't expect them to be provided for you.
- Be careful about the language and phrasing in your monitoring reports, especially if they go to the site.
- If there is a problem to be dealt with, discuss it with the appropriate people while you are at the site. Don't hit them with it later.
- Document problems, but do it in a professional manner. Be sure to document the resolution to the problem.
- Be sure when you gather your papers to leave that you are not taking the site's copies of documents with you by mistake.
- Do not discuss grants and other financial information with anyone except the investigator without the investigator's permission.
- Be careful to leave things at a site in the same way you found them.
- Take some doughnuts or fruit in with you occasionally.
- Take the coordinator out for lunch once in awhile—especially if he or she is doing a wonderful job.
- Say thank you when someone makes your job easier.

APPENDIX C

Sample Forms, Checklists and Logs

Form FDA 1572 - Statement of Investigator

Form FDA 3674 - Certification of Compliance

Site Information Sheet

Elements of Consent

Activities for Preparation, Monitoring and Closeout of a Clinical Trial

Site Evaluation

Study Documents (based on ICH GCPs)

Study Closeout

Error Query/Correction

Query Resolution

Study Monitor Visit Log

Study Personnel Log

Study Subject Visit Tracking Log

Study Document File Verification Log

Site Visit Report

Investigational Drug Dispensing Record

Inventory of Returned Investigational Material

Performance Evaluation Visit Report—Monitoring

DEPARTMENT OF HEALTH AND HUMAN SERVICES
FOOD AND DRUG ADMINISTRATION

STATEMENT OF INVESTIGATOR

(TITLE 21, CODE OF FEDERAL REGULATIONS (CFR) PART 312)

(See instructions on reverse side.)

Form Approved: OMB No. 0910-0014
Expiration Date: March 31, 2022
See OMB Statement on Reverse.

NOTE: No investigator may participate in an investigation until he/she provides the sponsor with a completed, signed Statement of Investigator, Form FDA 1572 (21 CFR 312.53(c)).

1. NAME AND ADDRESS OF INVESTIGATOR

Name of Clinical Investigator			
Address 1		Address 2	
City	State/Province/Region	Country	ZIP or Postal Code

2. EDUCATION, TRAINING, AND EXPERIENCE THAT QUALIFY THE INVESTIGATOR AS AN EXPERT IN THE CLINICAL INVESTIGATION OF THE DRUG FOR THE USE UNDER INVESTIGATION. ONE OF THE FOLLOWING IS PROVIDED *(Select **one** of the following.)*

☐ Curriculum Vitae ☐ Other Statement of Qualifications

3. NAME AND ADDRESS OF ANY MEDICAL SCHOOL, HOSPITAL, OR OTHER RESEARCH FACILITY WHERE THE CLINICAL INVESTIGATION(S) WILL BE CONDUCTED **CONTINUATION PAGE for Item 3**

Name of Medical School, Hospital, or Other Research Facility			
Address 1		Address 2	
City	State/Province/Region	Country	ZIP or Postal Code

4. NAME AND ADDRESS OF ANY CLINICAL LABORATORY FACILITIES TO BE USED IN THE STUDY **CONTINUATION PAGE for Item 4**

Name of Clinical Laboratory Facility			
Address 1		Address 2	
City	State/Province/Region	Country	ZIP or Postal Code

5. NAME AND ADDRESS OF THE INSTITUTIONAL REVIEW BOARD (IRB) THAT IS RESPONSIBLE FOR REVIEW AND APPROVAL OF THE STUDY(IES) **CONTINUATION PAGE for Item 5**

Name of IRB			
Address 1		Address 2	
City	State/Province/Region	Country	ZIP or Postal Code

6. NAMES OF SUBINVESTIGATORS *(If not applicable, enter "None")*

CONTINUATION PAGE – for Item 6

7. NAME AND CODE NUMBER, IF ANY, OF THE PROTOCOL(S) IN THE IND FOR THE STUDY(IES) TO BE CONDUCTED BY THE INVESTIGATOR

FORM FDA 1572 (3/19) **PREVIOUS EDITION IS OBSOLETE.** **Page 1 of 2**

8. PROVIDE THE FOLLOWING CLINICAL PROTOCOL INFORMATION. *(Select **one** of the following.)*

☐ For Phase 1 investigations, a general outline of the planned investigation including the estimated duration of the study and the maximum number of subjects that will be involved.

☐ For Phase 2 or 3 investigations, an outline of the study protocol including an approximation of the number of subjects to be treated with the drug and the number to be employed as controls, if any; the clinical uses to be investigated; characteristics of subjects by age, sex, and condition; the kind of clinical observations and laboratory tests to be conducted; the estimated duration of the study; and copies or a description of case report forms to be used.

9. COMMITMENTS

I agree to conduct the study(ies) in accordance with the relevant, current protocol(s) and will only make changes in a protocol after notifying the sponsor, except when necessary to protect the safety, rights, or welfare of subjects.

I agree to personally conduct or supervise the described investigation(s).

I agree to inform any patients, or any persons used as controls, that the drugs are being used for investigational purposes and I will ensure that the requirements relating to obtaining informed consent in 21 CFR Part 50 and institutional review board (IRB) review and approval in 21 CFR Part 56 are met.

I agree to report to the sponsor adverse experiences that occur in the course of the investigation(s) in accordance with 21 CFR 312.64. I have read and understand the information in the investigator's brochure, including the potential risks and side effects of the drug.

I agree to ensure that all associates, colleagues, and employees assisting in the conduct of the study(ies) are informed about their obligations in meeting the above commitments.

I agree to maintain adequate and accurate records in accordance with 21 CFR 312.62 and to make those records available for inspection in accordance with 21 CFR 312.68.

I will ensure that an IRB that complies with the requirements of 21 CFR Part 56 will be responsible for the initial and continuing review and approval of the clinical investigation. I also agree to promptly report to the IRB all changes in the research activity and all unanticipated problems involving risks to human subjects or others. Additionally, I will not make any changes in the research without IRB approval, except where necessary to eliminate apparent immediate hazards to human subjects.

I agree to comply with all other requirements regarding the obligations of clinical investigators and all other pertinent requirements in 21 CFR Part 312.

INSTRUCTIONS FOR COMPLETING FORM FDA 1572
STATEMENT OF INVESTIGATOR

1. Complete all sections. Provide a separate page if additional space is needed.
2. Provide curriculum vitae or other statement of qualifications as described in Section 2.
3. Provide protocol outline as described in Section 8.
4. Sign and date below.
5. FORWARD THE COMPLETED FORM AND OTHER DOCUMENTS BEING PROVIDED TO THE SPONSOR. The sponsor will incorporate this information along with other technical data into an Investigational New Drug Application (IND). INVESTIGATORS SHOULD NOT SEND THIS FORM DIRECTLY TO THE FOOD AND DRUG ADMINISTRATION.

10. DATE *(mm/dd/yyyy)*	11. SIGNATURE OF INVESTIGATOR Sign

(**WARNING**: A willfully false statement is a criminal offense. U.S.C. Title 18, Sec. 1001.)

The information below applies only to requirements of the Paperwork Reduction Act of 1995.

The burden time for this collection of information is estimated to average 100 hours per response, including the time to review instructions, search existing data sources, gather and maintain the data needed and complete and review the collection of information. Send comments regarding this burden estimate or any other aspect of this information collection, including suggestions for reducing this burden to the address to the right:

Department of Health and Human Services
Food and Drug Administration
Office of Operations
Paperwork Reduction Act (PRA) Staff
PRAStaff@fda.hhs.gov

"An agency may not conduct or sponsor, and a person is not required to respond to, a collection of information unless it displays a currently valid OMB number."

DO NOT SEND YOUR COMPLETED FORM TO THIS PRA STAFF EMAIL ADDRESS.

FORM FDA 1572 (3/19) **PREVIOUS EDITION IS OBSOLETE.** **Page 2 of 2**

Form Approved: OMB No. 0910-0231. Expiration Date: 5/31/2026. See PRA Statement below.

FDA

DEPARTMENT OF HEALTH AND HUMAN SERVICES
Food and Drug Administration

Certification of Compliance

Under 42 U.S.C. § 282(j)(5)(B), with Requirements of ClinicalTrials.gov Data Bank

(For submission with an application/submission, including amendments, supplements, and resubmissions, under §§ 505, 515, 520(m), or 510(k) of the Federal Food, Drug, and Cosmetic Act or § 351 of the Public Health Service Act.)

SPONSOR / APPLICANT / SUBMITTER INFORMATION

1. Name of Sponsor/Applicant/Submitter

2. Date of the Application/Submission

3. Address

Address 1 *(Street address, P.O. box, company name c/o)*

Address 2 *(Apartment, suite, unit, building, floor, etc.)*

City

State/Province/Region

Country

ZIP or Postal Code

4. Telephone and Fax Numbers *(Include country code if applicable and area code)*

(Tel): ______

(Fax): ______

PRODUCT INFORMATION

5. **For Drugs/Biologics:** Include Any/All Available Established, Proprietary and/or Chemical/Biochemical/Blood/Cellular/Gene Therapy Product Name(s).
For Devices: Include Any/All Common or Usual Name(s), Classification, Trade or Proprietary or Model Name(s) and/or Model Number(s)

Continuation Page for #5

APPLICATION / SUBMISSION INFORMATION

6. Type of Application/Submission Which This Certification Accompanies

☐ IND ☐ NDA ☐ ANDA ☐ BLA ☐ PMA ☐ HDE ☐ 510(k) ☐ PDP ☐ Other

7. Include IND/NDA/ANDA/BLA/PMA/HDE/510(k)/PDP/Other Number *(If number previously assigned)*

If BLA was selected in item 6, provide Supplement Number

8. Serial Number Assigned to Application/Submission Which This Certification Accompanies

CERTIFICATION STATEMENT / INFORMATION

9. Check only one of the following boxes *(See instructions for additional information and explanation)*

☐ A. I certify that the requirements of 42 U.S.C. § 282(j), Section 402(j) of the Public Health Service Act, including 42 CFR part 11, do not apply because the application/submission which this certification accompanies does not reference any clinical trial.

☐ B. I certify that the requirements of 42 U.S.C. § 282(j), Section 402(j) of the Public Health Service Act, including 42 CFR part 11, do not apply to any clinical trial referenced in the application/submission which this certification accompanies.

☐ C. I certify that the requirements of 42 U.S.C. § 282(j), section 402(j) of the Public Health Service Act, apply to one or more of the clinical trials referenced in the application/submission which this certification accompanies and that the requirements of 42 U.S.C. 282(j), including any applicable provisions of 42 CFR part 11, have been met.

Certification Statement / Information section continued on page 2

CERTIFICATION STATEMENT / INFORMATION *(Continued)*

10. If you checked box C, in number 9, provide the National Clinical Trial (NCT) Number(s) for any "applicable clinical trial(s)," for which you (the sponsor/applicant/submitter) are the "responsible party" under 42 U.S.C. § 282(j)(1)(a)(i), section 402(j)(1)(a)(i) of the Public Health Service Act referenced in the application/ submission which this Certification accompanies. (Add continuation page as necessary.)

NCT Number(s):

Continuation Page for #10

The undersigned declares, to the best of her/his knowledge, that this is an accurate, true, and complete submission of information. I understand that the failure to submit the certification required by 42 U.S.C. § 282(j)(5)(B), section 402(j)(5)(B) of the Public Health Service Act, and the knowing submission of a false certification under such section are prohibited acts under 21 U.S.C. § 331, section 301 of the Federal Food, Drug, and Cosmetic Act.

Warning: A willfully and knowingly false statement is a criminal offense, U.S. Code, title 18, section 1001.

11. Name and Title of the Person who Signs Number 15

Name	Title

12. Address

Address 1 *(Street address, P.O. box, company name c/o)*	
Address 2 *(Apartment, suite, unit, building, floor, etc.)*	
City	State/Province/Region
Country	ZIP or Postal Code

13. Telephone and Fax Numbers *(Include country code if applicable and area code)*

(Tel):

(Fax):

14. Date of Certification

15. Signature of Sponsor/Applicant/Submitter or an Authorized Representative *(Sign)*

Sign

This section applies only to requirements of the Paperwork Reduction Act of 1995.

*****DO NOT SEND YOUR COMPLETED FORM TO THE PRA STAFF EMAIL ADDRESS BELOW.*****

The burden time for this collection of information is estimated to average 15 minutes and 45 minutes (depending on the type of application/ submission) per response, including the time to review instructions, search existing data sources, gather and maintain the data needed and complete and review the collection of information. Send comments regarding this burden estimate or any other aspect of this information collection, including suggestions for reducing this burden to:

Department of Health and Human Services
Food and Drug Administration
Office of Chief Information Officer
Paperwork Reduction Act (PRA) Staff
PRAStaff@fda.hhs.gov

"An agency may not conduct or sponsor, and a person is not required to respond to, a collection of information unless it displays a currently valid OMB number."

FORM FDA 3674 (05/23) **Page 2 of 4**

Site Information Sheet

Protocol ____

Investigator ____

Address ____

____

____

Telephone ______________________ Fax ______________________

Email ____

Directions to the site ____

____

Coordinator ____

Telephone ____

Pharmacist ____

Telephone ____

Other personnel ____

Best days, times for monitoring visits ____

Other pertinent information ____

____

____

Elements of Consent

Required elements

- ☐ Statement that the study involves research.
  - ☐ Explanation of the purpose of the research.
  - ☐ Expected duration of subject's participation.
  - ☐ Description of procedures to be followed.
  - ☐ Identification of any procedures that are experimental.

- ☐ Description of reasonably foreseeable risks and discomforts to subject.
- ☐ Description of benefits which may be reasonably expected.
- ☐ Disclosure of alternate procedures or treatment.
- ☐ Statement re: confidentiality of reports
  - ☐ Statement that FDA may inspect the records.

- ☐ Statement re: compensation for any research-related injury.
- ☐ Contact person for questions about the research and subject rights.
- ☐ Contact person in the event of research-related injury.
- ☐ Statement that participation is voluntary.
- ☐ Statement that refusal to participate will not result in the penalty or loss of any benefits to which the subject is otherwise entitled.
- ☐ Statement that the subject may discontinue at any time without penalty or loss of any benefits to which the subject is otherwise entitled.

Additional elements (include as appropriate)

- ☐ Statement that the treatment may involve risks to the subject (or embryo or fetus) which are currently unforeseeable.
- ☐ Circumstances under which the subject's participation may be terminated by the investigator without regard to the subject's consent.
- ☐ Any additional costs to the subject.
- ☐ Consequences for withdrawal and procedures for orderly termination.
- ☐ Statement that significant new findings will be provided to the subject.
- ☐ Approximate number of subjects involved in the study.

Activities for Preparation, Monitoring and Closeout of a Clinical Trial

Following is a list of activities from which personal checklists can be developed. Activities shown are generic and may vary from company to company.

Study Planning Activities

In-house

- ☐ Develop study timelines (IRB Approval, FDA-mandated waiting periods, bulk drug manufacturing, etc.)
- ☐ Update Investigator Brochure, when necessary (yearly or when changes are appropriate) Chemistry, Path/Tox, Pharmacology, and Clinical. (Date of last update ____________)
- ☐ Obtain or assign unique protocol numbers.
- ☐ Evaluate and finalize study budget(s).
- ☐ Determine if or which studies will be contracted to outside vendor and initiate, contract, or coordinate with CRO or company personnel according to company policy.
- ☐ Provide CRAs or CRO with protocol summary to help identify potential investigators.
- ☐ Order bulk drug supplies.
- ☐ Prepare initial IND submission (if appropriate).
- ☐ Determine laboratory needs (central vs local).

Field

- ☐ Interview potential investigators.

Pre-Study Activities

In-house

- ☐ Circulate draft protocol for review or through review process.
- ☐ Finalize and approve protocol (date of approval: ________________).
- ☐ Update IND.
- ☐ Get release from path/tox (e.g., all required pre-clinical activities are complete and no safety concerns exist).
- ☐ Submit request for investigational drug supplies.
- ☐ Write informed consents.
- ☐ Obtain investigator identifier numbers (if necessary).
- ☐ Request or design CRFs.
- ☐ Send draft CRFs for review.
- ☐ Finalize and order CRFs/EDC system.
- ☐ Obtain Use Patent Review.
- ☐ Prepare Investigator/Study Coordinator Training Manuals, if appropriate.

- ☐ Plan Investigator meeting, if appropriate.
- ☐ Prepare randomization list.
- ☐ Coordinate investigator meeting/start-up dates with field monitors.
- ☐ Establish study files.
- ☐ Design/set-up logs, tracking systems etc.

Field

- ☐ Evaluate and select investigators.
- ☐ Final site evaluations (pre-study visit).
- ☐ Collect and submit all regulatory-/company-required documents.
  - ☐ Signed protocol
  - ☐ 1572
  - ☐ Lab normal ranges and certification
  - ☐ CVs
  - ☐ IRB approval(s)
  - ☐ Informed consent approval
  - ☐ Letter of agreement/contracts
  - ☐ Ancillary Personnel/ Signature Form
  - ☐ Financial Disclosure information

Study Initiation

In-house

- ☐ Send study package(s) to field monitors (Protocol, Brochures, Consents, 1572, contracts/agreement letters, etc.)
- ☐ Submit appropriate documents to Regulatory Affairs and/or place in study file.
- ☐ Submit initial grant payment request, if appropriate.
- ☐ Send laboratory normal ranges to Biostatistician/Data Management.
- ☐ Ship clinical supplies (notify field monitor (CRA) when drug is shipped).

Field

- ☐ Conduct site initiation visits.
  - ☐ Confirm receipt of clinical supplies with each site
  - ☐ Review protocol requirements
  - ☐ Review sponsor policy on CRF/EDC completion and correction
  - ☐ Confirm presence of all required documents
  - ☐ Ensure establishment of study files
- ☐ Establish monitoring visit frequency and communicate to site.

Study Monitoring

In-house

- ☐ Assure all amendments or deviations are approved and filed with regulatory affairs, the investigators and internal study files.
- ☐ Assure IRB approval was received for changes/amendments.
- ☐ Monitor grant payments/adjustments.
- ☐ Document and file annual IRB approvals.
- ☐ Assure receipt and filing of CVs for investigators/subinvestigators added after study initiation.
- ☐ Assure 1572s are updated as required.
- ☐ Assure annual IND update is completed.
- ☐ Assure Investigator Brochure is updated annually or as needed and that revisions are sent to all investigators.
- ☐ Monitor site visit reports for any required action.
- ☐ Maintain current study enrollment and progress data according to company SOPs.
- ☐ Assure all adverse events are reported according to regulation and company policy.
- ☐ Provide field monitors with current study status prior to site visits.

Field

- ☐ Check with in-house colleagues to review site status prior to visit.
- ☐ Visit sites as scheduled/required.
- ☐ Review protocol compliance, especially inclusion/exclusion requirements.
- ☐ Assure required corrections are made.
- ☐ Review CRFs and compare to source documents.
- ☐ Ensure all protocol deviations are documented and reported appropriately.
- ☐ Review drug accounting, storage, dispensing.
- ☐ Check for new adverse events.
- ☐ Collect any outstanding data from previously reported adverse events.
- ☐ Assure that any safety update letters sent to site have been sent to the IRB.
- ☐ Review study files for extraneous documents and to ensure required documents are present.
- ☐ Meet with investigator and study coordinator to review study status, answer questions, etc.
- ☐ Document visit on written report.
- ☐ Confirm date of next visit with site.
- ☐ Written report of visit findings to investigation (optional).

Study Termination

In-house

- ☐ Notify regulatory department when all patients are off drug and study is terminated.
- ☐ Send randomization sheets to investigators, if appropriate (only after all

study documents are in-house).

- ☐ Send clinical data and statistical summary to investigators, if appropriate.
- ☐ Prepare final study reports.

Field

- ☐ All CRFs collected, corrected and in-house.
- ☐ No outstanding data for serious adverse events, protocol deviations, deaths or pregnancies.
- ☐ Drug collected, inventoried and returned to sponsor.
- ☐ Investigator files complete and investigator instructed regarding storage.
- ☐ Drug reconciled from inventory and shipping invoices.
- ☐ Investigator briefed on procedure if notified of FDA audit.
- ☐ IRB notified of termination.
- ☐ Study file complete and ready for audit.

Site Evaluation

CRA should evaluate each item below, making notes.

Investigator

- ☐ Qualifications
- ☐ Licensure
- ☐ Specialty
- ☐ Clinical trial experience
  - ☐ Number of previous trials
  - ☐ Number of similar trials
  - ☐ Enrollment in previous trials (numbers, time to enroll)
- ☐ FDA audits
- ☐ Number of trials assigned and status

Staff

- ☐ Study coordinator
- ☐ Other specialized personnel
- ☐ Training and licensure
- ☐ Experience
- ☐ Turnover
- ☐ General interest and attitude
- ☐ Number of trials assigned and status

Facility

- ☐ Appropriate for trials
- ☐ Ample storage for study supplies
- ☐ Appropriate drug storage
- ☐ Special storage equipment available (freezer, centrifuge, refrigerator, etc.)
- ☐ Special equipment available
- ☐ Active practice
- ☐ Facilities tour taken
- ☐ Study records storage, study records format (electronic or paper based), study records access
- ☐ Staff working areas
- ☐ Monitoring area
- ☐ Patient treatment areas

IRB

- ☐ Local IRB available
  - ☐ Frequency and timing of meetings
  - ☐ Average time to approval
  - ☐ Responsiveness
- ☐ Use central IRB

Laboratory/Tests

- ☐ Local lab available
- ☐ Necessary tests can be done
- ☐ Timeliness
- ☐ Certification
- ☐ Have experience with central lab

Protocol feasibility

- ☐ Experience with similar studies
- ☐ Interest level
- ☐ Availability of potential subjects
- ☐ Competing studies (in practice and in community)
- ☐ Timing appropriate
- ☐ Study coordinator availability
- ☐ Can attend investigator meeting

Study Documents
(based on ICH GCPs)

Protocol ______________________________

Investigator ______________________________

Pre-Study

- ☐ Investigator Brochure
- ☐ Signed protocol and amendments (if any)
- ☐ Informed consent form
  - ☐ Any other information to be given to subjects
  - ☐ Any advertising materials for recruitment
- ☐ Dated, written IRB approvals for:
  - ☐ Protocol [Date:]
  - ☐ Amendments, if any [Date:]
  - ☐ Consent and any other material to be given to subjects [Date:]
  - ☐ Advertising, if any [Date:]
  - ☐ Subject compensation, if any [Date:]
- ☐ CVs for investigator, subinvestigators
- ☐ Laboratory certification and normal ranges
- ☐ Study manual, if available
- ☐ Shipping records
- ☐ Decoding procedures for blinded trials
- ☐ Financial disclosure sheets
- ☐ Contract
- ☐ Sponsor-specific documents

During the conduct of the trial

- ☐ Investigator Brochure updates
- ☐ Protocol amendments and/or revisions
- ☐ Consent revisions
- ☐ Dated, written IRB approvals of:
  - ☐ Protocol amendments [Dates:]
  - ☐ Revised consents [Dates:]
  - ☐ New or revised subject materials [Dates:]
  - ☐ New or revised advertising [Dates:]
- ☐ CVs for new investigators and/or subinvestigators
- ☐ Laboratory updates of certification and/or normal ranges
- ☐ Shipping documentation (receipt of trial materials)
- ☐ Monitoring visit log
- ☐ Communications with sponsor (letters, telephone reports, etc.)
- ☐ Signed consent forms
- ☐ Source documents

- ☐ Signed, dated, completed case report forms (CRFs)
- ☐ Documentation of CRF corrections
- ☐ Notification to sponsors and IRB of serious adverse events and related reports
- ☐ IND safety reports received from the sponsor
- ☐ Interim and/or annual reports to the IRB
- ☐ Subject screening log
- ☐ Subject identification code list
- ☐ Subject enrollment log
- ☐ Investigational product accountability
- ☐ Signature sheet (all persons making CRF entries or corrections)
- ☐ Record of retained body fluids and/or tissue samples, if any

After study completion or termination

- ☐ Drug (device) accountability
- ☐ Documentation of drug/device return or disposal
- ☐ Completed subject identification code list
- ☐ Final report to the IRB [Date:]

Comments ____

____

____

Checklist should be kept in front of study file and updated as appropriate.

Study Closeout

Protocol ______________________________

Sponsor ______________________________

Investigator ______________________________

Date ______________________________

- ☐ Study documents file is complete (refer to Checklist: Study Documents).
- ☐ Final report has been made to the IRB and the sponsor.
- ☐ All case report forms (CRFs) are complete and have been submitted to the sponsor.
  - ☐ All CRF corrections/queries have been addressed.
  - ☐ Any patient diaries, etc. have been submitted, as required.
  - ☐ All adverse event follow-up is complete.
- ☐ All source documentation is in order.
  - ☐ If not with study files, location of materials is noted in the document file.
- ☐ Study personnel form is complete.
- ☐ Subjects' signed informed consent forms are filed.
- ☐ Drug dispensing and disposition forms are complete.
- ☐ Study drug has been returned as per sponsor instructions.
- ☐ All other study materials (extra CRFs, etc.) have been returned to the sponsor.
- ☐ Investigator Brochure is filed with other study materials.
- ☐ All study materials are filed together as per archival procedures.
  - ☐ Location of materials is noted in site records.

Error Query/Correction

Protocol____________________ Protocol date __________ Sponsor ____________________

Patient	Visit	Page	Field	Problem	Correction	Initials

Query Resolution

Protocol____________________ Investigator _______________ Subject Number ____________________

Page No.	Field	Issue	Resolution	Date	Initial

Study Monitor Visit Log

Protocol ______________ **Protocol date** ______________ **Sponsor** ______________

Name	Job Title	Date(s) of Visit	Signature	Study Coordinator Initials

Use addional sheets as needed. Keep with study documents file.

Study Personnel Log

Protocol____________________ **Protocol date** __________ **Sponsor** ____________________

Name	Job Title	Initials	Start Date of Study Responsibility	End Date of Study Responsibility	Signature

Use additional sheets as needed. Update when personnel changes occur.
Keep with study documents file.

Study Subject Visit Tracking Log

Protocol ______________________ Sponsor ______________________

Subject	Consent Date	Baseline	Week 1	Week 2	Week 4	Final Status	Comments

Study Document File Verification Log

Study Document File Review	**Initial / /**	**Initial / /**	**Initial / /**	**Initial / /**
Signed, IRB-approved protocol or cover sheet				
Signed, IRB-approved amendments ■ Amendment #, date ■ Amendment #, date ■ Amendment #, date				
IRB-approved informed consent document				
Signed, completed FDA 1572 form (Statement of Investigator)				
IRB approval letter, verifying approval of both the protocol and consent document				
IRB approval of advertising and subject recruitment materials, including any subject compensation				
Investigator Brochure (or package insert, for marketed products)				
Verification of laboratory certification and laboratory normal ranges				
Study Manual, if available				
Shipping records for investigation product				
Decoding procedures for blinded trials				
Financial disclosure forms				
CVs/licenses				
Sponsor-specific documents and communications				
Reviewer initials				

Attach a separate sheet with comments if any problems found.

Site Visit Report

Person Making Report________________________ **Title**_______________

Reason for Contact ____

Method of Contact ☐ **Phone** ☐ **Visit Date of Contact** _______________

Study (Protocol) Identification______________________________________

Site (Investigator) ID____

Site Persons Contacted____

Facilities/Staff	**Yes**	**No**	**N/A**	**Comments**
Changes in Staff?	*			
Are the investigator and staff fulfilling study obligations?		*		
Changes in facilities/ Equipment?	*			
Adverse Events	**Yes**	**No**	**N/A**	**Comments**
Have any serious medical events occurred since last visit?	*			
If yes, were required forms completed and submitted?		*		
Any outstanding data or forms for this or previous events?	*			
Was the IRB informed, if required?		*		

Study Conduct	**Yes**	**No**	**N/A**	**Comments**
Are protocol requirements being followed?		*		
Consent for all patients available and signed prior to enrollment?		*		
Site Conduct	**Yes**	**No**	**N/A**	**Comments**
Were CRFs reviewed?		*		
Source documents reviewed?		*		
Were CRF problems discussed w/staff?		*		
Was patient eligibility confirmed?		*		
Is recruitment on schedule?		*		
Were corrections made?		*		
Were any protocol deviations noted?	*			
Is the investigator accessible during visits?		*		
Are changes, events, etc. being communicated to the IRB?		*		
Were all completed CRFs collected?		*		
Drug Supplies	**Yes**	**No**	**N/A**	**Comments**
Is investigational product stored properly?		*		

Drug Supplies	Yes	No	N/A	Comments
Are dispensing procedures satisfactory?		*		
Is investigational product being accounted for properly?		*		
Are study supplies adequate?		*		
Documentation	**Yes**	**No**	**N/A**	**Comments**
Signed protocol		*		
1572		*		
CVs for PI and sub-investigators		*		
Approved consent		*		
IRB approvals		*		
Agreements/contracts?		*		
Signed amendments		*		
Lab normals/ accreditation?		*		
Current Investigator Brochure		*		
All pertinent correspondence on file?		*		
IRB Correspondence-Annual, SAEs?		*		
Any unresolved issues from previous visits?	*			

Administration	Yes	No	N/A	Comments
Were results of visit discussed with investigator and staff?		*		
Will findings be provided to site in writing?				
Was appointment made for next visit?		*		

* Requires a comment. Add additional pages if necessary.

Comments ____

____

____

____

Signed ____

Investigational Drug Dispensing Record

Protocol Number ______________________________

Protocol Title ______________________________

Investigator ______________________________

Subject Number/Initials ______________________________

Treatment Code (if applicable) ______________________________

Complete the following information using a new line each time medication is dispensed or returned. Use a separate sheet for each subject.

Date Medication Dispensed or Returned	Lot Number and Identification Code	Quantity Dispensed (Number of tablets)	Quantity Returned (Number of tablets)	Initials	Comments

Inventory of Returned Investigational Material

Sponsor/Address ______________________________

____

Protocol Number ______________________________

Protocol Title ______________________________

Investigator/Address ______________________________

____

Contact Person/Telephone Number ______________________________

The following investigational material is being returned.

Drug	Lot Number	Code Number	Full Containers	Partial Containers	Empty Containers	Total Containers

Comments ______________________________

Performance Evaluation Visit Report - Monitoring

Name of Clinical Research Associate (CRA)	
Accompanied by (please print)	
Date of Visit	
Investigator/Protocol Identifier	
Project Manager	
Location (City, State/Province, Country)	
Purpose of Visit	Performance Evaluation Visit

CRA Demographics			
CRA experience level	0-2 years	2-5 years	>5 years
CRA experience in therapeutic area under study	Low	Medium	High
Complexity of the project	Simple	Average	Complex
Site Factors			
Investigator clinical research skill level	Low	Medium	High
Study Coordinator clinical research skill level	Low	Medium	High
Pharmacist* clinical research skill level	Low	Medium	High
Total patient enrollment	Low	Average	High
Rate of enrollment	Slow	On schedule	Fast
Comments on Demographics and Site factors			

*Pharmacist or designated investigational product (IP) dispenser

0. Visit Review – Preparation	Yes	No	NA
0.1 Was a visit confirmation letter sent to the site?			
0.2 Did the CRA send all appropriate documentation to the accompanying Evaluator prior to the visit?			
0.3 Were the Project Manager (PM), Sponsor and site informed of the accompanied visit?			
0.4 Was the site adequately informed as to what would be required of them during the visit?			
0.5 Was the CRA knowledgeable regarding site staff?			
0.6 Was the CRA's knowledge of the protocol/therapeutic area adequate?			
0.7 Was the last visit report reviewed prior to this visit?			
0.8 Did the CRA have a plan for the visit?			
0.9 Was the visit scheduled per sponsor contract?			
0.10 Did the CRA prepare for the visit by bringing study-related monitoring tools such as monitoring notes, tracking logs, forms, etc.?			
0.11 Were there any outstanding items from the previous site visit?			
If Yes, please specify:			
Comments on Visit Preparation			

1. Informed Consent Forms (ICF), Assent and HIPAA/EU Directive Authorization	Yes	No	NA
Did the CRA:			
1.1 Check that all previously unreviewed HIPAA/EU Directive authorizations were completed according to applicable regulations?			
1.2 Verify that the correct version of the ICF was being used?			

1. Informed Consent Forms (ICF), Assent and HIPAA/EU Directive Authorization (Continued)	**Yes**	**No**	**NA**
1.3 Verify that all versions of the ICF/assent were properly completed and present for all subjects?			
1.4 Verify that the consenting process at this site meets regulatory requirements?			
Comments on ICF, Assent and HIPAA/EU Directive Authorization			

2. Case Report Form (CRF), Source Document (SD) Review and Serious Adverse Events (SAEs/SUSARs)	**Yes**	**No**	**NA**
Did the CRA :			
2.1 Review CRFs and source documents in a thorough, organized manner?			
2.2 Verify complete and consistent documentation for AEs, concomitant medications, physical examinations and functional tests?			
2.3 Check that subject eligibility, visit dates and procedures met protocol requirements?			
2.4 Identify issues with ICHGCP compliance?			
2.5 Report protocol waivers/violations/deviations as per the study procedures?			
2.6 Review documentation for date and time of laboratory specimen collection and investigator review/signature?			
2.7 Issue appropriate queries?			
2.8 Verify all outstanding data queries as resolved?			
2.9 Communicate all the issues appropriately with the site staff?			
2.10 Verify completion of all required CRFs?			
2.11 Transmit CRFs according to the monitoring plan?			

Comments on Comments on CRF, SD Review & SAE's/SUSARs

3. Serious Adverse Events (SAEs) and Serious Unexpected Suspected Adverse Drug Reactions (SUSARs)	Yes	No	NA
Did the CRA:			
3.1 Identify any unreported SAEs during this visit?			
3.2 Verify that all previously reported SAEs and SUSARs were submitted as required by Local Regulatory and Ethics committee requirements?			
3.3 Verify complete and consistent documentation for SAEs/SUSARs?			
Comments on SAEs and SUSARs			

4. Investigational Product (IP) Accountability and Supply Management	Yes	No	NA
Did the CRA:			
4.1 Request access to Pharmacy/IP records prior to the visit?			
4.2 Use the IP Accountability process as outlined in the checklist?			
4.3 Verify that all required documents for IP release were on file?			
4.4 Verify that the blinding information was intact and that it was stored appropriately?			
4.5 Assess subject's compliance by comparing logs/labels to the CRF and source data?			
4.6 Verify that receipt records, accountability logs (including a Master IP Accountability log) and/or destruction records were completed, up-to-date and accurate?			

4.7 Verify that general study supplies and IP supplies are adequate, found to be unexpired and being checked at each visit?			
4.8 Verify that proper storage, handling and transporting methods are being employed at this study site?			
4.9 Confirm that the appropriate temperature logs were completed and adequate?			
4.10 Conduct an organized, thorough review of the IP, document all discrepancies and communicate these to the site?			
4.11 Follow up on discrepancies recorded during the previous visit(s)?			
Comments on IP Accountability and Supply Management			

5. Regulatory File Review	**Yes**	**No**	**NA**
Did the CRA:			
5.1 Sign the Site Visit Signature log?			
5.2 Review the regulatory file?			
5.3 Check that regulatory documents were filed and up to date?			
5.4 Copy appropriate documents for the sponsor/ central files?			
5.5 Review regulatory documents in a complete and organized manner?			
5.6 Identify outstanding issues?			
5.7 Resolve the issues identified?			
5.8 Give the site staff a method for rectifying outstanding issues?			
Comments on Regulatory File Review			

6. Laboratory and Specimen Handling Procedure	Yes	No	NA
Did the CRA:			
6.1 Check that handling, storage and shipment of samples was in accordance with the requirements of the laboratory manual?			
6.2 Check and confirm that laboratory reference ranges and certifications were on file and current?			
6.3 Check the supply of all laboratory materials and kits?			
6.4 Check expiration dates for laboratory kits?			
Comments onLaboratory and Specimen Handling Procedure			

7. Study Staff, Patient Enrollment and General Conduct	Yes	No	NA
Did the CRA:			
7.1 Meet and discuss the findings of this visit and any required follow-up actions with the Principal Investigator?			
7.2 Meet and discuss the findings of this visit and any required follow-up actions with other appropriate site staff?			
7.3 Answer questions from study site staff?			
7.4 Discuss site recruitment?			
7.5 Communicate clearly and concisely?			
7.6 Behave in a professional and courteous manner during the visit?			
Comments on Study Staff, Patient Enrollment and General Conduct			

8. Post Visit activities	Yes	No	NA
Did the CRA:			
8.1 Conduct the visit to an acceptable standard?			
8.2 Accomplish objectives for the visit?			
8.3 Write the visit report within appropriate time-lines?			
8.4 Write the visit report to an adequate standard?			
8.5 Document all required follow-up actions and resolutions?			
Comments on Post Visit Activities			

Overall Performance/Achievement of Objectives:		
Exceeds Expectations	Meets Expectations	Needs Improvement

Training Given on the Day:

Areas For Development /Further Training Needed/Actions Agreed:

CRA Comments:

CRA ____________________ Date ____________________

Regional Manager or designee ____________________ Date ____________________

APPENDIX D

Job Descriptions and Academic Programs

CRA Job Summary

Clinical Research Associate (CRA)—Entry Level

Clinical Research Associate (CRA)—Advanced Level

Academic Programs

CRA Job Summary

This document describes two levels of CRA responsibilities. For simplicity, they are called CRA 1 (entry level) and CRA 2 (advanced).

CRA 1	CRA 2
Investigator Selection	
• Will not be involved in this activity. Will work with Investigators/CROs selected by the Sponsor.	• In consultation with the Sponsor/CRO select investigators appropriate for the therapeutic area and protocol. Note: May also be involved in CRO evaluation/selection.
Pre-Study	
• Meet with Investigator and staff and review study requirements (protocol, CRFs, sponsor policy and procedures, investigator responsibilities, staffing and patient recruitment). • Conduct study initiation visit. • Confirm appropriateness of the IRB. • Collect and forward all required study documentation to Sponsor. • Document visit.	• Assess study site to ensure facility, patient population and staff are sufficient to support the protocol. • Negotiate study budget and/or indemnification agreement. • Assist in planning and conducting Investigator Meeting and/or Start-up Meeting. • Meet with PI and staff and review study requirements (protocol, CRFs, Sponsor policy and procedures, investigator responsibilities, staffing and patient recruitment. • Conduct study initiation visit. • Confirm appropriateness of the IRB. • Collect and forward all required study documentation to Sponsor. • Document visit.

CRA 1	CRA 2
Study Monitoring	
• Conduct routine monitoring visits to include: – Review protocol compliance – Review CRF/source documents – Resolve questions/issues with Investigator/Staff – Check/inventory clinical supplies – Review communication with the IRB – Review drug accountability • Confirm Informed Consent. • Correct previous errors. • Submit all collected documents and site visit report to Sponsor. • Log and track study progress.	• Conduct routine monitoring visits to include: – Review protocol compliance – Review CRF/source docments – Resolve questions/issues with Investigator Staff – Check/inventory clinical supplies – Review communication with the IRB – Review drug accountability • Confirm Informed Consent. • Correct previous errors. • Submit all collected documents and site visit report to Sponsor. • Log and track study progress.
Study Close Out	
• Review and collect remaining CRFs. • Retrieve clinical supplies and any other study materials. • Review investigator's study file to insure that all documents are in order and ready for audit or inspection. • Review file (document) retention schedule/policy. • Submit documentation for study closeout. • Arrange any final payments. • Review publication policy/procedure. • Review any follow-up requirements that may be required (IRB notification, ongoing medical events).	• Review and collect remaining CRFs. • Retrieve clinical supplies and any other study materials. • Review investigator's study file to insure that all documents are in order and ready for audit or inspection. • Review file (document) retention schedule/policy. • Submit documentation for study closeout. • Arrange any final payments. • Review publication policy/procedure. • Review any follow-up requirements that may be required (IRB notification, ongoing medical events).

Clinical Research Associate (CRA)

Advanced Level

Position Description

The Clinical Research Associate, independently or in consultation with the Sponsor/CRO will:

- Locate and select clinical investigators appropriate to the therapeutic area and phase of the study.
- Assess potential study sites to ensure the facility, staff and patient population are sufficient for study conduct.
- Negotiate the study budget (grant) and any other contract agreements required by the Sponsor/CRO, if required.
- Plan or assist in conducting study start-up meetings.
- Meet with Clinical Investigators and their staff prior to study initiation to insure all aspects of the study are understood by the investigator and staff, confirm the appropriateness of the IRB and insure that all documentation required to initiate the study is complete.
- Monitor study progress to assure compliance with protocol requirements,
- FDA regulations and Good Clinical Practice by conducting site visits as directed by the Sponsor/CRO.
- Monitor and track patient enrollment and study progress.
- Perform site audits to include source document review.
- Ensure the timely, accurate and complete collection and submission of study data.
- Identify, address, and resolve issues and problems as they might occur.

At study completion:

- Ensure collection of all data and remaining study supplies for return to the Sponsor/CRO.
- Ensure that appropriate study documents are complete and properly filed.
- Prepare the site for possible FDA inspection.

- Assist the Sponsor/CRO in problem solving and provide consultation on monitoring and study related activities.
- This position requires 70% travel.

Educational Requirements
Must have a minimum of a Bachelors Degree, preferably in a relevant biological or health science.

List of Academic Programs That Train Clinical Research Professionals*

United States

Ph.D. Programs
Baylor College of Medicine, Houston, Texas
University of Colorado, Denver CO

M.S. Programs
Albert Einstein College of Medicine, Yeshiva University, New York, NY
American University of Health Sciences, Los Angeles, CA
Campbell University, Research Triangle Park, NC
Duke University, Durham, NC
Massachusetts General Hospital, Institute of Health Professions, Boston, MA
Mayo Clinic, Rochester, MN
New York Medical College, Valhalla, NY
University of Louisville, Louisville, KY
University of North Carolina Wilmington, Wilmington, NC
University of Pittsburgh, Pittsburgh, PA
Virginia Commonwealth University, Richmond, VA

Post-baccalaureate Certificate Programs
American University of Health Sciences, Los Angeles, CA
Boston University, Boston, MA
Duke University, Durham, NC
Eastern Michigan University, Ypsilanti, MI
Jefferson Medical College, Philadelphia, PA
LaSalle University, Philadelphia, PA

Massachusetts General Hospital, Institute of Health Professions, Boston, MA
Mayo Clinic, Rochester, MN
Medical College of Pennsylvania/Hahnemann University, Philadelphia, PA
Mercer County Community College, Trenton, NJ
University of California—San Diego, LaJolla, CA
University of California—Santa Cruz, Santa Cruz, CA
University of Chicago, Chicago, IL
University of Cincinnati, Cincinnati, OH
University of Louisville, Louisville, KY

B.S. Programs
George Washington University, Washington, DC
Campbell University, Buies Creek, NC
University of North Carolina Wilmington, Wilmington, NC

Associate Degree Programs
Durham Community Technical College, Durham, NC
George Washington University, Washington, DC

Outside the United States

Australia
Monash University, Sydney
University of Canberra, Canberra

Canada
British Columbia Institute of Technology, Burnaby, British Columbia
Humber College, Toronto, Ontario
University of Western Ontario, London, Ontario

United Kingdom
Institute of Clinical Research, Maidenhead, UK
John Moores University, Liverpool, UK
University of Leeds, Leeds, UK
University of Oxford, Oxford, UK

*Does not include K30 Programs designed for individuals with MD or PhD degree

INDEX

A

Absorption, Distribution, Metabolism and Excretion (ADME) 68
Academic Sites 190
Acres of Skin 39, 419
Active Comparator Control 141
Adaptive Design 146
Additional Elements of Consent 117
Adverse Drug Reaction (ADR) 310
Adverse Event (AE) 7, 10, 310, 314, 316, 318, 319, 320, 321, 322, 323
Advertising 100, 102, 203, 330, 332, 355
Artificial Intelligence (AI) 336
Association of Clinical Research Professionals (ACRP) 24
Audits 27, 375, 376, 377, 378, 379, 380
Automated Validity Checks 173

B

Basic Elements of Consent 117
Belmont Report 26, 38, 39, 43, 50, 421
Benefit vs. Risk 96
Bias 26, 89, 109, 114, 137, 142, 143, 144, 149, 151, 155, 212, 236
Bioavailability Studies 55, 67
Biological Products 46, 64, 85, 86, 107
Biologics 46, 64, 79, 82, 146
Biologics License Application (BLA) 82
Bioresearch Monitoring (BIMO) 378
Black List 388
Blinding 143, 159
Bureau of Chemistry 34

C

Career Preparation 24
Case Report Form (CRF) 3, 4, 6, 8, 18, 19, 28, 119, 153, 163, 168, 169, 170, 171, 172, 173, 174, 178, 219, 226, 231, 240, 241, 244, 245, 246, 248, 254, 261, 263, 264, 265, 266, 269, 270, 271, 276, 286, 287, 288, 303, 317, 319, 352, 353, 359, 371, 398, 399, 401, 402, 404, 407, 461
CCEA (complete, consistent, enduring and available) 226, 271
Center for Biologics Evaluation and Research (CBER) 82
Center for Devices and Radiological Health (CDRH) 79
Center for Drug Evaluation and Research 420
Center for Drug Evaluation and Research (CDER) 420
Class I devices 79, 80

Class II devices 80
Class III devices 80, 81
Clinical Investigators 45, 47, 48, 49, 107, 181, 199, 330, 339, 376
Clinical Research as a Care Option (CRAACO) 336
Clinical Research Associates (CRA) , 1
Clinical Research Coordinator (CRC) 221, 258
Clinical Study Report 13, 15, 243, 368
Clinical Trial Management System (CTMS) 337
ClinicalTrials.gov 87, 194, 337
Closeout Procedures 359
Common Elements of a Protocol 155, 156
Common Rule 50, 51
Compliance 33, 47, 48, 50, 162, 325, 342, 347, 350, 353, 354, 356, 358, 376, 379
Concomitant Medication 19, 103, 156, 162, 172, 265
Conducting Clinical Trials 406
Confidentiality 38, 47, 98, 117, 132, 176, 194, 195, 196, 226, 268, 297, 298, 424
Conflict of Interest 102, 106, 111, 212, 341
Continuing Review 104
Contract Research Organization (CRO) 5, 6, 8, 9, 16, 22, 25, 26, 55, 56, 61, 69, 90, 97, 101, 103, 170, 192, 216, 218, 220, 224, 231, 240, 254, 255, 257, 293, 295, 297, 302, 313, 359, 361, 365, 368, 369, 376, 416, 423, 460, 462, 463
Contracts 232, 235, 237, 238, 424
Control Groups 140
Controlled Substance 185
COVID , 1, 10, 11, 12, 13, 14, 15, 16, 17, 24, 47, 49, 85, 204, 213, 269
CRA Personality 20
CRF Design and Development 168, 169
CRF Layout 171
CRF Review 18, 19, 245, 246, 248, 261, 264, 265, 271, 276, 303
Crossover Design 145

D

Data Monitoring Committee (DMC) 108
Data Safety Monitoring Board (DSMB) 93, 108
Data Safety Monitoring Committee (DSMC) 108
Decentralized Clinical Trials 146, 151, 177
Dechallenge 321
Declaration of Helsinki 33, 38, 43, 50, 420, 421
Dedicated Research Sites 189
Delegation of Authority (DOA) 119
De Novo Classification 81
Devices 46, 79, 82, 176
Disqualification of Investigators 186
Disqualified/ Restricted/ Assurance 48
Diverse and Equitable Participation in Clinical Trials (DEPICT) Act 42
Diversifying Investigations Via Equitable Research Studies for Everyone (DIVERSE) Trials Act 42

Drug Accountability 360
Drug Discovery 64
Drug Dispensing 263
Drug Importation Act 34

E

Early Study Termination 357
Electronic Case Report Form (eCRF) 6, 8, 19, 153, 168, 170, 173, 226, 248, 249, 253, 254, 261, 264, 265, 266, 272, 273, 274, 275, 287, 317, 399
Electronic Clinical Outcome Assessment (eCOA) 176, 177
Electronic Data Capture (EDC) 8, 153, 173, 281
Electronic Informed Consent (eIC) 130, 133
Electronic Medical Record (EMR) 120, 266, 298, 382
Electronic Patient-Reported Outcomes (ePRO) 148
Electronic Signatures 45, 273, 385
Electronic Source (eSource) 9, 10, 11, 201, 266, 268, 272
Error Patterns 174
Errors 286, 287, 371, 373, 397, 398, 410
Establishment Inspection Report (EIR) 386
Estimating Enrollment 325
Exceptions to Informed Consent 126, 127
Expected/Unexpected 313
Expedited NDA Approval Process for Life-Threatening Illnesses 40
Expedited Review 105
Exposure in Utero 316

F

Facebook 335, 355
FDA Audits of Investigative Sites 379
FDA Compliance Program 48, 379
FDA Guidance
- For IRBs 107
- On Conduct of Clinical Trials of Medical Products During the COVID-19 Public Health Emergency 133
- On Electronic Source Data in Clinical Investigations 272
FDA Inspections 48, 59, 121, 378, 381, 384, 385
FDA Modernization Act (FDAMA) 41
Federal Policy for the Protection of Human Research Subjects (Common Rule) 50, 51
Final Visit Report 363
Financial Disclosure 45, 59, 104, 209, 210, 211, 212, 230, 236
Flesch-Kincaid Grade Level 116
Follow-Up Letter 294, 301, 307
Food and Drug Omnibus Reform Act (FDAMA) 42
For-Cause Audits 375, 376, 377
Form 483 (Notice of Observations) 386
Form 1571 (Coversheet for IND Submissiions) 312
Form 1572 (Statement of Investigator) 47, 54, 101, 183, 199, 207, 209, 210, 212, 230, 236, 258, 296, 310
Form 3454 (Certification of Absence of Financial Interest) 212

Form 3455 (Disclosure of Financial Interest) 212
Form 3500A (IND Safety Report) 312, 313
Fraud 397, 402, 403, 408, 409, 410

G

Genotoxicity Studies 68, 73
Good Clinical Practice (GCP) 1, 33, 46, 50, 164
Grants 60, 207, 209, 232, 233, 235, 237, 238, 422, 426
Guide to Clinical Studies and Developing Protocols 154, 341

H

Hamilton Depression Rating Scale for Depression (HAM-D) 140
Health and Human Services (HHS) 34, 421
Health Insurance Portability and Accountability Act (HIPAA) 118, 119, 226, 267, 297, 298, 421
Historical Control 142

I

ICH E6(R2)—Guidelines for Good Clinical Practice 45, 46, 113, 114, 121, 310, 366
ICH GCPs 269
Incentive Payments 340
Independent Ethics Committee (IEC) 93
Informed Consent 2, 3, 6, 8, 13, 14, 19, 34, 38, 43, 47-58, 73, 93, 96-135, 149, 160, 161, 166, 183, 184, 186, 201, 209, 230, 242, 251, 262, 277, 283, 298, 326, 330, 331, 338, 339, 361, 364, 367, 381, 384
Informed Consent Review 261, 262
Institutional Biosafety Committee (IBC) 83
Institutional Review Board (IRB) 94, 105, 107, 283
Integrated Approaches to Testing and Assessment (IATA) 201
Intent-To-Treat (ITT) 149, 151
Interactive Response Technology (IRT) 411
Interactive Voice Response System (IVRS) 6, 9, 16, 55, 249, 254, 290, 293, 294, 411
Interactive Web Response System (IWRS) 6, 9, 249, 254, 290, 293, 294, 411
International Council for Harmonization 1
International Council for Harmonization (ICH) 1, 8, 26, 33, 45, 46, 47, 50, 52, 55, 89, 113, 114, 118, 121, 226, 229, 241, 243, 269, 300, 310, 366, 368
International Council on Harmonization (ICH) 420–422
Investigational Device Exemption (IDE) 13, 107, 147, 276, 414
Investigational New Drug Application (IND) 6, 13, 37, 39, 53, 54, 63, 66, 68, 69, 74, 76, 77, 83, 101, 107, 157, 183, 276, 310, 311, 312, 313, 318, 323, 361, 375, 414
Investigational Product (IP) 289
Investigator 2, 3, 4, 6, 14, 27, 28, 29, 47, 48, 50, 54, 55, 57-

61, 69, 81, 91-239, 244-248, 252-278, 281-300, 301-394, 401, 402, 403, 404, 405, 408, 413, 420, 426
Investigator Meeting 212, 213, 214, 215, 217, 218, 219, 220, 221, 222, 225, 237
Investigator Reporting 103, 315, 317
Investigator Responsibilities 48, 59, 165, 184, 207, 226, 289
Investigator Site File (ISF) 248, 359
IRB 219
IRB Audits of Investigative Sites 378
IRB Membership 102, 105
IRB Registration 106, 107
IRBs 420–422

J

Jewish Chronic Disease Hospital Study 39

K

Kefauver-Harris Amendments (Drug Amendments of 1962) 37
Kelsey, Francis 37
Kopcha, Michael 65

L

Last Value Carried Forward (LVCF) 149
Legally Acceptable Representative (LAR) 121, 128, 129, 131
Long Form Consent 122

M

Machine Learning (ML) 412, 416
Medical Device Classification 79, 82
Misconduct 397, 401, 402, 408, 410
Missing data 149, 151
Missing Data 13, 149, 151, 171, 173, 281, 282, 286
Moderna 85
Monitoring Log 231, 248, 249, 250
Monitoring Plan 8, 239, 240, 243-246, 251, 253, 254, 260, 263, 278-285, 294
Monitoring Visit Reports 8, 229, 299, 300, 385
Multinational Trials 88

N

National Commission for the Protection of Human Subjects of Biomedical and Behavioral Research 38
National Institute of Allergy and Infectious Diseases (NIAID) 49
National Institutes of Health 420, 421
National Institutes of Health (NIH) 41, 49, 83, 86, 98, 108
New Drug Application (NDA) 7, 33, 36, 40, 41, 63, 72, 73, 74, 75, 77, 212, 236, 362, 376, 380, 388, 394, 403, 409
NIH 422
NIH-Regulated Research 49
No Action Indicated (NAI) 187, 387, 394
Noncompliance 27, 57, 276, 285, 347, 348, 352, 353, 356, 377, 378, 394, 410
Nuremberg Code 36, 38, 50, 421
Nurse Practitioner (NP) 181, 182

O

Obtaining Informed Consent 121
Office for Human Research Protection (OHRP) 33, 129

Official Action Indicated (OAI) 187, 387, 394
OHRP 420, 420–422, 420–422, 420–422
Outcome Measures 150
Over-the-Counter (OTC) 162, 351

P

Parallel Design 145
Part-Time Sites 189
Patient Report Outcomes (PRO) 6
Payments to Research Subjects 338
Performance Evaluation 301
Per Protocol (PP) 149, 151
Pfizer/BioNTech 85
Pharmacokinetic Studies 68
Phase 1 54, 64, 67, 69-72, 77, 84, 138, 154, 178, 339, 352
Phase 2 40, 54, 67, 70, 71, 72, 77, 84, 110, 138, 154, 165, 415
Phase 3 42, 67, 72, 73, 74, 77, 82, 84, 85, 87, 138, 156, 157, 165, 166, 196
Phase 3b 70, 74, 77
Phase 4 40, 74, 76, 77, 84, 305
Physician Assistant (PA) 181, 182
Placebo Control 141, 205
Placebo Effect 139, 140, 141, 151
Placebo Response 139, 151
Preclinical Research 64
Preclinical Studies 64, 66, 67, 68, 72, 76
Premarket Approval (PMA) 80, 81
Premarket Notification (510k) 80
Preparing for a Monitoring Visit 253
Prescription Drug User Fee Act (PDUFA) 40, 41, 43, 72
Pre-Study Visit 188, 205, 208
Primary Outcome Measures 150
Principal Investigator (PI) 120, 181, 182, 196, 197, 198, 201, 203, 204, 213, 214, 246, 320, 322
Protected Health Information (PHI) 118
Protocol Adherence 261, 263
Protocol Amendments 19, 103, 104, 166, 167, 361
Protocol Complexity 165, 178, 353, 354
Protocols 6, 9, 40, 53, 69, 72, 74, 93, 105, 137, 153-159, 165-168, 177, 178, 224, 239, 241, 247, 257, 279, 287, 297, 301, 303, 314, 315, 322, 324, 341, 350, 353, 365
Protocol Summary 155, 157, 194, 331

Q

Quality Management 241-243, 245, 279, 280, 365- 368, 373
Queries 6, 8, 10, 19, 26, 168, 173, 174, 176, 239, 253, 254, 261, 266, 286, 287, 288, 306, 360, 366, 371, 372, 399, 411

R

Randomization 9, 143, 144, 151, 155, 159, 160, 197, 219, 226, 248, 251, 254, 263, 284, 290, 294
Readability and Comprehension 116
Real-World Data (RWD) 76
Rechallenge 321
Recordkeeping and Retention 185
Recruitment 3, 6, 11, 12, 18, 29, 38, 87, 94, 101, 102, 188,

191, 192, 195, 203, 209, 225, 239, 246, 248, 325, 330, 334, 335, 336-341, 354, 355, 369, 412, 413, 414
Remote Regulatory Assessments 378
Remote Monitoring 9, 10, 11, 14, 18, 20, 26, 27, 240, 243, 245, 253, 269, 274, 276, 278, 285, 416
Repeated-Dose Studies 73
Repeated-DoseToxicity Studies 73
Reproductive Toxicity Studies 73
Restricted and Disqualified Investigators 187
Retention 22, 30, 50, 185, 201, 231, 272, 325, 342, 344, 346, 347, 353, 354, 355, 362, 363, 364, 412
Risk-Based Monitoring (RBM) 278-280, 283-285
Routine Audits 375, 376, 378

S

Safety Monitoring 12, 93, 97, 108, 109, 147, 309
Safety Reports 186, 309, 312, 313, 318, 361
Sample Collection 294
Sample Size 137, 138, 139, 151, 158, 164
Scientific Review Committee 107, 108
Screening Procedures 12, 161
Serious Adverse Event (SAE) 7, 19, 27, 248, 254, 255, 261, 314, 317, 319, 360
Short Form Consent 121
Site Evaluation Visits 102, 188, 195
Site Management Organization (SMO) 191, 192
Site Metrics 368
Society of Clinical Research Associates (SOCRA) 28, 30
Source Data Verification (SDV) 8, 9, 18, 19, 244, 245, 246, 271, 281, 282
Source Document Review (SDR) 264
Spilker, Bert 154
Sponsor 218, 221
Sponsor Audits of Investigative Sites 375
Sponsor Responsibilities 318
Standardization of CRFs 169
Standard Operating Procedure (SOP) 5, 6, 382
Statistical Significance 140
Study Closeout 231, 357
Study Design 137, 157, 159
Study Initiation 209, 223, 237
Study Monitoring 239
Study Objectives 159
Sub-Investigator 57, 167, 181, 182, 192, 196, 201, 322
Subject Compliance 164, 290, 325, 347, 353, 356
Subject Enrollment 160, 203, 245, 249, 330, 341, 353
Subject Selection 97, 155, 160, 330

T

Teratology 68, 73
Time Management 247
Tokenization 76
Toxicology 66, 68, 69, 73
Tuskegee Syphilis Study 39, 420
Twitter (now X) 335

U

Unanticipated Adverse Device Effect (UADE) 319

Unresolved Adverse Event (UAE) 316

V

Vaccine Adverse Event Reporting System (VAERS) 84
Vaccines 16, 24, 64, 67, 82, 84, 85, 86
Voluntary Action Indicated (VAI) 187, 389, 396
Vulnerable Subjects 49, 98, 110

W

Wiley, Harvey 35

X

X (formerly Twitter) 335

Y

YouTube 335, 355